SOCIAL AND BEHAVIORAL SCIENCE FOR HEALTH PROFESSIONALS

Brian P. Hinote

Middle Tennessee State University

Jason Adam Wasserman

Oakland University William Beaumont School of Medicine

Foreword by William C. Cockerham, University of Alabama–Birmingham

ROWMAN & LITTLEFIELD

Lanham • Boulder • New York • London

Executive Editor: Nancy Roberts
Associate Editor: Molly White
Senior Marketing Manager: Karin Cholak
Marketing Manager: Deborah Hudson
Interior Designer: Ilze Lemesis
Cover Designer: Chloe Batch

Credits and acknowledgments for material borrowed from other sources, and reproduced with permission, appear on the appropriate page within the text.

Published by Rowman & Littlefield
A wholly owned subsidiary of The Rowman & Littlefield Publishing Group, Inc.
4501 Forbes Boulevard, Suite 200, Lanham, Maryland 20706
www.rowman.com

Unit A, Whitacre Mews, 26-34 Stannary Street, London SE11 4AB, United Kingdom

British Library Cataloguing in Publication Information Available

Library of Congress Cataloging-in-Publication Data
Names: Hinote, Brian P., 1976– author. | Wasserman, Jason Adam, author.
Title: Social and behavioral science for health professionals / Brian P. Hinote,
    Jason Adam Wasserman; foreword by William C. Cockerham.
Description: Lanham: Rowman & Littlefield, [2017] | Includes bibliographical
    references and index.
Identifiers: LCCN 2016032736 (print) | LCCN 2016034057 (ebook) | ISBN
    9781442249707 (cloth: alk. paper) | ISBN 9781442249714 (pbk.: alk.
    paper) | ISBN 9781442249721 (electronic)
Subjects: | MESH: Social Medicine—trends | Health Behavior | Health Status
    Disparities | Socioeconomic Factors
Classification: LCC RA418 (print) | LCC RA418 (ebook) | NLM WA 31 |
    DDC 362.1—dc23
LC record available at https://lccn.loc.gov/2016032736

Dedication

To my family, especially Tyne, Eliot, and Ethan, without whose unconditional support and encouragement this work would have never been possible. All my love.

—Brian

To Nicole and Ellie for the early mornings, late nights, and countless weekends. I love you both.

—Jason

Contents

Foreword xi

Preface xiii

  Threshold Concepts xiv

    Threshold Concepts and Health Practitioners xv

    Key Threshold Concepts for Each Chapter xvi

Acknowledgments xxiii

PART I Foundations of Social Science and Health 1

CHAPTER 1 Introduction to Health and the Sociological Imagination 3

  A Multidimensional Approach to Health and Health Care 4

  The Sociological Imagination 8

  Bringing the Sociological Imagination into Focus 9

  Critically Analyzing Health and Health Care 13

  The Paradox of American Health Care 14

  Health Care as a Social Institution 16

  Organization of the Book 17

  Activity—Exercising the Sociological Imagination 19

CHAPTER 2 The Shifting Landscape of Health and Medicine: Past, Present, and Future 21

  Introduction 21

  Medicine before Modernity 22

    Premodern Thinking 23

    Humoral Medicine 24

  The Advent of Modernity 26

    The Birth of Modern Medicine 27

    The Rise of Modern Clinical Practice 29

    Education for Medical and Allied Health Professions 29

    The Business of Modern Health Care 31

  A Shifting Landscape of Health and Disease 32

    Disruptive Illness: Chronic Disease and Incalculable Risk 33

    Changing Disease Profiles 34

    The Consequences of Incalculability 37

The End of Modern(ist) Health Care: Clinical Practice in the Chronic Illness Era   40

Conclusion   43

Activity—Exercising One's Epistemology: Seeing Disease through Premodern, Modern, and Postindustrial Frameworks   44

CHAPTER 3   The Logic and Methods of Empirical Research   47

The Statistical Imagination   48

What Is Science?   51
The Scientific Method   52

In Pursuit of Causality   55
Covariation   55
Eliminating Spuriousness   56
Time Order   58

Classic Experimental Design   59

Clinical Trials   62

Other Research Designs   64
Quasi-Experimental Methods   64
Correlational and Cross-Sectional Methods   65
Preexperimental Methods   66
Qualitative Methods   66

Research Translation: From Findings to Practice   67
Does the Study Add to Our Understanding?   68
Who Is Being Studied?   68
Is the Research Design Appropriate?   69
Is Systematic Bias Avoided or Minimized?   69
Statistical Considerations   71

Research Ethics   72

Conclusion: Evidence-Based Medicine and the Statistical Imagination   74

Activity—Thinking Critically about Research   75

PART II   Social Epidemiology and Determinants of Health   77

CHAPTER 4   Social Class and Health   79

The Social Determinants of Health   80

Socioeconomic Status   84
Social Class as a Fundamental Cause of Health and Disease   88
Neighborhood Disadvantage and the Role of Clinical Practice   91

Conclusion   95

Activity—The Flint Water Crisis: The Many Dimensions of Class and Health   96

CHAPTER 5 A Matrix of Health Inequalities 99

Age 100

Gender 108

Race and Ethnicity 113

Culture 119

Conclusion: A Matrix of Inequalities 124

Activity—Historical Memory, Inherited Culture, and Distrust of Health Care: The Tuberculosis Outbreak in Marion, Alabama 127

CHAPTER 6 Health Behavior and Lifestyles 129

A Renewed Emphasis on Health Behavior 130

Explaining Health Behavior 133
    The Health Belief Model 135
    Alternative Models 136
    Process Models 139
    A Health Lifestyles Paradigm 143

Implications for Health Care Practice 147

Activity—Habitus and Health Behavior: How Can You Get Janek Polakow to Diet and Exercise? 149

PART III Social Science in Clinical Practice 151

CHAPTER 7 Power, Medicalization, and Clinical Practice 153

Introduction 153

Medicalization 154

Power in the Clinic 158
    Two Forms of Power 158
    The Clinical Functions of Power 161
    Medicalization, Social Control, and Overdiagnosis 165

Conclusion: Dilemmas of Difference 172

Activity—Risks, Benefits, and Perspective: Navigating the Autism Spectrum 174

CHAPTER 8 The Illness Experiences of Patients and Families 177

The Illness Experience of Patients 178
    Grief in Health Care 181
    Illness and Identity 184

Families and Caregiving   188
    Caregiving Burden   188
    The Stress Process Model   190

Conclusion: Disease and Illness, Patients and Persons   195

Activity—The Illness Experience of Patients and Families   197

CHAPTER 9   The Social Dynamics of Clinical Communication   199

The Social Structure of Clinical Encounters   201
    The Influence of Age   202
    The Influence of Gender   203
    The Influence of Socioeconomic Status   205
    The Influence of Race/Ethnicity   206
    The Influence of Culture   208

Narrative and the Art of Clinical Practice   210

Basic Interviewing Techniques   213

Conclusion   218

Activity—Eliciting Patient Narrative: Role-play Activities   220

CHAPTER 10   Health Professions and Interprofessional
Teamwork   223

Introduction: Specialization and Complexity   223

Professions in Transition   225
    The Emergence of Professional Medicine   227
    The Deprofessionalization of Medicine   228
    Emerging Professions   230
    Problems within a Complex Professional Landscape   232

Best Practices for Interprofessional Teamwork   234

Just Culture and Medical Error   239

Conclusion: Beyond Checklists   241

Activity—Teamwork and Just Culture: The Case of "Psycho Mike"   244

CHAPTER 11   Bioethics, Social Science, and Clinical Practice   245

Introduction   245

The Emergence of Bioethics   247

Principles of Biomedical Ethics and Beyond   250
    The Four Principles of Biomedical Ethics   252
    Other Forms of Ethical Reasoning and Decision-Making   256

From Theory to Practice   260
  A Framework for Practical Bioethics   260
  The Social Psychology of Clinical Ethics   263

Conclusion: The Bioethical Imagination   265

Activity—Navigating Bioethical Decisions   266

PART IV   Health Systems and Policy   269

CHAPTER 12   Health Care Systems and Policy   271

Introduction   271

System Goals   274
  Costs   274
  Access   276
  Quality   278
  Health Care System Models   283
  The Mutual Aid Model   284
  The State Model   285
  The Professional Model   288
  The Corporatist Model   289

Health Care in the United States   290
  Provider-Induced Demand and Overtreatment   290
  Patient-Induced Demand and Overtreatment   293
  Bureaucratic Complexity   295

Conclusion: The End of Modern Health Care   297

Activity—Matching Health System Design to the Health and Illness Landscape   298

CHAPTER 13   Conclusion   301

References   307

Index   329

Foreword

Brian Hinote and Jason Wasserman fill an important gap among textbooks with the publication of *Social and Behavioral Science for Health Professionals*. Up until now, there was not a single textbook in the United States providing in-depth coverage of the social determinants of health written for students and practitioners in the health professions. No books whatsoever were in this category. What passed for behavioral science in the existing medical and health literature for professional students was typically a blend of psychology and psychiatry. If there was any sociology, it was minimal. Yet interest in sociology is increasing because of the growing recognition—supported by ample evidence—that social factors can cause health problems. Sociology is now included in the Medical College Admission Test (MCAT). This is a relatively new development. Previously, social variables were either ignored or considered simply as background information for biomedical explanations of health afflictions. We currently know that this is not the case as a considerable literature has emerged in recent years documenting a causal connection between social factors, health, and disease (Cockerham 2013).

According to the National Research Council and the Institute of Medicine, the most important social factors determining health are income, accumulated wealth, education, occupational characteristics, and social inequality based on race and ethnic group membership (Woolfe & Aron 2013). Other social variables such as gender, age, neighborhood characteristics, culture, health policy, and the social aspects of health care delivery are important as well. Such variables can have direct effects on both unhealthy and healthy lifestyles, high- or low-risk health behavior, and on living conditions, food security, levels of stresses and strains, social disadvantages over the life course, environmental factors that influence biological outcomes through gene expression, utilization and access to health services, and other outcomes.

However, understanding the role of social factors in health and the onset, course, and consequences of a disease is only part of the challenge for health professionals. The often missing link is an awareness of how to apply this knowledge to the reality of health care. And it is in the application of this knowledge that the book by Hinote and Wasserman excels. By bringing together the subject matter of medical sociology, health psychology, bioethics, and other fields under one umbrella, the authors demonstrate how insights from these disciplines can be *applied* to a variety of health-related situations. This is seen especially in the chapters on social class and health, health inequalities, health behavior and lifestyles, medicalization and clinical practice, the illness experience, clinical communication, health professions and interprofessional teamwork, and bioethics and clinical practice. Other chapters discuss health and the sociological imagination, the changing landscape of health and medicine, and health systems and policy. Altogether, the authors provide an excellent compendium of topics relevant to students undergoing training in medicine, nursing, dentistry, pharmacy, public health, and other health-related fields including medical sociology and health psychology.

A particular advantage of this book is that it focuses on health issues representative of the early twenty-first century in the United States. The context of medical practice and the work roles of various health professions have changed significantly since the mid-twentieth-century era of physician dominance. The federal government and health insurance companies now have a major presence in decision-making about patient care. The cost of care has skyrocketed compared to the past, nurse practitioners can prescribe drugs, pharmacists are required to have doctorates, medicine is feminizing as seen in the increase in women physicians and physician assistants, and there is greater equality in the doctor–patient relationship. Yet old problems persist, such as the effects of poverty and adverse living conditions on the health of the poor and the high number of people still without health insurance. These and other situations are covered in this novel and insightful textbook that represents a significant advance over what has previously been available for students in the health professions.

William C. Cockerham, PhD
Distinguished Professor of Sociology
University of Alabama at Birmingham

Preface

While not always recognized as such, work in health and medicine has always been, in no small part, a social and behavioral science. As the more widely recognized cliché goes, "medicine is both art and science." In this, people mean to say that while practitioners utilize their scientific understanding of biology, chemistry, physiology, and anatomy, applying those disciplines to the sick, suffering, and disabled requires a sort of clinical judgment that is intuitive, drawn from the wisdom of experience, and oriented toward weaving together the idiosyncrasies of individual patients, their values, family situation, work demands, and so on. Science is rational and universal, thereby applicable to all bodies, but art works in a more nuanced and creative way from individuality. The collaboration of the two constitutes clinical practice, and standing at this juncture is social and behavioral science. Understanding who the patient is; the social environments in which they live and in which they became sick; attempting to manage their illnesses; and engaging their values and dispositions as well, this is the work of social and behavioral science.

The "idiosyncrasies" of individual patients, it turns out, are often patterned and predictable social characteristics and behavioral tendencies. Knowledge of how social factors are associated with disease patterns in populations and communities, or how individuals experience illness and its burdens, gives practitioners a starting point for understanding how diagnoses can be informed by social–psychological considerations, and how treatments should match a patient's life experiences and circumstances to be most effective. Moreover, developing strong social skills promotes good interpersonal communication with patients and colleagues, and helps establish rapport and trust in both clinical and professional relationships. All are essential to promoting good (and effective) patient care, developing healthy organizations, and promoting optimal health systems and divisions of labor. Put simply, social and behavioral science directly informs health care and clinical practice at many levels.

Medical, nursing, and allied health education are increasingly integrating the fundamentally important roles of the social and behavioral sciences, long recognized in academic circles, into their curricula. The expansion of courses in various professional programs to include fields like sociology and psychology attest to this shift, as does even a cursory review of the most recent core competencies and content standards articulated by the major accrediting bodies in these fields.[1] But perhaps the most striking change concerns the Medical College Admissions Test (MCAT), which now devotes one of its four subsections to social and behavioral science content. This change has provided "sociology departments an unprecedented opportunity to instruct premedical students on contextualizing human difference and being sensitive to the diverse trajectories of people in the health care system" (Olsen 2016:72). Similarly, nursing programs increasingly require courses in the social and behavioral sciences to satisfy degree requirements. And perhaps most importantly, Olsen's (2016) study demonstrates the effects that sociology can have on premed students as they struggle with the limitations of biology in explaining human behavior and disorder, and begin to develop a sense of their own professional identity. However, while Olsen (2016) articulates well the value of sociology for premedical students, the broader landscape suggests that a wide range of clinicians are increasingly looking for not just sociology, but pragmatic training in the social and behavioral sciences more broadly defined. This book

---

[1] We provide a web supplement which maps the content of this book to these standards, across various professional groups.

therefore speaks to a wide range of current practitioners, and those in training, and we intentionally eschew the traditional disciplinary boundaries of sociology proper, instead letting the needs of practitioners dictate the content of the book.

Among a range of sociological topics, we include in this book a chapter on bioethics; cover the history of medicine and health professions; discuss interviewing strategies that emerge from the counseling literature; and detail material on behavioral change theories that more typically reside in psychology, in order to respond to the needs of both current and future practitioners who are increasingly populating our courses and for whom traditional social science content is not always best suited. In addition to new considerations and professional developments regarding what content is relevant, the question then becomes how best to teach it.

Threshold Concepts

There is an old debate about the extent to which social science, in general, and the social sciences related to health and medicine, in particular, *should* focus on applied issues. This is obviously important for this book since our audience constitutes not professional social and behavioral scientists, but those who will work in diverse fields like medicine, nursing, dentistry, and allied health. The idea that the social sciences should strive to apply and inform real-world contexts hardly seems controversial. But the backlash against the American Sociological Association's choice of "Public Sociology" for their annual meeting in 2007 is only one example of how contested the status and role of *applied* work can be. Professional discourse about the difference in "sociology *of* medicine" and "sociology *in* medicine" also shows that there are particular, strongly held, long-standing notions about what sociology is and how it should interact with the world (Clair et al. 2007; Straus 1957, 1999). The same can be said for other social science disciplines as well, where an allegiance to *pure academia* and the needs of the *real world* are not always aligned.

Like many others, we find this debate not only tiresome, but also premised on a false dichotomy. First, there is no reason that the diverse and expansive terrains of social science cannot fully accommodate both theoretical and applied work. Second, there is no reason to think that work that is applicable cannot also be fully academic. Indeed, many would argue that even the most theoretically inclined academic has an obligation to articulate why their work matters. Third, and most importantly for this book, the false dichotomy between academic and applied work in the social sciences presumes that theoretically rich concepts are somehow not easily applied in real-world contexts. There is an implicit assumption that the kinds of robust concepts that are truly definitive of social and behavioral science fields, in their applied versions, must be reduced or deflated in some way. We find the opposite to be true in our work. That is, the most robust theoretical concepts in our fields of training are, in fact, the *most* applicable because they speak to the widest range of experiences within the health professions. The transposable nature of such concepts not only allows them to organize and make sense of a wide range of health care practices, but also stimulates the ability of practitioners to see their professional experiences in new ways. That is, the core ideas of the social and behavioral sciences are most transformative because they expand how practitioners think about and engage in their work. Perhaps ironically, this makes them the most useful in applied contexts.

More recent work in medical and allied health education supports this perspective. The amount of technical and factual knowledge that practitioners should possess is ever expanding. Educational institutions try to keep pace by cramming more information into curricula, but there is an upper limit of what can be accomplished with this approach. There are only so many hours in a day and only so many years of training that people are willing to undergo before they simply will choose another field. Medical and allied health education needs a new, more efficient way to do things. One popular approach that is gaining traction centers on moving away from thinking of curriculum as a list of things to learn, focusing instead around key *threshold concepts*.

Threshold concepts are rich, transformative, and integrative. That is, they are robust and widely applicable to a range of experiences, and they change how someone sees the world. One can therefore carry them over into any number of new contexts, obviating the need to teach every single piece of knowledge in every hypothetical applied scenario. Put another way, rather than having students learn everything about medicine, nursing, and allied health, which has become daunting if not impossible, education should focus on teaching students to think in a variety of ways like doctors, nurses, and allied health practitioners. Thinking can be brought fruitfully into any number of situations.

Threshold Concepts and Health Practitioners

We recognize that health practitioners are not typically full-fledged professional social or behavioral scientists. Our goal in this book therefore is not to provide an array of facts or research findings about health and health care, but to illustrate flexible ways of thinking that can be adapted to any number of areas of health and health care (Wasserman 2014). We present a lot of facts and findings related to health and medicine from our various fields of expertise, but always with the goal of illuminating deeper concepts that are transposable to multiple dimensions of health and illness. In keeping with that goal, we have not provided a glossary, but rather a list of threshold concepts corresponding to various chapters of this book. As such, it should not be used like a glossary, which one might turn to only in the event that you do not know the meaning of a word. Rather, it will be helpful to read about and reflect on the threshold concepts in advance of each of the chapters in which they appear.

While we also articulate specific learning objectives for each chapter, the threshold concepts in each are designed to help students, "[see] things in a new way" (Meyer & Land 2003). Glynis Cousins (2006) has summarized several key features of threshold concepts (see also Meyer & Land 2006)We describe four critical features below, along with how we broadly see the application of each to the social science of health and health care:

1. They are *transformative* in that they engender a conceptual shift that changes how one perceives a particular phenomenon. We hope that learning about the social dimensions of health and illness expands and fundamentally changes how you see these things. In particular, we hope you gain an appreciation for the various ways that social and behavioral phenomena cause disease, affect treatments, and characterize the numerous social interactions that constitute the process of health care.

2. They are *irreversible*. Once the learner experiences a transformative shift, it is not easily undone. Threshold concepts affect our ways of seeing the world, rather than just the facts we consume. We therefore do not often dismiss or forget them as we do with facts, because they are internalized into our fundamental understandings of what we observe. While eventually you may forget much, or even most, of the factual information we present in this book, we hope that you internalize a way of seeing that includes the social features of health and illness.

3. They are *integrative*. Each threshold concept integrates various elements of the world; they bring together things that we might otherwise see as separate and unrelated. Each of these concepts brings together various aspects of health and illness or social forces underlying them: for example, where the experience of illness cannot be fully understood apart from one's social relationships, or where the micro-level phenomena of clinical practice cannot be fully understood apart from the larger macro-level social structures in which they are nested.

4. They are *troublesome*. Threshold concepts often present counter-intuitive understandings of phenomena and disrupt our perceptions of how things are, by expanding our thinking about them. This is perhaps the most important for this book, particularly where we hope that every chapter challenges historical assumptions about health and health care practice and causes you to reconsider the boundaries of your professional work (see Cousins 2006).

Below we describe these threshold concepts and the chapters in which they most clearly reside (though many are threaded throughout the entire book). Here, we do not provide full descriptions or explanations because these concepts are robust and not easily summarized. Rather, we try to provide a foundation for understanding the transformative, irreversible, integrative, and troublesome nature of each concept that will be elaborated in each chapter.

Key Threshold Concepts for Each Chapter

Sociological Imagination (Chapter 1): The sociological imagination (Mills 1959 [2000]) refers to the ability to connect larger social and historical forces to our most intimate and personal experiences, and at the same time to understand how our individual actions reflect and reinforce our social worlds. Put another way, it is the ability to see how macro- and micro-levels of social life are interwoven, how social structures affect our choices, and how our choices affect social structures. For health practitioners, this means seeing how social forces constrain or enable patients' behavioral choices, how clinical practices involving individual patients and practitioners are conditioned by the historical development of modern society and Western science, and how interactions with those patients not only affect their lives and their families, but also contribute to the broader social patterns of health care. The sociological imagination is troublesome because it calls into question why we act as we do, and forces us to consider the extent to which we exercise our own agency, and the extent to which our choices are strongly shaped by the social world around us. This confrontation transforms how we see the world; it causes us to consider new possibilities for action where we may have previously acted out of unconscious habit.

Reflexivity and Disruption (Chapter 2): Culture always conditions the ways that we think about and understand the world, and new ways of thinking eventually undercut earlier ideologies that dominate particular eras of human history. This occurs because the problems we face, and the technologies we employ to face them, change over time. While premodern approaches to health and medicine drew on intuitive ways of thinking about health and disease, modern rationality eventually undercut and displaced those ideas, a process facilitated by the development of science and scientific evidence bases. More recently, in the contemporary era of late modernity, chronic illnesses have become more salient and have multiple, often hidden, causes. As a result, modernist approaches are limited in their ability to fully engage the complexities of health and disease. In sum, societies routinely proceed through periods where dominant ways of thinking and their established institutions become mismatched to the state of the times and therefore become less and less effective. This forces us to reconsider not only *what we are doing*, but also *how we are thinking* about particular problems. That is, such a situation forces us to embrace *reflexivity*: not just to think up a new solution, but to think about our thinking. When new ways of thinking and engagement emerge that are better matched to the challenges a society faces, they "disrupt" institutions that are organized around old modes of thought. When we understand how socially constructed ideologies underpin all areas of social life, and how new challenges can enable or even force us to think in new ways that widely undermine a variety of social institutions, we gain a new perspective and deeper appreciation of the challenges and conflicts that we see all around us.

The Statistical Imagination (Chapter 3): In our lives and work, thinking critically about the world around us requires that we visualize the ways that social structures are shaped and in turn contribute to the shape of the social world. The sociological imagination asks us to envision things for which we have evidence, but that we cannot see directly because they occur across larger populations. The *statistical imagination* draws on this same paradigm, but with a more specific focus on how thinking critically about the evidence and explanations we use to substantiate our claims about the empirical world. Ritchey (2007:3) defines the statistical imagination as "an appreciation of how usual or unusual an event, circumstance, or behavior is in relation to a larger set of similar events and an appreciation of an event's causes and consequences." For our purposes, understanding the roles played by probability in research, along with the ability to think probabilistically about how researchers produce their results, is critical to evaluating the kinds of clinical and epidemiological evidence that practitioners must interpret. For example, suppose in your clinical practice you work with postpartum women. You read the results of a study in which the researchers mailed surveys to women who had experienced stillbirths and found that only a very small percentage of them reported symptoms associated with *complicated grief* (a form of grief that is protracted, unremitting, and considered in need of professional attention). Someone lacking a good statistical imagination, who is unable to think critically about the forces shaping this result, might be influenced to pay less attention to signs of complicated grief as a result of this study. Someone with a well-developed "appreciation of an event's causes" (like the relatively low proportion of women in the sample with complicated grief), however, might realize that women who are experiencing complicated grief are also less likely to return a paper survey. That is, there is a *selection bias* that shapes this event, such that the result probably does not reflect complicated grief in the general population. The statistical imagination is the ability to think about what causes data to appear as they do, so that important findings can be distinguished from less important or artificial results.

Social Determinants of Health (Chapter 4): The phrase *social determinants of health* has become widely used and variously understood. The WHO states that "social determinants of health are the conditions in which people are born, grow, live, work and age. These circumstances are shaped by the distribution of money, power and resources at global, national and local levels." More specifically, it refers to factors such as environment, interpersonal relationships, and group memberships ranging from more intimate (e.g., family) to increasingly remote (e.g., social class), which affect health in various ways. In this book, social determinants of health represent threshold concepts insofar as they require one to consider social contexts that condition physical experiences, including access to positive and negative health resources, and affect the ways that individuals come to think about and act in the world (through the process of socialization). This is transformative for thinking about disease, particularly where we tend to have a vision of disease causation and experience that is insufficiently restricted to the individual or, at best, their family circumstances. Particularly in the chronic illness era, where so many diseases emerge from hundreds of thousands of micro-decisions (about eating and exercising, for example), a clear vision of disease causation and experience requires understanding the ways that social life is structured to advantage or disadvantage individuals in their health pursuits. As a supplement to this concept, we also discuss the notion of *fundamental cause*, as a way to articulate the ways in which diseases result from influential social factors.

Disparity (Chapter 5): According to the Centers for Disease Control and Prevention, health disparities are defined as, "preventable differences in the burden of disease, injury, violence, or opportunities to achieve optimal health that are experienced by socially disadvantaged populations. Populations can be defined by factors such as race or ethnicity, gender, education or income, disability, geographic location (e.g., rural or urban), or sexual orientation. Health disparities are inequitable and are directly related to the historical and current unequal distribution of social, political, economic, and environmental resources." What is especially transformative and disturbing about health disparities is that they result from situations and conditions of the social order that all of us participate in, but no single person controls. This makes disparity an incredibly challenging concept that can feel insurmountable to address, yet they require human remediation because they are human constructions. Moreover, understanding the relationship between individuals and social disparities is complex, but important. For example, individual practitioners do not create larger social health disparities, but they can in small but important ways either exacerbate or counteract them.

Habitus (Chapter 6): Pierre Bourdieu (1990:53) defines *habitus* as a system of "durable, transposable dispositions," inculcated through socialization and conditioned by our experiences, which shape our inclinations to behave in particular situations, even when presented with a range of diverse behavioral options. Chapter 6 of this book centers on the notion of lifestyles, which refers to the patterned ways of living that intersect with individuals' identities and which they take up and practice over time. Lifestyles can be more or less unhealthy, and they are behavioral profiles that are either constrained or enabled by available material and nonmaterial resources (e.g., time, money, sense of control, etc.). Habitus helps us understand the ways that material social contexts (availability of healthy food, health insurance with good access to medical professionals, etc.) come together with attitudes toward health, and how each influences and reinforces the other. That is, someone who lives in a food desert, with limited access to healthy food choices, is not only physically limited in their ability to eat healthy foods, but over time, they develop particular patterns of eating that are less healthy. In other words, these are habituated. Even if healthy food becomes available, and as a result of this habituation, they may not select it because it doesn't appeal to their tastes and preferences. In turn, it becomes difficult for food outlets to justify stocking healthy foods when they are not often purchased, which perpetuates the food desert and further shapes dispositions toward less healthy options, and so on. These processes help explain why efforts at nutrition counseling and preventative medicine in the clinical encounter often meet with limited success. These types of interventions address individuals as rational decision-makers, but all of us make most of our daily decisions out of habit, not through rational deliberation. Moreover, this concept explains how health-related patterns and gradients of health develop and why they are so persistent.

Medicalization and Overdiagnosis (Chapter 7): When we talk about social influences, we imply that there are powerful external factors that change how we think and behave. This is a challenging idea, particularly because we typically see power as overt and obvious (i.e., repressive power). As a result, we overlook how many of our actions are influenced though subtle, social forces that are nonetheless powerful. Understanding the notion of *disciplinary power* allows us to understand how social forces influence our daily lives in ways that are not always obvious but are far more pervasive. Health care practitioners, for example, are not often physically forced to practice in certain ways (though repressive power can be influential where financial incentives influence behavior). More often, practitioners have internalized particular ways of thinking about health and illness that affect the choices they make. For example, medicalization refers to the process by which conditions that were not considered health or medical issues come under the purview of health and medicine (e.g., alcoholism). While it can be significantly fueled by repressive power (e.g., money), at its core medicalization requires a shift in the thinking of health practitioners, patients, and society at large, such that they conceive various conditions as medical problems. That is, medicalization requires we *think* of alcoholism as a medical condition. Once we think in this way, we naturally behave accordingly. Understanding the functions of disciplinary power transforms our recognition of how pervasively influential social forces can be, and how power dynamics can permeate every aspect of our social lives, including health care practice.

Verstehen (Chapter 8): *Verstehen* is a German word that literally means "interpretive understanding." However, following Max Weber, we use the term to refer to the sociological skill of "taking on the role of the other." If we examine a situation as external onlookers, we can see interesting and important things about others' lives. For example, we might understand that someone in a lower-SES bracket experiences particular challenges balancing work and caring for a sick family member. But *verstehen* requires that we go further to also attempt to understand the way they see their circumstances, the attitudes and values that form the lens through which they see the world. This gives us access to not only the material, objective challenges they face, but also those built into their social and emotional experiences. For understanding how patients and families experience illness, this is essential. These experiences are not only constituted by the objective conditions of one's life (social class, for example), but also by how they understand their situation, whether it accords with their expectations for their own life, whether it limits their pursuit of things that are important to them, and so on.

Discourse and Narrative (Chapter 9): Commonplace understandings of discourse or narrative often reduce it to a set of practical communicative functions. We think of it as a means of conveying information, but we often fail to appreciate the deeper way in which ideologies, beliefs, attitudes, and fears are built into in the way one speaks, the things they say, and how they assemble and communicate their stories. Discourse concerns both the *structure* and *content* of someone's thought and narrative, and how they put that together into communication. Importantly, ideologies and attitudes are woven not only into the narrative constructions of a speaker, but also form the lens through which a listener understands that narrative. For health and medicine, then, promoting good communication involves more than just ways of speaking to a patient or strategies for getting them to articulate their full story, although those are important. Good clinical communication actually begins at a deeper level of understanding how interpersonal discourse is a microcosm of not only individual attitudes and fears, but also broader social structures. That is, various features of their social positions and experiences manifest in a patient's narrative about their illness. Moreover, the discourse that co-occurs between patients and providers can reflect, and be confounded by, social structural phenomena such as race/ethnic or class inequality. Broader social conditions like class and race often emerge as problematic communication when providers and patients come from significantly different backgrounds. As a result, best practices in clinical communication, which primarily center on eliciting an undisrupted and therefore complete narrative from the patient, must also proceed from understanding the larger sociological barriers that can corrupt those processes.

Professionalization and Deprofessionalization (Chapter 10): While in everyday life we use the term loosely to refer to just about any type of work, from a sociological standpoint, a *profession* represents a unique kind of work characterized by a high degree of autonomy and self-regulation. Professions are accompanied by a social contract whereby society agrees to protect the practice terrain and economic interests of a professional group, in exchange for some level of service commitment. For example, physicians are expected to provide the best treatment to a patient, not the most profitable, and they are also granted the professional autonomy to set practice standards collectively and make medical decisions. Because, in the sociological sense of the term, the extent to which a particular occupation can be considered "professional" depends on social agreements and societal forces, different occupations become more or less professional-*ized* over time. These processes of professionalization and deprofessionalization depend on the power and solidarity wielded by practitioners, whether they have a significantly marketable commodity that relies on a highly specialized set of expertise, and the extent to which they are positioned to serve social functions relative to other contending occupations. For example, it wasn't until medicine developed the expertise to actually cure infectious disease that allopathic physicians gained enough power to successfully negotiate the ability to self-regulate and enforce licensure for medical practitioners. These protections helped medicine professionalize, but more recently, the ability of other kinds of practitioners (e.g., nurse practitioners and physician assistants) to provide medical care, along with the management of medicine by administrators and corporations, has promoted a shift toward deprofessionalization in medical fields. The key, however, is recognizing the social forces underlying these shifts, since these will influence future professional transitions, including the extent to which other health occupations achieve professional status.

Bioethical Imagination (Chapter 11): The *bioethical imagination* refers to the practitioner's skills in bringing various social contexts and psychological factors together with normative considerations in the process of coming to an ethical decision (De Vries et al. 2007). Recall that the sociological imagination requires us to understand how macro-level social structures manifest in micro-level events, and how those more personal moments also reflect and reinforce larger social patterns and trends at macro-levels of scale. Similarly, the bioethical imagination requires that we understand how various sociological and sociohistorical conditions shape individual experiences of health and illness, and thereby intersect moral decisions like when to end curative treatments and shift toward exclusively palliative care. It requires that we take on the role of the other (i.e., *verstehen*, see Chapter 8), so that we understand that the values and attitudes of individuals who are different from us, particularly patients, constitute a lens through which they view their bodies and illnesses. Similarly, we also must understand how our unique training conditions how we see our own roles vis-à-vis patients, and the ways that these too form a lens through which we make sense of moral dilemmas as practitioners. Accordingly, social constructions and individual preferences intersect in complicated ways when health and illness meet moral decision-making. The bioethical imagination is the ability to see beyond the individual, private moment in which someone confronts an ethical choice in the course of their illness experience, to see how the larger social contexts in which they live and make decisions affect how they understand the situation and the moral decisions they are likely to make.

Systems (Chapter 12): A system is a set of interdependent social features that may include physical or normative boundaries, particular sets of functions and processes, along with various actors performing various roles. Importantly, systems often emerge to confront social problems or fill some sort of social need, but they are shaped by social and cultural forces such that the contours of particular systems tend to reflect the values and ideologies of the societies in which they are built, or of particularly powerful groups within those societies. Health care systems are incredibly complex, particularly in the United States where care often appears, particularly to the patient, fractured and chaotic. In fact, U.S. health care can be characterized as a set of overlapping systems that are coordinated more or less successfully at different moments and for different populations. Still, the shape of the health care systems reflects various features of American culture, including individualist values and tremendous rates of inequality. We sometimes misunderstand systems as emerging from various independent decisions, or even worse, we take systems as given rather than constructed. However, a deeper social scientific perspective entails the recognition that health care systems emerge in response to both professional and epidemiological shifts, that they are patterned on particular sets of social and cultural values, and that once established, they tend to self-perpetuate and change only slowly. The latter is especially challenging where the epidemiological landscape is shifting more rapidly than health care systems can effectively respond.

None of the concepts described here are unique to health and medicine, but all are critically important for thinking about these phenomena with more nuanced social and behavioral science perspectives. We might say that the overarching threshold concept is the sociological imagination itself, as it is important for understanding the rest. The core concepts of each chapter trend more heavily toward the macro (disparity, social determinants, etc.) or the micro (discourse and narrative, *verstehen*, etc.). Yet none ever solely resides at only one level of scale. For example, social disparities have real implications for individuals, and understanding the role of the other (*verstehen*) requires that we peer into the larger social contexts in which they have been socialized. Similarly, social determinants of health affect the illness experiences of individual patients while discourse and narrative are imbued with a number of social constructions such as ideologies that emerge from macro-level forces. The sociological imagination basically requires an understanding of all of these processes and their interconnectedness.

Often being socially or culturally competent in the health care setting is reduced to having a good bedside manner or collegial personality. But illness is both pathological and social in character. Moreover, it requires interpersonal engagement not only as a superficial feature of provider–patient interaction (i.e., as something that happens *while* patients are diagnosed and treated), but as a core component of diagnosis and treatment. After all, a significant portion of the diagnosis is made based on what a patient tells us. On top of all of that, the complexity of health care today requires greater engagement in the form of interprofessional teamwork. At each turn, a good understanding of the social conditions and dynamics that cause illness, affect patient care and interprofessional teamwork, and create the systems of health care in which you work is important for being an effective practitioner. While each chapter of this book will give a number of details, elaborate relevant research findings, and the like, fundamentally each is designed to illustrate the deeper social complexities involved in each area. Each of the threshold concepts identified above is an effort to call your attention to those core ideas.

Brian P. Hinote
Jason Adam Wasserman

Acknowledgments

Nancy Roberts and Rowman & Littlefield not only have been especially wonderful to work with in bringing this book to print, but their enthusiasm for the project also boosted our efforts, and our insights, tremendously. Thank you not only for supporting, but also cultivating, our vision for this book.

Ernest Krug and Mark Haimann provided their seasoned clinical perspectives along with helpful comments on early drafts of the manuscript. Stephen Loftus also provided extremely helpful guidance on threshold concepts, as well as incisive comments on parts of the manuscript.

Bill Cockerham, Jeffrey Michael Clair, and Kenneth L. Wilson have provided mentorship and support over the years that has been immeasurable in its effect and which, while perhaps undetectable to the reader, we can see and feel on every page of this work. Special thanks to Bill and Jeffrey for comments and feedback on the content included in the manuscript and for support and encouragement through the process.

Bill Canak and Grace Budrys provided thoughtful feedback and comments on very early drafts of the manuscript, while Michael Flannery shared important thoughts on the historical development of medicine. Amy DeBaets, Matt Sims, Gustavo Patino, Malli Barremkala, and Dwayne Baxa were invaluable sounding boards as we developed various cases for use at the end of the chapters, and Bob Noiva provided excellent counsel on issues related to mapping to the core competencies and content standards of the various disciplines and professional associations.

We also appreciate the efforts of the following reviewers who read the entire manuscript and made helpful and constructive suggestions: Lara Foley, University of Tulsa; Janet Hankin, Wayne State University; Duane A. Matcha, Siena College; and Teresa Scheid, University of North Carolina at Charlotte.

Special thanks to Brad Bartel, the members of the Non-Instructional Assignment (NIA) Committee, the Office of the Provost, and the Office of Student Success at Middle Tennessee State University, in addition to John Omachonu of Kennesaw State University, for material and nonmaterial support that was invaluable to completing this project.

Finally, there have been many students who, in the classroom, unknowingly served as sounding boards for developing and refining ways of articulating the concepts and issues explored in this book. Thank you all.

PART I

Foundations of Social Science and Health

Introduction to Health and the Sociological Imagination

LEARNING OBJECTIVES

After reading this chapter, students should be able to

- Articulate the dual processes of differentiation and specialization in health care practice, discuss why multidisciplinary perspectives that incorporate social and behavioral factors are important for contemporary patient care, and provide real-world examples of these factors.

- Define the sociological imagination and discuss its promise for improving contemporary health and clinical practice.

- Discuss several classic studies in social science and health/medicine and how they illustrate the contribution of social forces to the shape of health and health care.

- Identify multiple contradictions in U.S. health care today, how some practitioners feel limited amidst the shortcomings of the current system, and envision ways that the health care system might be transformed to respond to those challenges.

The notion of health, and the many practices, activities, and systems that surround it, has fundamentally transformed in recent decades. Not too long ago, health simply was considered the absence of something—a disease, an injury, or a disability. Health was largely the homeostatic condition opposite these defects or deficiencies. But as the twentieth century disappeared into the pages of history, so too did modern definitions of health and disease, along with ideas of how to embrace the former and evade (or at the very least, delay) the latter. We will explore these transformations in greater detail throughout this book, paying special attention to the dramatic shifts in how laypersons, researchers, and clinicians think about health and disease as concepts and conditions, and what this means for health care practitioners in the twenty-first century. Shifts in the landscape of health and health care are important because they necessitate a shift in how twenty-first-century health and medical professionals train and practice. In many ways, we are at the beginning of something new, at a time when health professionals require updated and versatile tools to enter fields that are increasingly multidisciplinary and complex. A more robust understanding of how social factors influence illness experience, disease processes, patient–provider relationships, and health systems has become a necessary part of the practitioner's toolkit.

This book aims to bring the insights of multiple social and behavioral science disciplines to our understanding of health and health care delivery in order to highlight the core challenges and contemporary issues of today's health care practice. This work emerges from multiple ideas and events that have converged in recent years. First, as professors and researchers we noticed greater emphasis on interdisciplinary perspectives reflected in the core competencies of major professional associations across a broad spectrum of occupational groups. For example, there is now greater emphasis on *concepts in social science*; *interpersonal and communication skills*; *social and cultural sensitivity*: *social factors* and *population health*; *health policy* and *health systems*; and various other skills that fall outside of the more traditional focus on biomedical processes, which essentially view the body as a machine. Second, and largely in response to these new professional trends, we watched as universities and other training schools began to place their premedical, health science, or allied health professional students into introductory sociology and psychology courses, or began to develop their own health-focused social and behavioral science offerings. Third, as scholars and educators working with students in the health sciences as well as health professionals in the workforce, our courses and research in recent years have focused upon the various ways that interdisciplinary social and behavioral science approaches intersect fields like epidemiology, clinical practice, medical education, and health care financing and policy.

So rather than developing or reformulating a sociology or psychology of health, or a philosophy or economics of clinical practice or health policy, this book introduces the most relevant insights from multiple disciplines in a way that emphasizes their application in contemporary health care delivery. In doing so, we not only draw from a range of diverse academic fields to specifically address the core competencies of multiple professional and credentialing associations (which are summarized in the instructor's materials provided online by Rowman and Littlefield.), but we also seek to show how interdisciplinary approaches like ours can help practitioners better understand their work and the various ways that they conduct it. We write this book for those of you training or working in one or more of many professional health science fields (e.g., medicine, nursing, pharmacy, dentistry, health care administration, and other allied health disciplines), and for anyone who seeks to develop a broader understanding of the ways that social and behavioral science insights intersect the structure and function of health care practice. This interdisciplinary approach—which at times draws together sociological and psychological approaches with epidemiology, economics, philosophy, and history—aims to increase the reader's understanding of the many factors that influence the delivery of health care.

A Multidimensional Approach to Health and Health Care

Along with many of our colleagues, we argue that an integrated, multidisciplinary approach is essential to understanding myriad health-related phenomena in the twenty-first century. And by extension, such an understanding is a very important part of how professionals go about their work; set goals for themselves and their broader professions; respond to new and not-so-new health threats as individual practitioners, teams, and institutions; collaborate and communicate successfully with both colleagues and patients in increasingly complex situations and organizations; and do all of this while continuously honing their skills in ways that help them do their work more effectively. We believe that this is true whether you are on the front lines of patient care, somewhere within the massive set of parallel systems that constitute American health care delivery, or simply a critical observer of health and health care as a patient or a citizen. Earlier we mentioned that interdisciplinary social and behavioral science content is now clearly represented in core competencies and content standards of virtually all of the medical and allied health professional associations. But beyond meeting educational standards for the purposes of credentialing, understanding the influential social and behavioral factors that affect every level of health care practice ultimately matters for patient care.

As only one brief example, let's consider the development of modern scientific fields. Expanding scientific knowledge throughout the nineteenth and twentieth centuries led to the proliferation of various health-related occupations, as well as new professional terrains and occupational groups. At the same time, many of these fields have become increasingly specialized, so that over time practitioners have focused upon narrower scopes of professional practice. Increasing complexity in the health care system is one end result of these dual processes of differentiation and specialization. The various fields that constitute modern "health care" are so differentiated and specialized that their independence from one another often serves to inhibit our abilities to provide comprehensive care for patients. In other words, the many highly specialized fields and occupations within contemporary health care delivery developed in a way that separated them from each other, so much so that today we often refer to various professions as *disciplinary silos*. To be clear, we are not saying that all fields are completely independent from others, but if you think about it from a developmental perspective, the histories of Western societies unfolded in a way whereby the body largely became the domain of allopathic medicine; the spirit remained the domain of the priest; the mind became the domain of psychiatry, psychology, and related fields; and on and on. Then, within medicine itself, these processes have left the heart to cardiology, the lungs to pulmonology, the skin to dermatology, and so on. We could analyze other allied health professions, and virtually any other field, in a similar way. There are, of course, general practitioners today, but there are far more medical specialists, earning more money and enjoying higher levels of professional prestige, thus reflecting a set of values and incentives that encourage specialization.

These disciplinary silos emerged to promote efficiency—where practitioners can become very good at their work, but their work focuses on a narrower piece of the overall health picture. At the same time, this division of labor also became an obstacle to "whole-patient" care. Ensuring a well-functioning health care system amidst such a complex professional environment requires an interdisciplinary understanding of how social, historical, and epidemiological forces shaped the landscape of the health professions, and how these larger processes manifest in interpersonal interactions between practitioners. In other words, understanding the big picture is more critical than ever when practices are set up in such highly specialized and concentrated ways. Bridging the silos is critically important to providing the best care to patients, promoting health in a way that is sustainable in the long term, and creating educational, insurance, reimbursement, and policy systems that support healthy populations in a cost-effective manner, while at the same time caring for individuals that inevitably fall ill or become injured.

Perhaps these ideas seem largely academic or esoteric at this point, so let us provide a more specific example that might help bring things into better focus. About four years ago, an otherwise healthy man in his mid-thirties presented to his primary care physician with mild chest discomfort and shortness of breath. Of course, any mention of pain or discomfort in the chest is taken quite seriously, to the point that any symptom resembling chest pain necessitates an immediate trip to the emergency room (ER). The patient underwent a number of screening procedures there, including blood work and an electrocardiogram, all of which were within normal parameters. He was admitted later that day at the advice of the ER physician and was assigned a cardiologist as his attending physician. Over the next few days, he underwent a battery of tests evaluating his heart that revealed nothing notable or abnormal. After many thousands of dollars and several days away from work and family, the discomfort persisted but the patient was discharged nonetheless, with his attending cardiologist and others recommending little more than taking a few more days away from work, and surmising that all of this might be "in your head."

A few months later a pulmonologist would discover that the patient was experiencing mild bronchospasms, associated with moderate-to-intense physical activity and aggravated by stress. This part of the patient's history is noteworthy, because he worked well over forty hours per week (albeit in a satisfying job), with twin 2-year-olds in his household (and all of the logistical and financial challenges that they entail), and tried to maintain an active leisure-time exercise regimen. This abbreviated story illustrates how the landscape of highly specialized health professions makes it easy for practitioners to overlook plausible alternatives that are outside of their narrow scopes of expertise. Here, a reputable cardiologist never considered or adequately investigated the possibility that the chest discomfort could originate outside of the heart, despite the fact that many of these other possibilities were only centimeters away. Further complicating the diagnostic process, these symptoms largely originated beyond the mechanics of the body altogether. Understanding the social and behavioral experiences of this patient was critical to the diagnosis. Finally, while the patient's illness was not life threatening in the long run and was manageable with lifestyle modifications, this case study illustrates the significance of underlying social and behavioral causes of health.

That such a relatively simple condition holds the potential to confound a hyperspecialized clinical gaze trained to focus on one somatic system demonstrates the need for health care providers to understand and utilize social and behavioral science in practice. All of this makes clear that contemporary health care delivery unfolds at the nexus of multiple fields. Health care practitioners must not only develop the ability to understand and envision the complexity of the human organism itself, but they must also comprehend the complexity of the interactions between the organism and other social and environmental conditions that influence patients' health, as well as the broader institutions of health care. Understanding the etiology of disease and a patient's prognosis also means considering the lifestyle factors that strongly contribute to this condition's development and subsequent management. Making sense of such a complex set of factors also means considering the various social and economic influences underlying the choices constituting a health lifestyle, as well as how a patient's living and working environments impinge upon his or her ability to adhere to medical advice and manage their condition. Therefore a purely biomedical approach to disease management is incomplete, in large part because what is required to effectively manage increasingly complex diseases stretches into the realms of psychology, economics, bioethics, sociology, and other fields. The social and behavioral sciences, therefore, offer a great deal to practitioners working in health and medicine. Beyond simply making patients feel better or more accompanied, in the contemporary era of complex, multifactorial illness, a good understanding of the social and behavioral contributions to health and disease is important for every element of patient care, including the core processes of diagnosis and treatment.

The various disciplinary approaches from which we draw in the chapters that follow help us move beyond thinking about health, disease, and health care as only individual phenomena. Certainly our primary experiences in the world as practitioners and patients are very personal. But these individualized perspectives can often limit our understanding of what is happening around us more broadly. In other words, our experiences are not always indicative of larger trends and do not, on their own, provide a window into the more macro-level processes that quietly influence our daily lives. One classic example that succinctly illustrates this point may be found in the work of sociologist Emile Durkheim (1897 [1951]), who studied suicide in nineteenth-century France. Prior to Durkheim's work, most explanations for suicide focused on the individual—the mental health of the person committing the act, or perhaps a biological defect. But when Durkheim examined suicide data at the aggregate (or group) level, he was able to discern patterns, which suggested that suicide cases often clustered into groups of individuals sharing similar attributes of one sort or another. Put another way, he was able to describe a set of social influences conditioning individual choices, thus creating room to describe and explain human behavior at multiple levels of analysis (i.e., the individual *and* the group levels).

This might seem somewhat simple today, but it is certainly not trivial. Durkheim's conclusions in this classic study are still important for a number of reasons. In particular, Durkheim's insight was that social groups are something much more than the sums of the individuals that compose them, and thereby exert unique and observable influences upon those individuals in ways that compel us to look toward the "bigger picture." Like Durkheim's analysis of suicide, we can discern that most of our world is patterned in very specific and observable ways, and thinking about the various foci of our work (e.g., health, disease, patients, etc.) in a deeper and more critical fashion allows us to better understand the individual case (i.e., the diagnosis, the patient, and our work as individuals) within the context of that bigger picture (i.e., disease etiologies, patient profiles, interpersonal interaction, professional collaboration, and health care delivery systems). With this more elaborate and accurate picture of the world, we can work more effectively and more conscientiously within it. By making sense of increasingly complex phenomena, creating a broader landscape from which to think about these ideas, and firmly connecting individuals to the larger groups to which they belong, the insights and perspectives that we outline in the following chapters will help you understand the *how* and the *why* of disease processes, clinical interactions, epidemiological shifts, diagnostic problematics, policy debates, and so on. As a result, we envision much of our contribution here as an important complement to your more discipline-specific training in the health and professional sciences.

The Sociological Imagination

The *sociological imagination* is one way of thinking that can help us match the complexity of contemporary health and health care, and is therefore a critical element in meeting the challenges of twenty-first century medical and allied health practice. It was named by C. Wright Mills (1959 [1977]), who was interested in understanding the rapid social changes taking place in the United States in the decades leading up to the 1950s. Because of the pace of that change and the increasing complexity of modern society, Mills suggested that the unfolding of this historical epoch was outpacing individuals' abilities to orient themselves to new arrangements. Remember that Mills wrote during the mid-1950s; imagine what he would say about the pace of change and level of complexity today! He also notes that individuals fail to comprehend their own experiences (good, bad, or neutral) within the context of broader shifts in society and history. But especially with regard to the problems that inevitably arise in our lives (called *private troubles*), he claims that many individuals fail to see their connection to broader events and arrangements in their society and surroundings (called *public or social issues*). We might think of these troubles as problems of biography or dilemmas existing at the *micro* (or smaller, individual) level, while issues are problems of society and history existing at the *macro* (or broader, large-scale community or cultural) level.

Making sense of an increasingly complex world, and our individual positions within it, therefore requires more than simply developing our capacities for reason, or gathering additional information. After all, rational thinking has dominated the structure and function of Western societies for several hundred years (see Chapter 2) and the amount of information available to us today is already overwhelming. Instead, Mills (1959 [1977]) argues, we must develop and embrace a perspective that allows us to see the various interconnections that exist between the individual and society, by connecting private troubles to public issues—that is, by seeing the interrelatedness of micro- and macro-phenomena. This sociological imagination holds *the promise* for tackling the complex challenges of contemporary society, including those of health and health care.

This is a very brief summary of Mills' discussion, but it provides us with important insights with which to facilitate a shift in our thinking about all sorts of ideas in health and health care. First, that which we experience in our personal lives commonly originates far beyond our own often-limited social milieu (i.e., physical surroundings, experiences, relationships, etc.). These perceived personal, individualized experiences are firmly connected to, and strongly shaped by, broader social, economic, and cultural arrangements. Second, we cannot understand our own lives as simply a matter of our isolated individual choices, nor the social world around us merely as the sum of other individuals' choices. Rather, we are shaped by the

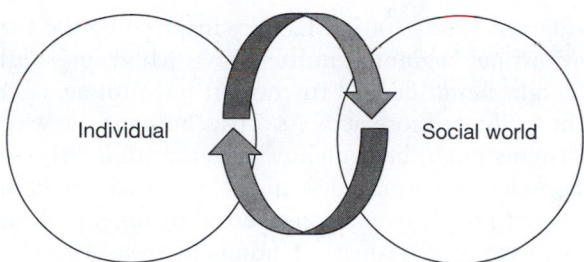

FIG. 1.1 A reflexive model of social reality.

social world around us, and we collectively reproduce or alter it, in turn. This is often called a reflexive model of social reality (see Fig. 1.1) and is a useful way to think about how our world works. Third, if we follow Mills down this road of thinking, we also see that both our perceptions of social problems and the range of possible options with which to solve them require us to consider not only the personal situations, conditions, characters, and behaviors of a subset of individuals but also the larger contours of society (i.e., history, social interaction, institutions, etc.; p. 9). Mills (1959:12) succinctly points out that the great issues and troubles of his time are framed in terms of the "psychiatric" in a misguided attempt to avoid engaging the much larger shifts often responsible for issues and troubles in the first place. Here he is suggesting that we too often mistakenly look to the individual alone to analyze larger issues requiring much broader perspectives of ourselves and the world.

Mills' (1959 [1977]) work is not only a seminal contribution to American sociology, but his ideas constitute an important part of how we discuss many of the ideas and phenomena that we present in subsequent chapters. In other words, we connect smaller-scale phenomena with much larger trends as a way to make sense of increasingly complex clinical, epidemiological, and policy issues. As a result, the usefulness of this imagination stretches far beyond the boundaries of sociology as an academic and applied discipline. This is exactly the type of critical thinking and analysis that paves the way to addressing complex issues in what is now often called *late modern* society, and these are valuable tools for health care practitioners seeking to understand a complex and shifting landscape of health and illness and working to treat patients with increasingly complex, multifactorial illnesses.

Bringing the Sociological Imagination into Focus

Let us briefly consider a few examples of how connecting smaller-scale, individual behavior to much larger phenomena can help us understand the bigger picture in ways that facilitate greater understanding of what is going on in the world, in our lives, and in our work. Keep in mind how Durkheim's (1897 [1951]) work demonstrates that something unique and much larger emerges when individuals come together to interact in social groups, and how those social forces can act back on individuals and groups. These dynamics are endemic to all social settings, whether in an experiment or study, in a classroom, or in disease epidemiology, or clinical medicine. Our first example in this regard is the work of Stanley Milgram at Yale

University (see Milgram 1965 [2008]). Largely inspired by the events surrounding the Holocaust in Europe, beginning in the 1950s Milgram sought to investigate how individuals might be influenced to commit harmful acts against others and what factors might facilitate those acts. As a psychologist, he was actually considering how the Germans might be somehow different than "the rest of us" in that their psyches or consciences permitted so many to participate in attempts to exterminate large groups of people over a long period of time. In doing so he assessed levels of obedience in samples of American adults by measuring the degree to which they would comply with instructions from an authority figure in a white lab coat directing them to administer increasingly powerful electrical shocks to other people, under the guise of testing principles of teaching and learning. While the subject receiving the shocks was actually complicit in the experiment and was not really being shocked at all, the participants believed they were causing significant harm to an unwitting counterpart in the experiment. Across a number of experiments, Milgram found that a significant percentage of people kept administering more and more severe shocks, despite (staged) protests from their counterparts.

More interestingly, while they never would have done so on their own, they kept shocking their counterpart because they were told to do so by an authority figure, despite the fact that person never actually, in any physical or material sense, forced them to do it. How likely someone was to proceed with increased electric shocks varied by context, with the likelihood being lower, for example, when the participant could see the person, and higher when they could not. Milgram's results from multiple iterations and scenarios across these studies suggest that those Germans were probably not very different at all. That is, just about anyone placed in the right surroundings with the appropriate mix of props and carefully worded directions originating from a defined authority figure is capable of doing quite unpleasant things to others and without need for any force other than the symbolic social force of authority. We will not describe Milgram's work in any further detail here (you can take a look at some of his study's video footage on your own time). For now, consider what this study signals about social factors within the health care landscape about authority, obedience, and the like. After all, one key influential factor was the white coat worn by the authority figure in these experiments.

Philip Zimbardo (2000) conducted a similar study in the 1970s, now known somewhat notoriously as the Stanford Prison Study (see also Musen 1988 [2004]). Like Milgram, Zimbardo was motivated by questions pertaining to how individual behavior can often take a turn toward the unpleasant or downright cruel, this time in the context of prisons. So Zimbardo and his colleagues created a mock prison in the basement of the psychology building at Stanford in which to place randomly assigned "prisoners" and "guards." Like Milgram's subjects, these volunteers knew that they were part of an experiment and could decline at any time to participate. Zimbardo reports that the experiment started uneventfully, but as participants slowly settled into their roles as part of dominant or subordinate groups, their individual behaviors began to more and more resemble that of actual prison inmates and correctional guards, sometimes in brutal fashion. Even Zimbardo, cast in this experiment as prison warden, describes how he himself was absorbed into the mock environment by virtue of his position and role in this "prison." While the study was designed to continue for two weeks, it had to be terminated after six days because the participants became so fully consumed by their roles (which were randomly assigned to them by researchers). The study demonstrated that individuals tend to conform to behavioral expectations (i.e., *roles*) associated with group membership (i.e., *statuses*). The force of these role expectations within a larger status system led individuals to act in ways dramatically different than they likely would behave if left alone, or in other contexts. Again, think about how this might inform the behavior of actors within health care settings where individuals assume the roles of physician, nurse, patient, loved one, administrator, and so on. How do various role expectations and status arrangements in health care affect how individual practitioners and patients behave?

Two other brief examples, the work of Jane Elliott (see Peters 1985, 1987) and Solomon Asch (1955), also illustrate the interrelatedness between social structure and individual behavior. Elliott's work unfolded in her classrooms, where she manufactured a sense of difference among schoolchildren by giving meaning to a previously meaningless attribute—eye color. In the social sciences, we refer to this process as the *social construction* of reality. In this case, the reality perceived by the children was constructed around the special and significant meanings given to something that is otherwise insignificant. Elliott shifted the meanings normally associated with race in 1960s America to eye color in her classroom, where children with brown eyes were assigned clearly defined behavioral attributes like laziness, dishonesty, ignorance, and violence, and those with blue eyes were assigned the opposites of these characteristics. In short, what unfolded over time was a situation in which otherwise friendly classmates began to react aggressively and antagonistically to one another in the classroom and on the playground on the basis of eye color. In addition, individuals in these dominant and subordinate groups (which, again, were completely fabricated by Elliott) also exhibited behavior consistent with their group membership, like performing assigned tasks and exercises more quickly and efficiently, or more slowly and inefficiently, according to their group membership and its assigned characteristics and meanings. These arrangements persisted for a week, at which time Elliott flipped the dominant and subordinate groups and subsequently observed similar behavior and self-identities shift toward the opposite direction (i.e., formerly subordinate individuals readily embraced their new dominant roles and positions, and vice versa). Elliott's work shows us how the social construction of the world around us (reinforced by group socialization and experience) can strongly shape not only our behavior but our self-identities as well (which are also socially constructed, by the way). With regard to health and health care, consider how various meanings and metaphors permeate discourses of disease and illness and how these shape our experiences of our work, our patients, our colleagues, and so on. For example, how do discourses about "battling" cancer shape our understanding of a variety of patient reactions to that disease, how they might implicitly frame less aggressive treatments or transitions in care at the end of life as "losing" (or even running from) said "battle"?

In a similar vein, studies by Asch (1955:31) explore the ways that "social forces constrain people's opinions and attitudes." In these experiments, Asch and his associates assembled participants for a study in "visual judgment" where they would simply compare the lengths of lines on two large white cards. On one was a single vertical line, and participants were instructed to match this line with one of three lines of distinctly different lengths on the second white card. The alleged subjects announced their selections one by one, all agreeing with one another, for multiple rounds of a seemingly boring experiment. However, many participants (in different trials) eventually diverged from the group's consensus, with much of their dissent persisting over multiple rounds of the experiment. What these dissenters did not know was that they were under scrutiny; all of the other participants were at the outset instructed to provide incorrect answers in matching the lines. Asch sought to transform the subject into a minority of one who was brought into a conflict between two opposing forces: sensory evidence on the one hand and the unanimous perspective of the group on the other. Of the 123 subjects initially studied, a sizable percentage conformed to the power of the group (about 37%) and reported answers that their own senses told them were clearly incorrect. Asch's conclusions emphasize that we often submit to group conformity, even when it conflicts with our own perceptions of the world. Moreover, the participants in the study did not report an answer they knew was false simply to go along with the group. Rather, they came to doubt their own perceptions; they figured that they must be wrong, even when they clearly were right. Think about that: we often trust the perspective of the social group over and above our own senses! Again, think about how this may shape practice in health care settings, where caring for patients, particularly those with complex or difficult illnesses, is often rife with conflict and debate, and where evidence is often far less clear than Asch's mismatched lines. We believe Asch probably says it best:

> Life in society requires consensus as an indispensible condition. But consensus, to be productive, requires that each individual contribute independently out of his [or her] experience and insight. When consensus comes under the dominance of conformity, the social process is polluted and the individual at the same time surrenders the powers on which his [or her] functioning as a feeling and thinking being depends. That we have found the tendency to conformity in our society so strong that reasonably intelligent and well-meaning young people are willing to call white black is a matter of concern. It raises questions about our ways of education and about the values that guide our conduct. (Asch 1955:34)

Certainly important dissenting voices on a health care team or from the patient themselves might easily be squelched in a health care environment, particularly when one adds in issues of status and hierarchy, power, authority, behavioral expectations, and so on, demonstrated by the above studies.

All of the studies briefly mentioned here help bring into better focus the ways that human behavior unfolds within broader and quite influential social contexts. We believe that this is important in itself, as a way to understand complex phenomena as mentioned above, and it is up to all of us to assemble the complex pieces of the social world around us to make more sense of our place within it. But perhaps the more important insight is that such realizations open up the possibility of doing things differently, of approaching a situation or problem creatively, or to choose a course of action that deviates from that which often invisible social forces otherwise often guide us. This is the sociological imagination in action—bringing into focus previously invisible connections, making sense of complex and sometimes counterintuitive observations, and illuminating creative paths forward. We now turn to look more deeply at how thinking in a social-scientific way, that is, using the sociological imagination, can help us better understand disease.

Critically Analyzing Health and Health Care

Throughout the history of health care, many individuals and groups have approached issues of health and illness in ways that would now be considered inter-disciplinary, with dramatic and far-reaching results. It seems somewhat paradoxical, then, that researchers and practitioners subsequently receded into their highly specialized disciplinary silos when there exists such a rich history of innovative thinking that traversed ground that separate disciplines eventually claimed for themselves. Importantly, practitioners in a variety of fields are embracing inter-disciplinary approaches once again amidst a complex health landscape for which the approaches of single disciplines are insufficient. Several thinkers in the 1800s provide us with insightful work analyzing the bigger picture of health and well-being, where physiology, medicine, politics, economics, ethics, philosophy, epide-miology, and health care intersect. Friedrich Engels provides one such book, *The Condition of the Working Class in England* (1845 [2009]), where he interweaves living and working conditions into the politics and economics of capitalism to paint a picture of overcrowding, pollution, poor sanitation, and underdeveloped urban infrastructure, and their effects on residents in nineteenth-century London. Among his contemporaries we also find Edwin Chadwick, who in his *Report on the Sanitary Condition of the Labouring Population and on the Means of Its Improvement* (1842) similarly integrates data and observations germane to the social and economic origins and correlates of sickness and death in Scotland, England, and Wales. Both utilize various research designs to investigate the complex ways that factors external to the individual can significantly impinge upon the longevity and well-being of specific human populations.

We should also briefly mention physicians John Snow, Rudolf Virchow, and Salomon Neumann, whose work in medicine proved influential long after it was carried out. Snow, who laid the foundation for modern epidemiology with *On the Mode of Communication of Cholera* (1849), investigated cholera in London by plotting infections geographically, collecting spatial and face-to-face information in neighborhoods, and systematically and critically scrutinizing his data to link environments, social behavior, and modes of cholera transmission at a time when the germ theory of disease did not yet exist. Snow's work contributed method-ologically to how we investigate and understand many diseases, but also showed how integrative approaches to health and disease can serve as the basis for positive interventions and change. After all, by understanding community dynamics Snow brought into focus a perspective unseen from within the walls of the clinic, but ultimately improved the treatment recommendations made by clinical practi-tioners. Similarly, Virchow (a pioneer in cellular pathology) and Neumann (in medical statistics) both firmly linked public health and epidemic disease outbreaks to complex sets of social and economic conditions among particular groups of people at risk for contracting specific diseases. The work of these thinkers and others sought to explain "the linkage between social conditions and medical problems, the idea that human disease is always mediated and modified by social activities and the cultural environment" and that clinical treatments would remain largely ineffective if we do not consider the larger, daunting influences of social context (Bloom 2002:11–12).

The physician Stewart Wolf and his colleague John Bruhn, a medical sociologist, provide us with one of the most famous illustrations of how invisible social forces shape health and disease trends in their study of Roseto, Pennsylvania, a town first settled by Italian immigrants in the 1880s (see Bruhn & Wolf 1979; Gladwell 2008; Wasserman & Hinote 2012). The mystery of Roseto was not a disease epidemic or previously unseen illness; the perplexing epidemiological trend of Roseto was that residents were dying of old age rather than the most deadly diseases of the mid-twentieth century, which were driving mortality nearly everywhere else in the United States. At the time, for example, heart disease was the leading cause of death among men below age 65. Wolf and Bruhn could not initially explain how residents were able to evade the widespread cardiovascular disease affecting towns only a few miles away, despite the fact that Roseto's inhabitants often smoked heavily and many were obese. It turned out that the key to health in Roseto could not be found among the individual choices of residents or in their DNA. The answer was in their social interactions; their extended family and kinship structures; the egalitarian nature of the community; and their highly integrated ethnic, civic, and religious ties. In Chapter 5, we will explore the deeper features of social life in Roseto that help explain health among its residents. But for now, Bruhn and Wolf (1979) show us, as have many others, that we cannot understand health by thinking about the lone actions of isolated individuals, or by a purely biomedical explanation of disease (see especially Engel 1977). Instead, we must look instead toward social influences, communities, and institutions, and what those mean for health care delivery and the health professionals working among them.

The Paradox of American Health Care

Today there are many others doing similarly important work in the areas of social epidemiology, health behavior, clinical practice, health care delivery, bioethics, and more, much of which we will discuss in the following chapters. A lot of this work examines the ways that *culture* (i.e., shared knowledge among the members of a social group) and *life chances* (i.e., arrangements of advantage and disadvantage) shape our health-related choices, and how the ways that institutions are constructed very clearly influence the how we think and behave within them, even as we carry out our work with patients and colleagues. We want to emphasize one recent study that specifically pertains to frontline health workers like the ones that make up our audience, as a way to begin thinking about how the work of American health care professionals reflects many of the realities we discussed above, and the insights still to come.

The work of Bradley and Taylor (2013) examines several contradictions in American health care and offers a useful introductory example of how we can use a sociological imagination to gain a sense of the big picture when it comes to some of our most pressing issues. Indeed, American health care is full of contradictions. Among the most notable we might include the following:

1. We spend more on health care in the United States than most of our industrialized peers, but we exhibit aggregate health indicators that lag behind these counterparts.
2. Our system is not really a system at all. It is by all accounts unsystematic in that multiple health care arrangements and programs exist side-by-side, with very different ways of working.
3. We have one of the largest and technologically rich health care sectors in the world, but nonetheless seem unable to address many of the health and disease issues that typically confront most Americans today, and as a result struggle to balance effectively the tripartite concerns of cost containment, access to care, and quality.

Bradley and Taylor (2013) interviewed patients, health workers, and administrators to better dissect these paradoxes and gleaned at least four key themes from their data. First, *the health care sector bears the brunt of an inadequate social service sector*. Because health is such a multidimensional concept today, and because American health care was largely structured to focus on the physical and biomedical aspects of health (in another paradoxical mismatch that we will discuss in Chapter 2), health care has difficulty addressing the core causes of patient conditions and complaints (i.e., social factors like poverty, lack of access to healthy foods, living and working conditions, environmental exposures, etc.). One survey of physicians noted their awareness of the effects of social environments on health, where 85% reported that unmet social needs directly contributed to poor health and that those needs are just as important as their medical conditions. They also reported that if they had the power to write prescriptions for what patients really need, the top prescriptions would be for fitness, nutritious food, employment assistance, education, and housing. Second, and in reality, *frontline personnel are forced to respond to these larger social concerns with limited resources*, and from the limited domain of clinical practice. Many professionals described the challenges associated with providing care in a way that meets the real and increasingly complex needs of patients amidst the rising tide of bureaucracy and paperwork. While they frequently recalled choosing their profession out of a desire to focus on patient care and to help make those patients better, they clearly expressed that their inability to treat patients effectively was very much related to administrative, legal, and financial realities.

Third, *the need for a more holistic approach is widely acknowledged but requires professional collaboration between health and social service sectors*. In other words, the increasing sophistication of medicine has led to a reductionist approach to clinical practice, and consequently today's health care structures are ill-equipped to deal with the physical, emotional, social, psychological, and spiritual connections to health and disease, especially following the rise of chronic disease and other more complex disorders. Finally, *barriers and difficulties in establishing relationships between social services and health care have many roots*. There are many barriers involved with pushing health care to where it should probably be—in a place where it can adequately care for patients in ways that tend to the real causes of their troubles. The authors specifically cite Roy Porter's (1997) account of nineteenth-century primary care: "The open secret of general practice, its strength and weakness, has been that many clients do not actually have a disease; they are sick, sad or solitary, they need solace." Bradley and Taylor (2013:57) go on to note that the providers interviewed reported that "this statement is as true today as it was in the nineteenth century, and the expectation that health services can address social needs is a key challenge in delivering timely, cost-effective health care." These conclusions illuminate previously invisible connections, make sense of sometimes illogical and contradictory observations, and stimulate the development of creative paths to move forward in addressing the needs of both patients and providers in contemporary health care. While we will return to a deeper exploration of health care systems in Chapter 12, this serves as a good example of the sociological imagination in action. These themes also suggest important avenues of research and debate for those entering the health professions, and they set the stage for our journey through the coming pages as we seek to empower you as professionals to think critically and creatively about your work and the systems and institutions that your work supports.

Health Care as a Social Institution

As we conclude this chapter, we want to take time to talk about how social scientists discuss the often-misinterpreted notion of the *social institution*. Essentially, when sociologists discuss institutions, they refer to a range of processes and structures that address some social need (Budrys 2005:2). Many laypersons and professionals alike use the term *institution* to refer to specific organizations like Johns Hopkins University Hospital or the Mayo Clinic, but unless otherwise noted, when we use the term institution we are talking about all sorts of organizations and systems, physical or ideological, that are connected to a specific sector of society, and that serve to shape and channel behavior toward specific ends. Sociologists typically refer to five primary institutions—education, family, religion, the economy, and politics—all of which encapsulate all sorts of individuals, groups, organizations, practices, structures, and purposes. There also exist so-called secondary institutions like health care, medicine, sports, and the like.

Grace Budrys (2005) argues that health care delivery has only recently been considered from this broader perspective, but like other institutions, the American health care delivery system shares a number of attributes with educational, familial, religious, political, and economic institutions. For example, it was constructed to meet specific societal needs, and in a way that very much reflects our values, expectations, behavioral expectations, and culture. While health care delivery is sometimes perceived as a purely rational, scientific endeavor, the structure and function of social institutions vary significantly across different societies, even those which seem to share underlying cultural assumptions. This is because the "building blocks" of culture, Budrys explains, are the bricks from which institutions are built. We think that this is a useful metaphor because it explains how institutions are put together, piece by piece—how they are *socially constructed* in very specific ways. American health care, as a social institution, was constructed like a house erected over multiple generations, with each set of inhabitants building upon, remodeling, or altering the bricks of those coming before them. The builders (i.e., individuals and groups with varying degrees of power and influence) used the bricks at their disposal that they wanted to see included in the finished product. But to complete the metaphor, we must also note that the social construction of institutions is never complete. We are constantly reproducing or reworking the form and function of social institutions. This is not to say that all of us as individuals have an equal say in how those institutions, including health care, should be organized, which is where the notion of power, another important sociological concept, comes in. Still, we believe that our readers will be in a good position to either reproduce existing health care arrangements, or change them by selecting and laying new bricks, or by remolding the bricks that make up the existing structure. We might argue that institutions rarely fail; instead, we fail to update them. This is one powerful reason why we think your exposure to critical approaches in the social and behavioral sciences is a worthwhile endeavor that has the potential to enrich your day-to-day work, your career, your personal experiences with health and health care, and, finally, the overall manner in which health care is provided.

The building block metaphor illustrates how institutions, cultures, and societies are put together, and how they reflect past experience, ideologies, history, social change, and so on—everything that makes up what we know as the world around us. Most importantly, however, this suggests that institutions are created by human social activity. And because human activity is ongoing, the social construction of institutions is a dynamic, rather than static, process that often proceeds alongside (or perhaps slightly behind) changes in other parts of society. This also means that, like that house in the examples above, institutions need to be maintained, and sometimes overhauled. These processes, although necessary, can be uncomfortable and unpredictable, and are inextricably connected to all sorts of other institutions and ways of life, which opens the door for any number of unforeseen difficulties to arise amidst these processes. So as you can imagine, dissecting and analyzing complex systems, not to mention reworking them, can be messy and frustrating business, which is a big reason why change is usually a very slow process. Still, these are worthwhile and absolutely necessary elements of designing and implementing approaches to health care delivery that achieve the objectives they were designed to meet—helping patients who are sick and promoting health and wellness.

Organization of the Book

As you can probably tell from our discussion thus far, this book aims to develop your capacities to see and understand the "bigger picture" when it comes to logic, history, disease trends, and health care delivery and policy. But we specifically aim to emphasize the importance of integrative, multidisciplinary approaches within the health professions, and to develop ways to help you conduct your work more effectively and conscientiously in today's health care landscape. In doing so, we dedicate

Part I of the book (Chapters 1–3) to discussing the history, logic, and methods of particular interest to health professionals, and build a firm foundation in social epidemiology (i.e., the various ways that social, economic, political, and environmental conditions manifest health or disease in human populations) in Part II (Chapters 4–6). If we recognize that these arrangements have considerable potential to affect health and well-being, then the next step is to consider what this means for the actual work of health professionals. This is the focus of Part III of the book (Chapters 7–11), which critically examines the clinical challenges associated with shifting definitions of illness and disorder. Here we also consider the important role played by provider–patient interaction and how this relationship has fundamentally transformed in recent years, along with the role of interprofessional collaboration and teamwork. We also discuss important ethical issues in health care and the practical challenges of working ethically in a complex health care landscape rife with perplexing moral dilemmas. Finally, in Part IV we will conclude by considering what recent epidemiological and institutional changes mean for American health care policy and our health care system, including health reform. Here we will wrap up by tying together the various ways that disease epidemiology, clinical practice, and health care delivery structures are connected to one another. In doing so, we pay particular attention to what this means for current and future health practitioners, and the ways that those clinicians and policymakers can critically engage the health care challenges of the twenty-first century.

But before we go any further, we want to outline a few points of interest, and of caution. First, we should acknowledge that exposure to new ways of thinking about complex ideas and phenomena can sometimes be quite uncomfortable. Many of us are remarkably content in how we look at the world around us, so the act of challenging many of the taken-for-granted notions of how things work can push us into uncharted territory. Again, this can be disquieting, but it can also be revelatory. This is because insights often come to us when we begin to free ourselves from the various ways that institutions and other structures influence our thinking, as we discussed above. And because we are all thinking, feeling, evaluating human beings, some topics might conjure up strong feelings, good or bad, in our discussions. This is not out of the ordinary. With that said, we strive to develop logical, well-argued, reasonable discussions of whatever phenomena we approach in the coming chapters. We hold our students and our readers to the same standard. We encourage you to focus less on how you feel about an issue and more on where your logic combined with the data take you. Most people, because of their background and socialization through family, peer groups, and education, possess a particular idea of how the world works, and they tend to gather as much information as they can to support that worldview. We say this not to imply that these people are wrong or backward, only that a good scientist does the opposite. As one of our colleagues pointed out many years ago, in matters of science what you *believe* or *think* matters less than what you can *demonstrate* using data, logic, and argument.

Second, the discomfort associated with assuming a critical perspective might be particularly discernible when we analyze those settings and institutions in which you actually work (or are training to work within). This logic might lead our readers to think that in pointing out the limitations of modern clinical practice or health policy, we have a negative opinion of the individuals and groups working within that system. This cannot be farther from the truth. In fact, by virtue of our training we intuitively look at the form and function of the system itself (i.e., clinical practice or health care delivery), while paying comparatively little attention to the motivations of the actors involved as individuals. This might seem strange, but we are sure that even poorly functioning or unresponsive health care *systems* are full of well-meaning, benevolent *individuals* doing the best that they can in their work. The legacy of sociology as an academic discipline involves identifying problems, critically engaging and reflecting upon them, and formulating ways to ameliorate their negative effects. Accordingly, a lot of work in health and health care delivery focuses on those problems, or the problematic elements or challenges facing the health professions. But don't get us wrong. There are many good things about American health care, and we certainly do not wish to omit the good things in emphasizing the not so good. Rather, we simply try to focus on the problems and challenges facing today's health care delivery and the professions within it, as a way to help you think more about how to approach those challenges critically and creatively.

Third, to aid our readers in discerning the core principles, themes, and major "take-aways" of each chapter, we will begin each chapter with a list of specific learning objectives to guide your reading and understanding as you move through each section. These will be useful in reflecting back on the material after reading, and then connecting core themes to other ideas and to your own work. Finally, we would like to include a note on references. Our work is inspired by many volumes of work by many different authors in many different disciplines, so to provide citations for most or all of the material that inspires our own thinking would create a reference list as lengthy as our manuscript itself. As a result, we will reference ideas that have a high degree of specificity in their origins, and those that represent seminal contributions to our fields of work and study. We also do this so that continually referencing numerous sources does not distract our readers from the major points of our writing. With that said, we encourage you to seek out other sources in these various areas of discussion and debate, both because more perspectives are almost always better when it comes to thinking about health and health care delivery, and because these ideas are constantly changing as the notion of health continues to transform, and as the building blocks of clinical practice and health policy are continually being replaced, remolded, or refurbished.

CHAPTER 1 ACTIVITY

Exercising the Sociological Imagination

Part 1

Create a chart with two columns, like the one below. On the left side, write a detailed description of the last time you went to a clinic for medical care (even if it was for just a routine checkup). The more detail you can provide, the better. After you finish the description, identify the social and psychological dynamics at different parts of the story (see the example below).

Example excerpt for this activity:

My Story	Social/Psychological Dynamics
I became worried because the pain was getting worse at night and I was sweating a lot while I slept, but I had no idea what it could be. Looking it up on the Internet only made it worse since it could have been any number of things from serious to trivial.	Ambiguous symptoms causing worry Seeking information on my own, rather than waiting for a professional
When I got to the clinic, I wasn't sure whether to go to the sick or well-patient side. On the one hand, this didn't seem like a contagious thing, but on the other hand, I wasn't there just for a well-visit/checkup.	My problem doesn't seem to fit the classifications of the waiting room
At the front desk, a woman greeted me and I signed in, and a little while later, a nurse took me back to the waiting room	Different people have different jobs/functions

Helpful Hints

1. Don't leave out things that have happened because they seem trivial or ordinary. Try to account for everything that has happened and that you have observed.

2. Discussing these with a group of people is more helpful because the similarities and differences make for a richer picture of the various social and psychological elements.

Part 2

Look back at your narrative and your analysis and reflect on the following questions:

1. Notice how various social and psychological elements of the experience occurred in your own mind or in interactions between you and the other people involved.

2. After reviewing the *micro-level* phenomena that you have identified above, identify and discuss the norms, social structures (e.g., class, race, gender, etc.), and historical conditions that are behind them.
   Example: The physician's white coat served to distinguish her from both myself as the patient and the other staff. This speaks to the role of power and hierarchy between doctors and patients, and also doctors and other professionals.

3. Review the material on paradoxes of U.S. health care (if necessary) and discuss ways in which you've seen some or all of those in your own experiences with health care or those of your friends and family.
   Example: My grandmother died from complications of diabetes. She received a lot of high-tech interventions at the end of her life that cost tens of thousands of dollars, but few efforts focused on preventing her from getting diabetes in the first place.

The Shifting Landscape of Health and Medicine
Past, Present, and Future

LEARNING OBJECTIVES

After reading this chapter, students should be able to

- Articulate how understandings of health and particular health care practices are linked to broader sociocultural ways of thinking (across the premodern, modern, and contemporary time periods).

- Critically evaluate the nature of modern health care practice and articulate its strengths and weaknesses.

- Identify how contemporary and future challenges for health and health care practice emerge from key shifts in the social and epidemiological landscape, specifically with regard to the complexity of chronic illnesses.

Introduction

It should be clear from Chapter 1 that health care delivery is a social institution; how it is constructed, how its actors behave, its clinical priorities and processes, and its way of understanding health and the body are all social in character. They are nested in broader cultural patterns, values, shared history, professional trends, and ways of thinking, and therefore shape the manner in which we conceptualize health and disease. Insofar as understanding the social character of health and health care delivery is essential for practitioners of all kinds, it is important to understand how modern medicine emerged from, and within, particular sets of social conditions. Perhaps more importantly, it is essential for health professionals to understand that many of the seemingly divergent challenges facing health professions today (indeed, many of those we examine in this book) share a common origin in the shifting social landscape upon which successful modern medical institutions were initially constructed. Assembling this complex picture, and finding within it our own professional work, not only highlights core features of health and health care, but is itself a good exercise of your sociological imagination.

In Chapter 1 we carefully point out that our audience includes very diverse groups of health professionals and practitioners, students studying in various health science fields, and even those with a general interest in how the social and behavioral sciences can inform discussions of health, clinical practice, and health policy. But in this chapter, we use the word *medicine* not to contrast the work of physicians against that of other practitioners, but because in the premodern era the variety of health professions we know today had yet to crystallize. While *health care* might seem a more inclusive term, it also tends to connote a kind of institutionalization that also did not occur until the modern era. Certainly, the professional health care landscape is now much more complex, but as a starting point we focus more directly on medicine as a way to trace the origins of the variety of clinical health professions that we recognize today.

We begin by discussing medicine and healing in the premodern era, which both illuminates the social nature of medical practice and sets the stage for the emergence of what we know today as modern clinical practice. We then discuss medicine as an institution of modernity, including how its successes after the discovery of the germ were born from applications of rational thinking, not just within the basic sciences but also in the organization and evolution of its corollary institutions (e.g., hospitals). Finally, we conclude with an examination of postindustrial shifts that are currently disrupting health and health care, and reveal several noteworthy elements of the fields in which you are likely to work, today and in the coming years.[1] Most students and some laypersons are familiar with challenges like cost containment, disparities in health care access, and difficulties delivering effective preventative care in clinical contexts. However, we believe that understanding the ways in which these seemingly divergent challenges and others emanate from similar underlying trans-formations in the landscape of health and illness is a necessary step in effectively confronting them. This is an endeavor for which health practitioners of all sorts ought to be on the front lines.

Medicine before Modernity

Understanding the premodern foundations of health care delivery is particularly important in two ways. First, premodern ways of thinking about and practicing medicine are relatively foreign to most people today, and recognizing this allows us to look objectively at the connections between health, clinical care, and social structures. This is an excellent precursor to examining those same connections for modern medicine, where the influence of social contexts can be more difficult to see, because we live and work within them, often uncritically. The obviously different ways of thinking about health and the body in the premodern era will therefore help delineate the boundaries of our own thinking. Second, understanding the sociohistorical foundations of premodern medicine is critical to understanding the nature of modern medicine and health care, which emerged at the end of the nineteenth century, in many ways in opposition to premodern ways of thinking.

While the end of the premodern period is generally marked around the 1500s with the dawn of the Enlightenment, medicine lagged behind, generally employing premodern practices well into the 1800s. What follows in this section will be less an account of the history of medicine in the premodern period than an overview, in very broad terms, of a premodern cosmology (i.e., an understanding of the universe) that underpinned ways of thinking about health and the body during that era, many

---

[1] We are borrowing from Christiansen's (2011) concept of *disruptive technology* here, and will illustrate in this chapter how changes in the nature of health and illness in the late industrial era are *disrupting* the patterns, practices, and even the ways of thinking that characterize modern medicine.

of which might seem silly to us today. But at the same time, premodern ways of thinking were at the heart of how all premodern social institutions and practices, including those of medicine, were organized. Understanding these elements of premodern society promotes our own ability to think critically about more recent health care delivery systems and clinical practice, which are also shaped in very specific ways by modernist thought. In other words, these elements are important in building our sociological and historical imaginations.

Premodern Thinking

To describe the "way people thought" across more than 2,000 years of history is difficult to say the least. As one might expect, there were countless divergent and opposing philosophies across this time period. At the same time, the premodern era can generally be characterized by an epistemology (i.e., a way of knowing the world) that relied heavily on *intuitive knowledge*. This intuitive way of understanding the world, including disease and sickness, took many forms. Early Greek inquiries can generally be described as an image-based naturalism that attempted to use thinking to understand cosmic processes based on earthly ones. Early Christian ways of knowing took a form we might describe as *revealed knowledge* where understandings of the world struck one in some sort of flash of insight (often attributed to revelations from God).[2] But for all of the variations in the philosophies and methodologies across the premodern millennia, there are important and informative commonalities.

Because knowledge was fundamentally intuitive or revealed, and because natural phenomena (including disease) could only be understood by appealing to the larger cosmological picture of the world,[3] institutions of premodern healing took a particular shape and character. For example, while there were eventually a handful of larger universities where one could study medicine (typically in Europe), the dominant form of education was apprenticeship, where trainees learned within a particular tradition of medical theory in what might be better termed a "discipleship." While today universities often ask students entering the health professions to articulate how health care is their "calling," or a form of work with a deep personal meaning to them, in the premodern period suitable students entering into an apprenticeship were judged as to whether they were literally *predestined* to enter the "healing arts," in the full cosmic sense of the term. As Paracelsus puts it:

> A good physician must be a born physician. Therefore no one should be surprised that the medical faculty is full of students who contribute nothing to its good reputation but only harm it and make it an object of contempt... And no more than an apple can be changed into a pear, will such people ever become good physicians. A life-long calling must be innate. ([1951] 1979:64)

---

[2] The most famous of these, perhaps, is Paul's revelation on the road to Damascus (see Badiou 2003 for an epistemological analysis of Paul's revelation).

[3] We are knowingly glossing over a difference throughout premodern medicine between empiricists and rationalists (Shyrock 1969). The former worked from the bedside of the individual patient (from symptoms) toward conclusions about disease and treatment. The latter worked from theories of the body and disease and applied these to patients. Both, however, utilized knowledge based on intuitive thinking (their own or that of hallmark figures of medicine like Galen).

Other notions of healing reflected the premodern cosmology as well. While there were general traditions into which groups of practitioners fell, and they shared their knowledge and practices with each other, ultimately each was left to navigate their practice based on their own intuitive skills. From a modern perspective, medicine as an institution was organized (or, more accurately, disorganized) in a way that more closely resembled religion than science.

Generally speaking, the premodern sense of the universe was monistic. That is to say, the world was conceived as a unity, without the fundamental separation between the material and spiritual realms (a division that constitutes an essential part of modern thinking). Premodern thought generally understood processes that were observable in nature to be instances of the same kinds of processes that occurred in the larger cosmic or spiritual realms. This fundamental cosmological condition forms the basis from which we can understand premodern medicine, which often seems incomprehensible to the modern person today. The Renaissance physician Paracelsus, for example, stated, in no uncertain terms, that anyone with a red beard was not fit to be a surgeon (Paracelsus [1951] 1979). This seems like random superstition until we understand that in the monistic premodern universe "red" was not simply an incidental adjective. Rather, it appears that for Paracelsus, "red" was inextricably linked to all sorts of qualities in the universe, including a number that were unbecoming of a healer—likely a propensity for aggressiveness where "red beards [might] sign a strong, war-like astrum" (Grell 1998:275). Similarly, disease was understood as a microcosm of a larger cosmic realm. Nowhere is this clearer than in the humoral theory of disease, which was the dominant way of conceptualizing health and illness in the premodern period.

Humoral Medicine

Humoral medicine originated with the early Greek thinker Hippocrates and was developed by his followers, who are believed to have written many of the works attributed to him (see Fig. 2.1; Porter 1997; Sigerist 1961). Insofar as it emerged from that larger premodern cosmology, humoral theory emphasizes the interrelatedness of the physical and nonphysical elements in the disease process. It supposes that the body is composed of four substances: blood, phlegm, black bile, and yellow bile. In simple terms, health is the result of a proper balance between these substances and disease was a result of their imbalance (though what constituted "proper" balance is not necessarily the same for all patients, but depended on a person's particular constitution and proper alignment with the state of the natural environment and cosmos). Additionally, each substance was located at the end of two polarities: (1) hot versus cold and (2) dry versus wet. At the individual level, these substances were associated with physical disease states and personality characteristics. However, each substance was also associated with universal elements such as fire, earth, air, and water, and additionally with states of nature (i.e., spring, summer, fall, and winter). The applications of this model of disease varied tremendously over time and across different practitioners, though its applications in the treatment of disease were most notably developed by Galen in the early Middle Ages.

Applying humoral theory to the disease process was not a straightforward process for a physician, but this model could provide guidance in what can best be

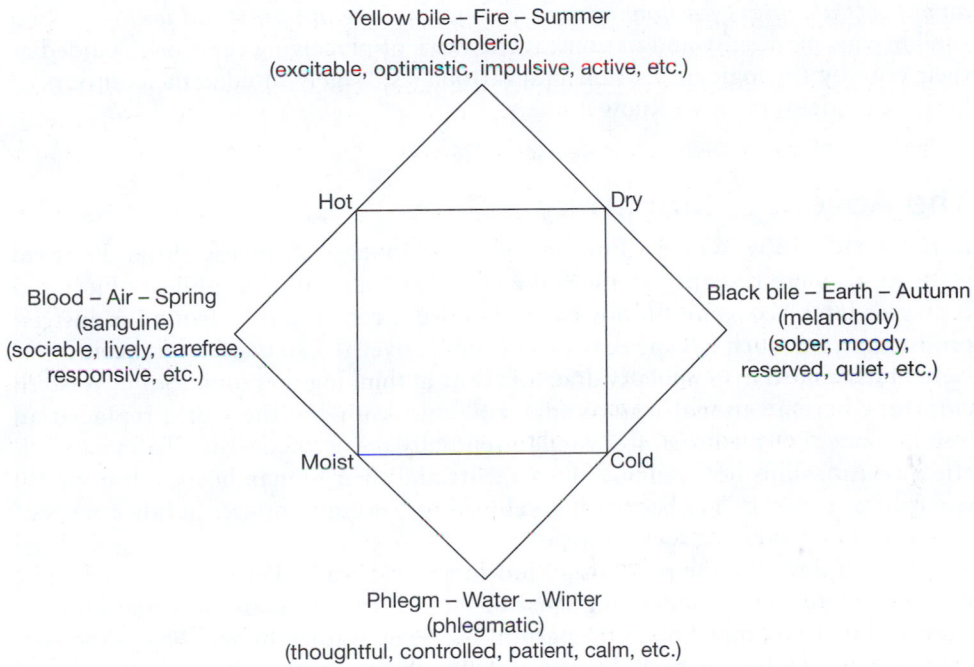

Yellow bile – Fire – Summer
(choleric)
(excitable, optimistic, impulsive, active, etc.)

Hot

Dry

Blood – Air – Spring
(sanguine)
(sociable, lively, carefree,
responsive, etc.)

Black bile – Earth – Autumn
(melancholy)
(sober, moody,
reserved, quiet, etc.)

Moist

Cold

Phlegm – Water – Winter
(phlegmatic)
(thoughtful, controlled, patient, calm, etc.)

FIG. 2.1 Humoral theory of medicine showing the interrelatedness of the individual temperament and body and the larger cosmos.

described as a process of divining imbalances, which might be interfering with the natural harmony between a person and the universe. A physician's role was to stare deeply and cosmologically at the person with a particular ailment, connecting their disease to any potential imbalances between their private constitution and that of the larger cosmos, as described above. That is, based not only on physical symptoms (e.g., excretions of humoral substances), but also on temperament of the patient, the season of the year, and so on, the physician could intuit the imbalance afflicting the patient. While some were more or less aggressive in their approach to treatment, physicians following the Hippocratic tradition generally saw their role as nudging the afflicted person back into proper alignment. This may entail any number of strategies.

While bleeding might seem wholly senseless to a practitioner today, from the perspective of a premodern physician we can see that such practices can have a clear internal logic. Take, for example, a premodern physician who is called to the home of a patient that has a hot fever and is sweating profusely. As noted in Figure 2.1, blood is a substance that is hot and wet. While taking account of that patient's personal constitution in relation to the season of the year, among other things, that physician might easily conclude that the patient has too much of that hot and wet substance in them. Taking out some of the patient's blood is a logical step, even if not founded on the same assumptions and knowledge as modern clinical practice. Of course, an actual practitioner's craft may vary tremendously from the simplistic hypothetical account above. *Nonetheless, when we work in a genuine way from the thinking of a premodern practitioner, we can see how the underlying culture of an era sets a context for how healing and health care are practiced within it.* In a similar way, modernity and its constituent ways of perceiving the world, guided at their core by the logic of instrumental rationality, largely molded the contours of health care delivery, as we know it today.

The Advent of Modernity

In the early 1500s, Western Europe began to undergo dramatic shifts. Political institutions were reshaped in the wake of democratic political philosophies, and centuries later, economies followed as they were reconfigured around industrial production. But such advances, which occurred over the span of several centuries, were underpinned by a similarly dramatic shift in thinking that took root in Western culture, where a rational way of analyzing and knowing the world replaced an intuitive one. For medicine, this would eventually mean uncovering the cause-and-effect relationships between infectious agents and their human hosts, but not until scientific approaches had been well developed for several centuries in other areas of social life (e.g., industry, agriculture, etc.).

We can describe the modern period in several ways. Perhaps most notably, however, there was an underlying sense in the cultural consciousness that humans were no longer wrapped up in the natural universe. Rather, human beings increasingly saw themselves as both distinct and exceptional within the natural order of things, and in pursuit of conquering nature and the challenges it posed. The growth in science and technology, in other words, fueled the idea that human ingenuity could (and should) harness and control the risks of the natural environment (i.e., the generally unpredictable phenomena of famine, disease, etc.). This marked a significant departure from the more humble orientation of premodern physicians, who typically believed that nature itself was the healing force and that they played a comparatively minor role in assisting a patient back into balance with larger cosmic forces. This shifting consciousness about the place of humans within the larger cosmos promoted, over time, the idea that a physician should cure, if not conquer, disease. Compare this sentiment to that of the premodern physicians who largely saw their task as humbly nudging the constitution of an afflicted person back into alignment with a more powerful and dominant cosmos.

However, before technology enabled modern medical practices to align with modernist ways of thinking, medicine often was practiced in a way that unconsciously drew ancient practices together with a new way of thinking about the universe, sometimes with grotesque consequences. Many practices like bleeding, purging, and blistering had been tempered by the requirements of humility at the heart of Hippocratic practice. This is not to say that aggressive bleeding and purging were not part of medical practice; Galen, in particular, had amplified an interventionist interpretation of the humoral medicine. However, the underlying epistemic shift in modernity empowered humanity to take responsibility for solving problems, including diseases. While "conquering" disease might have been considered hubris in the premodern era, in the new modern period, Western culture moved rapidly away from being resigned to the belief that cosmic forces were in control, and toward the idea that threats to survival in any form should be aggressively confronted with human ingenuity and effort, and thereby brought under control.

This is perhaps most clearly observed in the "heroic therapeutics" movement led by Benjamin Rush, among others (Shryock 1969). As Sharpe and Faden (1998:39) note, "In the late eighteenth and early nineteenth centuries, therapeutic activism found its most extreme expression in the so-called 'heroic medicine' championed by John Brown, Benjamin Rush, and others. When we look back at the history of iatrogenic harm in American medicine, it is this period that stands out most vividly for the violence of its remedies." These physicians were not without detractors, both from within the allopathic tradition, and most especially from "irregular" practitioners such as homeopaths and Thompsonians who espoused a nonaggressive form of practice and often carried over Hippocratic notions (Duffy 1993). Sharpe and Faden (1998:41) continue, "Rush, by contrast, specifically condemns the Hippocratic belief in the healing powers of nature and the physician as nature's servant as impediments to the progress of medicine." This sort of heroic intervention betrays a decidedly modernist disposition, even where scientific medical knowledge remained largely premodern. In a way, while knowledge and technology at this time lagged behind emerging ideas of therapeutic activism, we can appreciate how the modernist way of thinking about disease underpins the approach of Brown, Rush, and others, and still in many ways remains with us today.

This modern consciousness paralleled the development of medical science in important ways, not only with regard to scientific knowledge itself but also with respect to the social aspects of clinical practice. The premodern ethos entertained the reality of the mystical, such that cosmic processes were just as real in terms of understanding the nature of disease as were physical symptoms such as fever, rash, or vomiting. Where modern thinking is dominated by a human responsibility to manage risk and predictability, its concept of reality, and the focus of its endeavors, tends to center on material objects and empirical processes. This meant that treating disease became less about a practitioner's intuitive appeal to the heavens, and more about their ability to comprehend physical, observable disease processes unfolding within a particular patient. The physician's gaze therefore narrowed in scope from the entire cosmos, to the presenting patient and later to particular systems, organs, and symptoms within that patient. As Foucault eloquently puts it in *The Birth of the Clinic*:

> This new structure [of clinical practice] is indicated" by the minute but decisive change whereby the question: 'What is the matter with you?', with which the eighteenth-century dialogue between doctor and patient began" was replaced by that other question: 'Where does it hurt?', in which we recognize the operation of the clinic and the principle of its entire discourse. (1963:xviii)

The Birth of Modern Medicine

The beginnings of modern medicine are often traced to the discovery of the germ, primarily by scientists such as John Snow, Louis Pasteur, and Robert Koch in the mid-1800s. To be clear, these origins go back at least as far as Leeuwenhoek's work in the 1600s, and arguably much earlier if we consider pathogenic theories present in numerous ancient writings. Nonetheless, in the mid- to late 1800s, the technical capacities of medical science caught up to the rational modes of thought emerging from the Enlightenment, thereby fueling the development of the profession of medicine and eventually giving rise to the massive industry that we know today as health care. The entire social history of the development of modern medicine has been well documented elsewhere (see Duffy 1993; Porter 1997; Starr 1982), so here we should simply acknowledge that, broadly speaking, medicine is an institution developed by applying modernist rational thinking to every aspect of healing practice. In modernity, we observe and understand phenomena primarily in terms of their cause-and-effect relationships, we manage such phenomena by intervening in the causes in order to alter the effects, and the effects are the measurable outcomes (and hopefully successes) of our efforts. This is a rationalized, scientific way of thinking, but it is perhaps most easily recognized in the industry of health care delivery. Indeed, modernist logic fit well with the types of disorders that practitioners typically faced at this point in medical history. And just as in many other Western social institutions, it worked spectacularly well.

We can understand the fundamental logic of modern health care by understanding the logic of factory production because both share a modernist, and thus a highly rationalized, bureaucratized structure. The modern factory rationally broke down the task of production to maximize the efficiency with which goods could be turned out. The manager of a shoe factory makes decisions about how to divide the tasks that go into making shoes in order to produce shoes most efficiently. In particular, a factory manager will divide tasks such that one person puts on the soles of the shoes and another strings the laces, because that is more efficient. Even better, the manager will bring in new machines that can do the work faster and with fewer errors. We can evaluate whether the manager has done a good job simply by examining the profit margin, that is, how much return (i.e., the revenue from sales of shoes) the company obtained relative to their investment (i.e., the costs of materials and labor to produce the shoes). The product of these relatively straightforward calculations is an objective measure of success.

Modern health care delivery has similarly subdivided its tasks, personnel, and objectives (as noted in Chapter 1) according to the rationalized logic of modernity. For instance, we often utilize the principles of rationalized production to produce efficiencies that single human beings alone cannot easily achieve, like a highly differentiated and specialized division of labor, most or all of whom employ various technologies intended to expedite the proficiency and accuracy with which patients can be diagnosed, treated, and returned to their roles in society. Moreover, health care systems are highly bureaucratized structures that, while unique in many ways (as we will discuss later), similarly adhere to modernist principles of rationality, predictability, control, and efficiency, and we often evaluate health care through a modernist lens by assessing how well it produces these good outcomes (e.g., cures, treatments, satisfied customers, or some other target), at what rate, and at what cost. In short, the instrumental rationality emblematic of the modern period permeates not only *medical science* with its focus on the relationship between pathogens and tissues, but every other facet of health care, including *clinical practice*, *education*, *finance*, and *the health professions*. With the advent of modernist thinking, we no longer appeal intuitively to the larger cosmos, but focus on the cause-and-effect relationships both within the body of an afflicted person and within the systems of health care that have emerged over the last 150 years.

The Rise of Modern Clinical Practice

Today, health care is virtually synonymous with a clinical setting. When patients require diagnosis and treatment, they head to hospitals or office buildings where practitioners schedule or triage them into exam rooms equipped with all kinds of technology that enable the practitioner to detect the cause of their ailment and, hopefully, to intervene on it. In the premodern period, those that could access a physician got care at their homes. After all, there was no technology to speak of, so the practitioner could carry everything he needed in the iconic doctor's bag (compare this to the modern hospital room; see Photo 2.1). More importantly, the work of the premodern physician was not to look inside the body of a person, and certainly not to explore their physiology down to the cellular level. Rather, it was to connect their symptoms to a larger cosmological picture. The premodern physician worked from a raw form of bedside empiricism— that is, by looking deeply and thinking intuitively about the patient and the larger cosmos—rather than an analytic calculation of evidence from laboratory values and radiological images. For the latter, one needs not only a place to house the requisite technology, but to centralize care so that patients can be seen in quick succession. Clearly a practitioner traveling from patient to patient is not nearly as efficient as one moving from one exam room to the next. Thus, the clinic is a modernist institution in the way it is physically organized to adhere to the requisites of modernity, in particular in that it aims to achieve a factory-like efficiency of production. Perhaps most importantly, however, the development of the clinic represented an attempt to manage disease. Essentially, it is a place of quarantine. By virtue of its design, it removes those who are sick from normal social life. This is not only critical to the ability of clinical practitioners to treat disease, but also promotes the health and function of other areas of social life. As we discuss later, this is a model of health care provision that works extremely well for infectious diseases, but presents important challenges for treating chronic ones, which exhibit fundamentally different attributes and etiologies.

Education for Medical and Allied Health Professions

As noted above, the student–teacher relationship in the premodern period could best be described as a discipleship (though some were educated in larger university

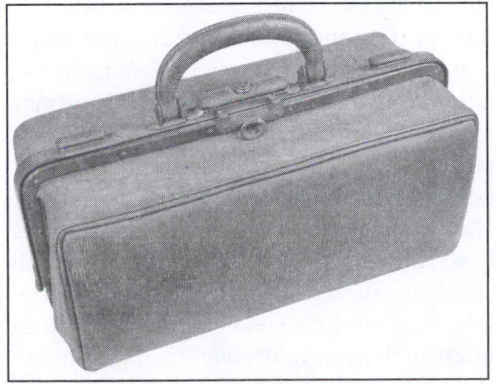 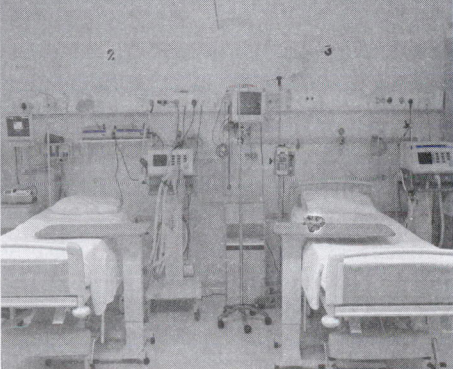

PHOTO 2.1 A doctor's bag and a modern hospital room illustrate the way technological advances limited the mobility of medical care.

settings, where medicine was taught more like philosophy or sociology is today). Beneath the weight of modern thinking, particularly where modernist logic values measurable inputs and outputs, educational systems transitioned from individualized apprenticeship relationships into standardized institutional programs. Only here, instead of the most efficient production of healthy patients, we see attempts to organize systems that result in the most efficient production of knowledgeable students.

Before the "discovery of the germ," medical treatments were incredibly varied and witnessed limited success. Without validation, the efficacy of treatments remained largely theoretical and therefore one learned medicine more as a philosophical tradition than as a science. However, as medical science advanced, it developed a product (i.e., health or, perhaps more precisely, cures) that it could reliably distribute to people. As scientific medical knowledge grew, it became increasingly necessary to educate practitioners in the science of physiology, pathology, anatomy, and the like. Moreover, knowledge in these disciplines was no longer a subjective, intuitive matter, but an objective, rational, scientific one. As such, this scientific knowledge could be transmitted to practitioners en masse. Apprenticeship systems therefore gave way to the classrooms of modern higher learning, where experts dispensed objective knowledge to student learners, usually in didactic lectures. That is, as medicine became more scientific, it drifted toward something that one simply had to learn, rather than something for which one had to be spiritually predestined.

Of course, incoming students for medicine and allied health programs often are asked why they believe their chosen profession is their "calling." But today, we think about this primarily in terms of how their life experiences have shaped them in ways that make them sensitive to the promise of medicine for the human condition. We no longer think, at least not typically, that the cosmos has predestined certain types of people for medicine and health practice. Certainly, today we look for students that have the appropriate facility with the sciences in combination with the proper dispositions toward the social and humanistic aspects of providing care. However, we largely believe that, provided one has these basic qualities, students can acquire the knowledge and skills to be a successful practitioner.

As medical practice came to be seen as something largely learned, rather than innate, regulating the quality of education that practitioners received became a major concern (at first for physicians, though developments in physician training have had tremendous impact on shaping educational systems for other health professions). In response to these growing concerns, the newly reorganized American Medical Association contracted an educator named Abraham Flexner to evaluate the state and quality of medical education at medical schools in the United States. The landscape of medical education witnessed dramatic reform following the Flexner Report in 1910, which included the closing of the majority of rural medical schools and all but two African American medical schools (Howard University and Meharry Medical College; Duffy 1993). These schools, according to Flexner, lacked adequate infrastructure and training of sufficient quality, though many were simply underfunded. The modernization of medical education had thus begun, and proceeded according to highly rationalized and universally applicable principles characteristic of the modern era. Once more, the effects were transformational.

In Flexner's wake, medical education morphed into the type of institution that still largely dominate the contemporary professional landscape (though we later discuss recent shifts in the landscape of medical/allied health education). The roots of prerequisite science courses can be found in Flexner's recommendation that, "admission to a really modern medical school must at very least depend on a competent knowledge of chemistry, biology (including botany), and physics" (1910:25). He added that competency in these areas for students wanting to enter medical education had to be certified at the college level, since, at the time, many medical schools had no requirements for college-level education. In light of Flexner's recommendation that medical schools also affiliate with hospitals, medical curricula also evolved into what are now referred to as their "traditional" form, made up of two years of basic science education, followed by two years of clinical education in a hospital setting.

The recommendations laid out in the Flexner report have dominated the structures and processes of medical education for more than 100 years and strongly influenced the structure and function of educational programs for other health care professions. Importantly for our purposes, we can understand the sociohistorical position of that report, as predicated on the development of modern medical science. Indeed, Flexner's study in many ways did for medical education what science did for medicine proper: it approached medical education in a relatively systematic way and its findings were generalized across the board, with the goal of improving the outputs of the process (i.e., better trained practitioners). More recently, however, medical and allied health educators are exploring new pedagogical approaches and programmatic arrangements in medical and health education. As we will later see, these are largely a response to the shifting landscape of contemporary health and illness, in the same way that the Flexner report was responsive to the advent of modern medicine at the dawn of the 1900s.

The Business of Modern Health Care

Health care systems are incredibly complex and the reimbursement systems in U.S. health care are particularly difficult to untangle. In Chapter 12 we will explore health care systems and policy in more detail, but here our purpose is simply to understand how basic reimbursement strategies were developed in ways that were responsive to modernist medical practices. As described above, modernist thinking values, and therefore emphasizes, the efficient production of measurable outcomes. As a result, ideas about the nature of the universe receded from a focus on the diffuse notions of a cosmic nature (e.g., the nature of God, what constitutes virtue, etc.), moving toward a focus on discrete, observable objects, or more accurately, things that can be objectified. In our shoe factory, discussed above, we can measure the efficiency of production by examining how much we invested in parts, hours, energy, and so on. All of these are objectified and therefore measurable. We can calculate how much each part of the shoe costs, how much each hour of workers' time costs, and so on. We can then compare this to the value of the end products— the shoes we make—which are also things for which a value can be objectively measured in terms of how much they cost to produce and for how much money they might sell in the marketplace.

Essentially, early health professionals organized themselves around the same core logic, a way of thinking quite similar to our shoe factory above. In particular, these professionals began to achieve more and more success in treating infectious diseases in the first half of the twentieth century. This was not coincidence; acute and infectious diseases are well matched with a modernist way of thinking (as we will see later, other types of disease are less well suited to this logic).[4] That is, the modernist focus on the cause-and-effect relationships between discrete objects matches the curative agenda of modern medicine. Modern medicine's earliest successes concerned attacking the ability of a pathogen to infect tissue, either by killing the pathogen (e.g., with antibiotics or antisepsis) or by blocking its ability to infect (e.g., vaccines). This was typically efficient, calculable, and predictable—the hallmarks of modernist logic.

The truly miraculous success of modern medicine at killing pathogens or preventing infection gave birth to an industry that for the first time in its history possessed a truly valuable commodity (Starr 1982). More importantly for the business of health care, medicine not only had a valuable commodity, but one that could be *objectively* valued. The ability to objectively value the inputs (i.e., treatments, labor costs, etc.) and outputs (i.e., cures) played a critical role in the "making of a vast industry" (Starr 1982). Costs of care could now be objectively calculated and billed accordingly. Thus, while reimbursement systems are incredibly complex in practice (and we will discuss these in a later chapter), it is important to understand that they all share common underlying goals in the objective commodification of health care. Even where the contemporary landscape of health has become more complex, reimbursement has largely remained structured around the dual objectives of diagnosis and treatment that originate in the modern period. The logic around which the business of health care organized in the late 1800s and throughout the 1900s was decidedly matched to the treatment of acute and infectious ailments, which are discrete, and lend themselves to objectively measurable treatments and outcomes that are clearly successful or unsuccessful. The paradigmatically different causal profile of chronic illnesses, however, has been particularly disruptive to the structure and function of these modernist systems since the epidemiological transition.

A Shifting Landscape of Health and Disease

As described above, medicine's ability to reliably treat infectious illnesses (either by killing pathogens or inhibiting or preventing infection itself) emerged from the scientific analysis of cause-and-effect relationships between discrete objects (i.e., agents, hosts, and environments). And indeed the ultimate success of modern medicine was built around an effective understanding of infectious diseases. But these infectious disease models inspired more than advances in medical science, antisepsis, and public health. They eventually constituted the foundation upon which every other realm of medicine would eventually be built, including medical education,

---

[4] In reality, modern medicine's success was made possible by modernist scientific ways of thinking, but we also have to recognize that these ways of thinking about the world shaped medicine in only one of many possible directions.

the business of health care, and the shape of medical and allied health professions. Indeed, it is difficult to overstate the success of modern medicine after the discovery of the germ. Through antibiotics, vaccines, and antisepsis procedures, both in clinics and more broadly in public health and sanitation programs, many diseases that had plagued humanity for millennia were, in a relatively short period of time, virtually wiped out from entire populations. In the annals of human achievement, perhaps nothing is more impressive and the impacts have been undeniable. Life expectancy in the United States, for example, rose from about 47 years to 76 years from 1900 to 2000. However, the success of modern medicine (and modern medical science) eventually gave way to a dramatic rise in the prevalence of chronic illnesses, which beginning in the early to mid-1970s became the most significant threats to health and mortality in developed countries.

We have discussed in the preceding section how the discovery of the germ and medical science's ability to kill it were at the foundation of the development of an entire modern health care industry, from medical and health education to clinical practice. Now we discuss how the rise of chronic illness epitomizes a shifting health landscape that defies modernist logic, and thereby exerts significant pressure on virtually every aspect of the health care industry built on that way of thinking. The challenge for health care professionals in the twenty-first century will be to rethink and perhaps reshape these institutions—including clinical practice, education, and the business of health care—such that the ways that those institutions are structured actually match the nature of chronic disease.

Disruptive Illness: Chronic Disease and Incalculable Risk

Across much of the twentieth century, modern medicine and the industries eventually built upon it were organized primarily around treating infectious illness and acute injury. As discussed above, this is evident in the structure of the clinic, medical education, and the organization of health care financing and reimbursement. Although these basic structures largely are still with us, we can see tremendous changes across the last four decades not only in the epidemiology of disease, with the rise in prevalence of chronic illness, but also in ways that health care is practiced within those modernist structures. In the early 1900s, many medical scientists were convinced of the imminent discovery of a "magic bullet," an antimicrobial compound that would treat all infectious diseases (Dubos 1959). The growing capacity of medicine to treat disease made heroes out of physicians and medical scientists like Paul Ehrlich, a physician scientist who discovered Salvarsan in 1909, the first (moderately) effective treatment for syphilis (Witkop 1999). The 1940 Hollywood film *Dr. Ehrlich's Magic Bullet* starring Edward G. Robinson glorified not only the figure of Ehrlich, but also the promise of medical science for eradicating disease. A 1955 *New York Times* article features Jonas Salk, who developed the first widely successful polio vaccine, noting that he "became almost a folk hero overnight." Although the vaccine was not widely released until 1957, the concern about polio was so great that the scientists working on it, including Salk, were prominent in the American consciousness.

Cinematic depictions of physicians and health care today tend to be quite different. *The Doctor* (1991), for example, tells the story of a physician confronting his own professional arrogance in the face of a cancer diagnosis. He goes on to confront the callous nature of the medical establishment and develops an appreciation for showing compassion and empathy to patients. The film *Awakenings* (1990) tells the story of neurologist Oliver Sacks' remarkable success treating patients with encephalitis lethargica. In what appears at first to be another modern medical miracle, Sacks is able to wake patients who have been catatonic for decades. However, the efficacy of the treatment eventually fades and the patients become catatonic again. The takeaway message of the film is not found in the cure of disease, but in what the experiences of illness tell us about our humanity.

In a succinct example of art reflecting culture, the changing themes of these films are emblematic of the state and nature of contemporary health care and disease epidemiology. Few people today believe cures for all diseases are forthcoming. In fact, a large part of clinical practice today concerns long-term management of disease, with no focus on cure. Throughout most of the 1900s, when the goal of medicine largely centered on curing infectious diseases (and practitioners very often reached that goal), comparatively little effort was placed on developing trusting, empathic relationships with patients. In fact, the heroification of physicians in the early 1900s demonstrates rather clearly that public trust was, by and large, not a problem for the field (See Loewen 1995:9 for discussion of the concept of heroification). But today, developing rapport and trust with patients has become critically important for many reasons, particularly since many patients will be treated regularly for illnesses that they will manage for the remainder of their lives. Additionally, rather than the lone "cowboy" practitioner, health care is more often delivered by "pit crews" comprising practitioners from different specialties and different health professions (Gawande 2011). This remarkable professional shift emerged after, and in many ways as a result of, another important transformation in disease epidemiology.

Changing Disease Profiles

The term *epidemiological transition* is credited to Omran (1971) to highlight the shifting rates of *kinds* of illness in populations, particularly those in developed nations. He notes that when populations age—that is, when life expectancy rises such that the average age of the population increases—we witness a decrease in death from infectious disease and a corresponding increase in death from chronic disease (see also Fig. 2.2 from McKinlay & McKinlay 1977). Recall that across the 1900s in the United States life expectancy increased from about 47 to 76 years. Omran (1971:532) notes that in the late phase of the "age of receding pandemics" life expectancy increases to 30 to 40+ [where] pandemics of infection, malnutrition, and childhood disease recede." However, increased life expectancy based on the successes with these afflictions ushers in the "age of degenerative and man-made diseases, [where] life expectancy reaches an unprecedented high of 70+ years [and] Heart disease, cancer, and stroke replace infection as prime killers" (Omran 1971:168).

We all recognize that chronic illnesses like diabetes and heart disease are fundamentally different than infectious diseases. The latter involve the infiltration of a tissue by a pathogen that is not native to its host. The pathogen can either be killed

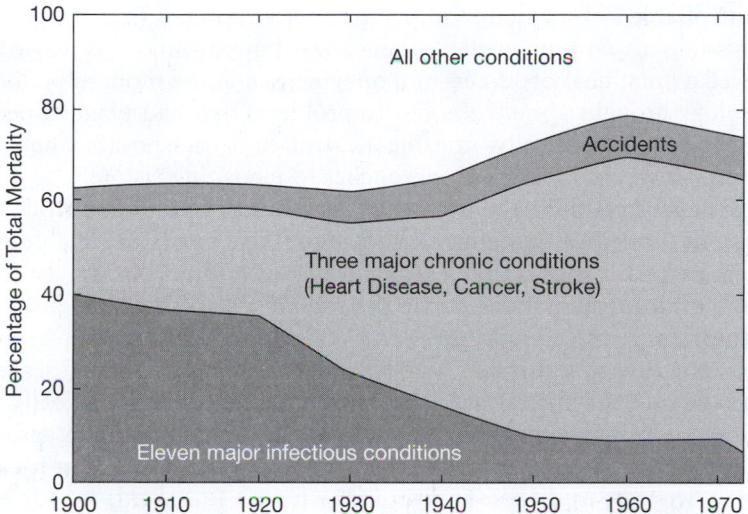

FIG. 2.2 Chart from McKinlay and McKinlay (1977) showing the proportional increase in deaths from chronic diseases versus infection diseases from 1900 to 1973.

Source: McKinlay, John B. & Sonja M. McKinlay. (1977). "The Questionable Contribution of Medical Measures to the Decline of Mortality in the United States in the Twentieth Century." *Milbank Memorial Fund Quarterly—Health and Society* 55, 405–28.

or its ability to infect the host can be blocked (in cases of vaccination). Either way, addressing the cause of infectious disease focuses on targets that are relatively discrete from their hosts. Chronic diseases, on the other hand, often emerge from hundreds of thousands of decisions a person makes across his or her life course (e.g., diet, exercise, etc.), while at the same time all of those decisions are nested in the constraints of the social environments in which that person lives. Moreover, chronic diseases typically are not the result of the presence of a foreign agent, but rather having too much or too little of various biomolecules that are indigenous to the human body. Cholesterol, for example, is synthesized by all nucleated cells in the body, but certain forms and levels are associated with coronary artery disease. While we attempt to set discrete benchmarks that constitute healthy or unhealthy levels (e.g., that fasting blood glucose over 126 mg/dL constitutes diabetes or that a body mass index greater than 24.9 constitutes overweight), these are notoriously fraught with diagnostic uncertainty. That is, where practitioners have no difficulty agreeing that someone with syphilis is sick and needs to receive penicillin, diagnosing and treating someone with mild to moderately high cholesterol is far more open to interpretation and variation (see Welch et al. 2011). This may seem odd today, but the benchmarks and guidelines for what is normal and abnormal are typically derived from population-level studies of risk and therefore often have a more ambiguous meaning for individual patients. The resulting ambiguity inherent in trying to diagnose and treat many chronic illnesses has not only challenged the institutions and practices of modern medicine, but it is reflective of broader shifts in society at large.

Recall from earlier discussion in this chapter that with modernity came the basic notion that human beings can and should confront the often unpredictable and uncontrollable risks posed by the natural environment (e.g., famine, disease, etc.). We also discussed how medical science was built around this way of thinking and achieved a great deal of success at managing risk in the modern period. Science and technology brought about solutions to problems that had plagued people since the dawn of time, and did so by utilizing a calculating, transposable, linear analysis of the world. However, modernist approaches to managing risk rely on a relatively high degree of predictability about how particular causes produce particular effects. To manage an infectious epidemic, for example, one needs to be able to predict that certain kinds of exposure (i.e., airborne versus bodily contact) leads to transmission and even further to determine the rate at which this happens (the "basic reproductive ratio," for example, gives an average number of subsequently infected persons per one case of a disease). Knowing the ways a particular disease is transmitted and the rate at which it will increase or decline epidemiologically allows us to manage the risk of transmission, even when we cannot cure the disease itself. We might quarantine a patient with rubella, for example, knowing that it can spread by airborne droplets and that on average, without intervention, for every one person infected, five to seven other people will be infected, meaning that the disease can spread relatively quickly in a population. If, however, we can isolate infected individuals (or better yet, cure them) such that we can drive the basic reproductive ratio below 1, meaning that, on average, less than one additional person is infected per case, then we can predict that the disease will die out in the population.

The ability to make such predictions is critical to the modern management of risk, including the risks posed by disease. As noted above, it has been tremendously successful at ameliorating the threats faced over thousands of years of human history. However, these successes have also yielded more complex problems, with consequences that are much less predictable. Ironically, it is the very successes of the modern industrial society that produce problems that a modernist way of thinking cannot solve. The social transformations that have come about as society confronts the limits of modernist thinking suggest that developed nations are moving into a postindustrial period (sometimes also referred to as late-modern or a second modernity). Ulrich Beck (1992, 1999), among other sociologists, have suggested that this represents a critical juncture for the organizations and functions of society at large. As we will see, the incalculability of chronic illness risk exerts significant forces of change in health care and various health professions.

The inability to accurately calculate risk has dramatic effects on modern society because it forces us to confront new complex problems with new, more complex ways of thinking. As modern successes have introduced problems that are unpredictable, *estimation* has increasingly replaced *calculation* in attempts to manage risk. Estimation can be thought of as our "best guess" about what to do in the absence of clear and convincing evidence. However, unlike calculation, which is an objective, scientific way of approaching a problem, estimation is a process that is easily affected by our individual biases, values, and subjective interpretations of whatever evidence is available. The objective nature of risk calculation drives wide consensus in society, because there is clear evidence about the best course of action around which everyone can organize. However, when we are resigned to estimating risk, in the absence of clear evidence about what to do, then social organization tends to fracture, and smaller enclaves form around divergent ideas about what is best to do.

Beck (1999) discusses the issue of nuclear power in Europe as emblematic of this shift toward a society characterized by risk estimation, rather than risk calculation. He notes that the fall out of a hypothetical nuclear power plant accident carries risks that are incalculable. Given the unpredictable way that radiation might spread and the variable effects it has on human life, there is no scientific consensus about the extent or magnitude of nuclear power risk and therefore no single locus of authority on the issue. Because of that, we see the splintering of different groups who are estimating the risks of nuclear power, using their individual values and subjective ways of understanding the world to make decisions about whether they feel it is safe. Someone with stronger environmentalist tendencies, for example, likely estimates that it is relatively dangerous. Another with a disposition more strongly guided by economic concerns may estimate that it is relatively safe. Because there is no authoritative consensus about its safety and no way to convincingly predict its risk potential, neither view can be convincingly invalidated.

The Consequences of Incalculability

In the face of risk incalculability, where people are left to estimate risk—and use personal values and attitudes to do so—social groups tend to organize around ideological enclaves. That is, we tend to affiliate more strongly with smaller groups of people who share our values and attitudes. Here the critical point is that in the face of unpredictability (meaning a lack of scientifically grounded consensus), people tend to reorganize themselves around shared values and attitudes. Where the same unpredictability attends chronic illnesses, we see similar and dramatic challenges emerge in health care delivery structures, which, after all, were built around managing the largely calculable risks of infection and acute injury.

The history of *patent medicines* (sometimes called "snake oil") makes clear that there have always been fads in health. People have always sought miracle cures to various ailments or magic compounds that will keep them from aging. But throughout the majority of the twentieth century, modern medicine enjoyed a great deal of authority over health knowledge. More recently, however, medicine's success at treating chronic illness has been tepid, at least when judged against its earlier success with infections. As a result, people gather information about how to be healthy from any number of sources with varying levels of scientific validity.[5] Instead of a cure, those with type 2 diabetes, for example, are resigned to taking

[5] As noted, there have always been a variety of sources of health knowledge ranging from patent medicines to folk practices and family traditions. Our point here is that the authority of these expands and contracts with respect to the authority of medical science. In earlier periods, before the discovery of the germ, when medical science could cure little, many medical and folk traditions emerged to form a highly pluralistic environment populated not just by allopathic practitioners, but also homeopaths, hydropaths, and so on. But these traditions waned under the authority of scientific medicine in the twentieth century. As Kaptchuk and Eisenberg (2001) note, "Specific historical events (e.g., the discovery of antibiotics or a linkage between acupuncture and endorphins) and general secular trends (e.g., confidence in scientific progress) undoubtedly affected utilization patterns and trends. It may be that the high prevalences in the 1920s and 1930s and in the 1990s and 2000s represent two peaks within oscillations." Note that the first of these spikes occurs before the major success of modern medicine at treating infection (the availability of penicillin), while the other occurs well after the epidemiological transition.

medication and adjusting their lifestyles to manage blood sugar for the rest of their lives. Perhaps more importantly, we should recognize that preventing chronic illness is both complex and unpredictable. Generally speaking, diet and exercise clearly contribute to good health, but what constitutes a healthy diet or the right kind and amount of exercise is highly contested. This is not to say that scientific evidence is lacking for the treatment and prevention of chronic illness, but that the evidence, which often is derived from population-level studies with varying and sometimes contradictory findings, has a more tenuous connection to individuals who are left to figure out for themselves what to do.

American comedian Lewis Black captured the perception of the average person trying to navigate health in the complex world of chronic illness:

> when I was a kid [they told] me eggs were good. So I ate a lot of eggs. Ten years later they said they were bad... so I stopped eating eggs and ten years later they said they were good again. Then I ate twice as many eggs and then they said they were bad... Then they said they're good, they're bad, they're good, the whites are good, the yellow [are bad]... Make up your minds! It's breakfast; I've got to eat! (Black 2000)

When we used this quote in a 2010 journal article, we noted that whole eggs were largely regarded as healthy again, with several large studies suggesting that the dietary cholesterol in eggs had little effect on the body's cholesterol levels (e.g., Hu et al. 1999; Wasserman & Hinote 2011). Yet later that same year a new study declared that in terms of cardiovascular health, "stopping egg consumption after a myocardial infarction or stroke would be like quitting smoking after lung cancer is diagnosed: a necessary act, but late" (Spence et al. 2010:e338). The media, which, of course, generates much of the health information that is actually consumed by the public, took the comparison one step further. For example, referring to an additional study by Spence et al. in 2012, the headline for one online article read, "Egg yolks almost as bad for your heart as smoking cigarettes, says study" (Murray 2012). Just below the title, the author continued, "Like Hollandaise sauce? Too bad—for your heart and blood vessels. Yolks are packed with cholesterol, causing blood-vessel-clogging plaque buildup, *just like smoking does*" (italics added). Joel Fuhrman, a physician, media personality, and proponent of a "nutrient dense" diet, noted that the comparison between eating eggs and smoking was "probably an overstatement," but largely concurred with the science of the Spence et al. (2010) study. At the same time, claims persist about the relative health effects of eggs on cardiovascular health. These come from sources as varied as the Harvard T. H. Chan School of Public Health website, which referenced the benefits of eggs and advises moderate consumption, to diet "gurus" such as Anthony Colpo (2012), who called the Spence et al. (2012) study, "one of the most appalling pieces of epidemiological hogwash I've seen for some time."

Our point here is not to debate the nutritional science behind egg consumption, but rather to point out that, from the perspective of the average consumer, managing the risk of eggs in particular, or diet or other lifestyle profile in general, has become a rather abysmal endeavor with few clear answers. More than that, recent work has shown that the public is increasingly demoralized by *medical reversal*, a situation where therapies commonly believed to be effective later are determined to be ineffective (Prasad & Cifu 2015). *As a result, people align themselves less with often elusive and frequently changing scientific consensus, and increasingly with lifestyle philosophies that accord with their values and attitudes.* Someone distrustful of medicine proper may seek out a nonprofessional like Anthony Colpo. His "research" appears to be largely conducted on himself and drawn from his own interpretation of particular selections from a vast and divergent scientific literature. Yet his self-presentation and renegade posture have appeal for those who feel alienated from or suspicious of traditional scientific and professional medical groups. Even a cursory review of how health is consumed in Western societies today shows that we get health information from not only medical professionals but also grocery stores, advertisements, and any number of health and nutrition businesses selling vitamins, supplements, smoothies and juices, and so on. Individual consumers are left to decide what sorts of diet they think are healthy: high-fat, low-fat, low-carb, high-protein, whole foods, plant-based, and on and on (see Wasserman & Hinote 2011).

Similar lifestyle philosophies emerge around exercise: yoga, CrossFit, Zumba, Pilates, and boot camps of any number of varieties. While most any kind of exercise is good for you at least in some respect, it is critical to note how connected these forms of exercise tend to be to the consumer's identity. That is, lifestyle patterns do not purely reflect an attempt to be healthy, but double as a way of expressing who we are. Whether we see ourselves as valuing "inner peace" or aggressively pushing ourselves to "extremes," there is a corresponding exercise program, usually with its own definitions of health and well-being, through which we can fulfill and grow our sense of our own identity. In short, the emergence of chronic illnesses as the most significant threats to mortality in developed nations initiated a shift toward the postindustrial, late modern health landscape that exists today. In this health landscape, diet, exercise, and other lifestyle factors appear to have an impact on the prevention and management of chronic disorders, but there is no publicly trusted scientific consensus on which kinds of lifestyles will *predictably* prevent chronic disease. As people go about estimating risk as we describe, they do so in ways that accord with their values, attitudes, and identities, which often are not grounded in an objective type of means-end rational thinking that characterized the modern period.

Earlier we also described this type of means-end logic as transposable, in the sense that the conclusions it produces are largely applicable across human populations. In other words, practitioners typically treated or prevented simpler infectious disorders in similar ways across individual patients and groups (at least prior to another more recent shift in epidemiology toward increasingly complex, highly resistant infectious agents). In another important transformation in disease etiology, causal processes and subsequent case management are now, in contrast, increasingly individuated. That is, individuals with the same or similar diagnoses (e.g., cardiovascular disease, cancer, hypertension, diabetes, etc.) are now likely to exhibit very different etiological profiles, with different contributions from lifestyles, environments, somatic responses, and even genetics, thereby making the challenging task of disease management all the more complex and unique to the individual patient. In sum, we cannot overemphasize the myriad ways that health and disease in late modernity epitomize dramatic shifts in not just epidemiology, but also in our thinking and behavior. We will further unpack these complexities in other sections of this book. But for now you should recognize that as current and future health professionals you will work within these new and complicated realities, and must in your work confront the consequences of disease shifts, less calculable and individuated risk profiles, and increasingly complex clinical scenarios (not to mention perplexing bioethical issues), all of which we can trace to the transforming landscape of health and illness in a new period of late modernity. But what does this mean, in specific terms, for twenty-first century clinical practice?

The End of Modern(ist) Health Care: Clinical Practice in the Chronic Illness Era

We wrote this book on the premise that health and disease have transformed in very specific ways over the past several hundred years, but especially important to our current health care professional landscape are the changes in recent decades. Consequently, the behaviors, professions, organizations, and institutions that surround health and disease have also changed (or are in the process of changing), often in dramatic ways. Nonetheless, many vestiges of the modern period are still with us today in American health care delivery (e.g., the structure of the clinic, health/ medical education, and health systems/policy). But as history has turned the page into late modernity, many of these institutions, because they were organized around the logic and disease profiles of an earlier historical and epidemiological period, are mismatched with the types of challenges that you are likely to encounter, and hopefully critically engage, as you enter your respective fields of work.

As we discussed in Chapter 1, shifts in the landscape of health and illness necessitate a consequent change in how twenty-first century health and medical professionals train and practice in those fields. Asking (or forcing) you to conduct your work in a novel and ever-changing environment using approaches developed long ago that no longer respond well to the challenges of twenty-first-century health care delivery is neither sensible nor fair. This is why in this book we have chosen to join so many of our colleagues across multiple health disciplines to rethink approaches to health care that may have been responsive to the late modern health landscape, but are becoming outdated. This includes providing you with the tools to do great things in the future, most notably working to care for the sick and to promote good health, and to understand your work and the challenges and experiences within it in new ways. We move through multiple levels of health, disease, clinical practice, and health care in more detail in the coming chapters, but it is important to move into those specific areas with a clear understanding of why all of this is important to you as a health professional.

The modern clinic evolved alongside the treatment of infectious diseases. It is, by its nature, a place of quarantine, where sick persons are removed from their normal social environments. This is advantageous for treating acute injuries and infectious diseases not only because infection should be isolated, but also because more sophisticated technologies are not mobile and therefore need to be centralized. But what constitutes a functional structure for the clinic with respect to injury and infection presents formidable challenges for treating chronic diseases. After all, chronic diseases are more fully nested in local contexts (i.e., families, neighborhoods, etc. all the way to the levels of culture and institutions). They are not simply the product of a pathogen infecting a host, but rather the result of hundreds of thousands of lifestyle decisions that a person makes across his or her life course in combination with the social structures that condition those choices. Put simply, chronic illnesses are more intimately connected with social life. Where the structure of the clinic dislocates the patient from the social environment, it cuts off practitioners from a great deal of information that is highly relevant to the course of the disease and strategies for treatment. While providing preventative care has been a topic of increasing importance, it has remained incredibly difficult and, compared with the past success of modern medicine with infectious disease, has been largely ineffective. In particular, despite a rhetorical emphasis on lifestyle and disease prevention, by many measures health status in the United States has worsened over the last several decades (e.g., rising rates of obesity, diabetes, heart disease, etc.). The fundamental problem for clinical practice is that the clinic was never designed to undertake such preventative measures, which require an intimate knowledge of both patient behaviors and their social contexts (discussed in Chapters 4–6), something that the clinic was never designed to facilitate (we discuss ways to mitigate this limitation and others in Chapters 7–10).

While public health has a long history, and public health initiatives have been an important part of the larger picture of health care across the twentieth century, we have seen both a shift in their focus and an increase in their prevalence that corresponds with the shifting health landscape. Surrounding the discovery of the germ from the mid-1800s through the mid-1900s we see a corresponding "sanitary movement" and "bacteriological era," focused on preventing the spread of infection (Rosen 1993). There was a natural divide between public health and clinical practice in these periods, since the former focused on preventing the spread of germs and the latter on killing infections once they happened. Although they shared a mutual interest and health professionals crossed between both, there was less need for discourse between the two. However, the epidemiological transition has promoted increasing interdependence, not only where public health studies play a critical role in setting clinical practice guidelines (e.g., target values for BMI, cholesterol, etc.), but because the diagnostic and treatment process for chronic diseases necessitates the greater inclusion of social environment. After all, these environments play fundamental roles in causing illness (Link & Phelan 1995) and set a context for how well or poorly someone will be able to manage their illness, often over a relatively long period of time. To the extent that those in clinical practice become "community health investigators"—if only by exploring relevant features of a patient's social environment—they likely will be more effective in treating chronic illnesses.

The need for clinical sites to intersect more fully with local communities appears increasingly recognized. Hospital-run community health initiatives, wellness fairs, and charity-funded ambulatory sites nested within neighborhoods, all signal the impact the epidemiological ascendancy of chronic illness has had on the landscape of health care delivery and the limits of the traditional clinical model. The advent of the patient-centered medical home (PCMH) also reflects an implicit recognition of the complexity and multifactorial causes of chronic illness. The coordinated care inherent to the PCMH model provides not only a range of medical care services under a single roof, but specifically includes social support services. A white paper from the Agency for Healthcare Research and Quality authored by Taylor et al. (2011:5) highlights the concept of a "medical neighborhood" in which PCMHs play a central role:

> We conceptualize the medical neighborhood as a PCMH and the constellation of other clinicians providing health care services to patients within it, along with community and social service organizations and State and local public health agencies... Defined in this way, the PCMH and the surrounding medical neighborhood can focus on meeting the needs of the individual patient but also incorporate aspects of population health and overall community health needs in its objectives.

There are many different models of this type of health care provision. For example, many skilled nursing facilities also place heavy emphasis on social services and community relationships and we have seen a call for a return to physician home visits (and a small related industry), which had been nearly totally eclipsed by home care provided by other health professions. Although largely focused on less mobile, often elderly, patients, research on home visits suggests there are potential benefits for wider populations:

> One study found that home assessment of elderly patients with relatively good health status and function resulted in the detection of an average of four new medical problems and up to eight new intervention recommendations per patient. Major problems detected included impotence, gait and balance problems, immunization deficits and hypertension. Significantly, these problems had not been expected based on information obtained from outpatient clinic encounters. Other investigators have demonstrated the effectiveness of home visits in assessing unexpected problems in patient compliance with therapeutic regimens. Finally, specific home-based interventions, such as adjusting the elderly patient's home environment to prevent falls, have also yielded health benefits. (Unwin & Jerant 1999)

While there are any number of new and developing clinical models that we could discuss, our point here is to highlight that all of these represent various efforts to address the new complex paradigm of chronic illness, which requires practitioners (or teams of them) to be conscientious not only of the whole patient as an individual, but the neighborhoods and communities in which he or she lives.

As discussed above, the fracturing of scientific consensus resulting from the perceived ambiguity of chronic illness also has affected the shape of medical institutions. Not only do clinical practitioners have to be attentive to patients' lifestyles, but where patient consumers drive the health care industry, demand has forced many institutions to incorporate complementary and alternative medicine. Many major hospitals now have integrative medicine departments and employ massage therapists, acupuncturists, naturopathic practitioners, "energy medicine," (*reiki*) and the like. Despite often modest or conflicting evidence of effectiveness from traditional scientific investigations, patients value these services and will pay for them (total out-of-pocket costs for complementary and alternative medicines in 2007 totaled $33.9 billion; Nahin et al. 2009). This demonstrates that medicine is not immune to social and cultural forces even though it is sometimes conceived as rooted in objective science. Moreover, our characterization above about the fracturing of scientific consensus may have given the impression that "average people" are estimating risk in ways that separate them from those in scientific industries. But the more complex reality is that even scientific industries have witnessed tremendous change resulting from the incalculable (or certainly less calculable) nature of risk in the era of chronic illness.

We can see the effects of a shifting health landscape in a number of other areas that we will not detail here. In particular, medical, nursing, and allied health educational programs have witnessed a growing inclusion of social science and public health into their curricula, in response to the need for practitioners of the future to have greater understanding of the social factors related to health and illness. There is a changing landscape of health professions with new kinds of providers (e.g., physician assistants), or those with expanding roles (e.g., nurse practitioners) negotiating terrain in clinical care that used to belong squarely to physicians (we will discuss this further in Chapters 8 and 10). There also has been a pedagogical shift in medical and allied health education that broadly seeks to emphasize problem-solving skills and the ability to handle complexity and uncertainty, rather than merely the consumption of massive amounts of information and an overreliance on advanced technology. Case-based, problem-based, and systems-based curricula all represent attempts to move away from the modernist scientific approach to health and present health science in more authentic ways. This too mirrors the increased salience of chronic illnesses, which have more complex and multifactorial causes that cannot easily be partitioned along the lines of traditional scientific disciplines (chemistry, biology, physics, etc.).

Many of these shifts have also challenged us to adapt and reform health care finance and reimbursement structures. Reimbursements for the kinds of discrete and measurable interventions that attend acute injury or infectious disease treatment are easier to quantify. Similarly, what constitutes success is much clearer (e.g., the absence of infection or the healing of an injury). Where these can be more easily measured objectively, reimbursement levels are easier to delineate. What constitutes success with a disease that is managed over the course of years or decades is more difficult to objectify. Moreover, preventative care such as lifestyle counseling is highly subjective and its efficacy depends on not only how well the provider communicates and how well the patient understands, but the quality of the relationship between them. What one is paying for becomes much less clear with chronic illnesses (we discuss this more fully in Chapter 12).

Conclusion

It is difficult to understand the many challenges facing both individual practitioners and larger health care systems without understanding how all of these challenges emanate in one way or another from transforming paradigms of health and shifting conceptualizations of illness. The premodern history of medicine not only brings into focus many of the premises upon which modern medicine was built (sometimes in reactionary ways), but it helps us to see clearly how our own medical practices are tied to particular ways of thinking about health and the body. Premodern medical treatments were connected to a cosmology that emphasized the interconnectedness of the world, and a corresponding need for balance within it, and they treated disease accordingly.

It was a shift in this way of thinking toward modernist rationality—something that predated modern medicine proper by several hundred years—that ultimately gave birth to the kind of medicine we are most familiar with today. But it is important not to overlook that modern health care is equally tethered to particular ways of thinking, particular logics of disease, which, although well suited for infectious disease and acute injury, in many ways are a mismatch with the causal profile of chronic illnesses. Meanwhile the complexity and ambiguity surrounding chronic illnesses promote a fracturing of scientific medical authority on which the modern medical clinic depends. The results of this are evident in the challenges facing current and future health care providers. These challenges range from improving, if not restructuring, clinical practices at a local level to reorganizing macro systems of health care to accommodate diverse and even divergent philosophies about health and the body. While we will undertake a more thorough discussion of many of these challenges throughout the remainder of this book, clarity on how they radiate from the common epicenter of the shifting epidemiological landscape gives practitioners a deeper level of understanding that is not only necessary to address the challenges of treating individual patients, but also utterly essential to reshaping health care systems—something which must be significantly driven by providers themselves (see Chapter 12).

CHAPTER 2 ACTIVITY

Exercising One's Epistemology: Seeing Disease through Premodern, Modern, and Postindustrial Frameworks

Part 1

It is the year 571 and you are a physician in Verona, the second largest and most important city in the region (what is now Italy). Because it stands at the intersection of several main travel routes, there are frequently traders and merchants passing through. Early one morning, a representative of King Alboin knocks on your door and asks you to attend to one of the King's favorite merchants who commonly brings gifts from Northern Africa for Queen Rosamund. Upon seeing the patient, you observe that he is bent over at the waist with a great deal of pain in his lower abdomen. He complains of chills, but his forehead is hot to the touch. The chambermaid who had been sent by the King tells you that when he first arrived two days before he had diarrhea, but since then had not had a bowel movement. He had eaten voraciously immediately upon his arrival, but had not had an appetite since. When you ask him about his last meal he says, "The King always sends the finest cuts of meat and the most luxurious fruits. I have a special weakness for figs, particularly since, when I am between destinations, I am often resigned to eating dry, tasteless seeds and nuts."

1. Using the lens of the humoral medicine, explain this man's ailment.

    Helpful Hint: Try to focus on understanding the symptoms that are observable at the bedside and conceptualize them using notions of balance that are paradigmatic of that era (do not focus on trying to make a "diagnosis").

2. What might you recommend as a treatment for this man?

    Helpful Hint: For this activity, ignore whether the treatment you come up with is historically accurate. Instead, focus on whether it follows in a coherent way from a humoral notion of disease (as well as the monistic notion of the universe).

Part 2

Imagine that it is 1961 and you are a family practice physician in Kansas City, Missouri. You are in your office about to start your day when your nurse comes in and says, "You were supposed to see Mr. Cowgill for a physical first, but there's a new patient here in quite a bit of pain, and you might want to see him right away." When you enter the exam room, the man is lying on his back. When you ask him to sit up, he clutches his abdomen and winces, as he does so. "So moving seems to be especially painful?" you ask. "Yes, but it basically hurts all the time no matter what," the patient replies. You take a history and some basic vital signs, noting that the man has a fever and reports being constipated for nearly three days. His lower abdomen is also distended. As you write these notes in his chart, he mentions, "I'm a traveling salesman with Hoover Vacuum Cleaners. I've been on the road for six weeks, mainly through the Southwest and now I'm making my way back to Chicago. Sure was nice to get to Kansas City and get some real barbecue, though, after being in the middle of nowhere and eating at greasy roadside diners and the trail mix my wife makes for me. But I haven't been able to eat for two days now. I feel nauseous."

You diagnose the man with diverticulitis.

1. Using a modernist lens, explain your diagnosis including his symptoms to the patient.

    Helpful Hint: Focus on causes and effects. If needed, briefly research diverticulitis online. A basic website like WebMD will be sufficient for this case.

2. What might you recommend as a treatment for this man?

    Helpful Hint: Here again, you may need to quickly research treatments online, but a website with basic information will suffice for the purposes of this activity.

Part 3

It's 2016 and you're a nurse practitioner in an urgent care clinic in Santa Fe, New Mexico. A man comes in complaining of pain in his lower abdomen. As you take a history and basic physical, he mentions that he's been out with his friends hiking and camping in the Palo Duro Canyons in Texas for the past week. You ask about his diet generally, and what he had been eating while on his camping trip, and he tells you that he's vegan and ate mainly nuts and beans. "For years, I used to eat nothing but meat and cheese, but then I got serious about my health and started eating mostly raw foods." He tells you he started seeing a little blood in his stool during the last few days of the trip. He has a fever, his lower abdomen is distended, and he is in a great deal of pain, particularly when he moves.

You diagnose the man with diverticulitis and prescribe a moderate dose of acetaminophen–codeine combination painkiller, warning him to call you if the bleeding in his stool worsens. You also prescribe oral ciprofloxacin (antibiotic) and tell him to rest for the next week, advising that lifting heavy objects or anything above mild physical activity could cause a perforation in his colon.

The patient responds that he wants the painkillers, but doesn't intend to fill the antibiotic prescription because he believes taking antibiotics inhibits the body's natural healing abilities. "Besides," he says, "everyone's taking so many antibiotics these days that germs are morphing into superbugs."

1. Using the concepts of uncertainty and risk estimation, explain this man's reaction to your treatment plan.

2. How might you respond to the patient's hesitancy to take antibiotics?

    Helpful Hint: Rather than, or at least in addition to, trying to persuade him with evidenced-based medical principles, think about ways you can work from his own worldview as you communicate with him.

The Logic and Methods of Empirical Research

LEARNING OBJECTIVES

After reading this chapter, students should be able to

- Articulate the importance of acquiring and continually honing a statistical imagination.

- Describe the steps of the scientific method and their roles in the production, replication, and verification of scientific knowledge.

- Discuss the various components of research design, establishing causality, and detecting statistical associations using the classic experiment as a model of logical proof.

- Describe various observational alternatives to experimental design when the implementation of the latter is unfeasible or unethical.

- Translate research findings into practical strategies for evidence-based decision-making in the health professions.

- Articulate the key fiduciary responsibilities of medical and allied health researchers with respect to generating good science that improves public health.

In order to make sense of the increasing complexity and many challenges that you will inevitably confront in your work, it is first necessary to develop the capacity to evaluate evidence that you observe or that is presented to you by others. Thus far we have begun to build upon the idea of the sociological imagination, to apply it to health and clinical phenomena, and to help you cultivate your ability to see the various interconnections among these issues. To do so, you will need a handful of skills to facilitate your ability to critically assess research data, which typically pertain to the group (i.e., it represents a macro-level of analysis). Large-scale tendencies and themes are typically difficult to see from our often-limited perspectives as individuals. The skills informed by this chapter will help you critically evaluate empirical evidence and the claims that are made based upon it. This has significant implications for your work. After all, to see the bigger picture, we must be able to visualize the connections between large-scale group analyses and their relationship to evidence-based decision-making at the level of clinical and professional interaction (recall the concept of the sociological imagination from Chapter 1). The focus of this chapter centers on the tools needed to do this with respect to research evidence.

To be clear, what follows is not a substitute for the material covered in a wide array of research methods and data analysis courses or texts. In fact, we will provide a list of references at the end of this book, and we encourage you to utilize them in the future. Instead of a methods chapter then, we are more interested in cultivating a systematic, methodo-*logical* approach to thinking about and critically evaluating empirical claims and observations. This chapter empowers you with conceptual tools to think logically about empirical observations, including that which is systematically collected according to the rules of research (i.e., *data*) as well as the many taken-for-granted notions that exist in virtually all aspects of our lives and our professions. These tools should help you distinguish that which is appropriately measured, probably causal, sufficiently strong, and potentially applicable, from that which is sloppily measured, hastily interpreted, arguably spurious, observably weak, and perhaps irrelevant. In short, we hope to facilitate your active engagement with, and critical reflection about, research data, rather than leaving that work and its interpretation to the "intellectual elite" (Gregory & O'Toole 1987:134).

In this chapter, we first extend our discussion of the sociological imagination to its conceptual counterpart, the *statistical imagination*, which facilitates our ability to connect smaller, observable phenomena to larger sets of observations, by using the rules of probability, validity, and reliability (Ritchey 2007). Next, we focus on the purpose, goals, and methods of scientific research, including types of scientific inquiry and common research designs you will encounter during the course of your work, to enable you to assess their relative strengths and weaknesses. Finally, we briefly examine the ethical responsibilities and obligations associated with conducting health research. Along the way, we examine critical questions related to translating research to clinical practice. So while Chapter 1 introduced readers to the *need* for a sociological imagination to navigate the health professional landscape in the twenty-first century and Chapter 2 provided a sociohistorical context and discussion of contemporary shifts to illuminate *why* such thinking is necessary, this chapter provides a specific toolkit for thinking like a research scientist.

The Statistical Imagination

As an outgrowth of Mills' (1959) sociological imagination, which refers to the ability to visualize the connections between the individual and larger society (or the various links between smaller- and larger-scale phenomena), the *statistical imagination* refers to an appreciation of how usual or unusual an event, circumstance, or behavior is in relation to a larger set of similar events (Ritchey 2007). Put another way, the statistical imagination is all about keeping an eye on the "bigger *empirical* picture," thereby allowing us to examine a specific research finding, clinical situation, or phenomena of interest within the context of larger sets of findings, scenarios, and patterns of behavior. This is important because a balanced perspective of the world around us requires more than analyzing and reporting data. It also involves the ability to think through a complex problem—and a sea of often-conflicting research on a disease and its treatment—while maintaining a sense of proportion and appropriate perspective. This means developing a critical perspective toward our preconceived notions, habits, and practices, as well as our own research and that of others. When practiced, this capacity for critical evaluation helps us develop a nuanced view of a complex professional and health landscape, one that, as noted in Chapters 1 and 2, is only growing more complicated. The statistical imagination will help you cut through the noise and confusion of that complexity.

At its core, the statistical imagination helps us understand that most events are predictable, meaning that we can identify their probability of occurring over time. This is an important foundation because on its most basic level, the entire point of research is to (1) explain things, or make sense of the world around us, and (2) help us make predictions about what is likely to occur in the future under similar conditions. Research in health and health care does this where it develops evidence-based interventions aimed at ameliorating human suffering, providing safe and effective care to patients, streamlining health care delivery processes to maximize efficiency, and shaping health policy to improve public health.

To be methodologically unimaginative often leads to reactionary behavior in health care settings. For instance, viewing one set of research findings in isolation might lead you to conclude that an experimental drug therapy for diabetics is safe and effective, when in reality, it could pose more serious problems for patients than diabetes itself. An inability to systematically think through the validity of research in a critical way can, very literally, put people's lives in danger. We find a useful example to illustrate the points mentioned thus far in the work of Ben Goldacre, who writes about health care's "trick coin." Goldacre (2013) draws our attention to a large corporation facing more than 10,000 lawsuits over an artificial hip now no longer used because of a 40% five-year failure rate in patients. This means that within five years, four out of every ten treatments failed to work or caused adverse events, and internal documents showed that the manufacturer knew about its problems for some time but never made those concerns public. He goes on to note that the evidence bases for medical treatments may be undermined not only by a lack of transparency on the part of companies but also by *a simple trick of probability*. The best evidence available suggests that about *half of all clinical trials ever conducted on the treatments in use today* have never been published in academic journals (and the most questionable studies presumably are the ones least likely to be published). In particular, studies that find no effects (or negative, sometimes very serious effects) are less likely to be published than studies that find positive effects. The "trick," then, is this: if we toss a coin but hide the result at least part of the time it comes up "tails" (i.e., a negative, undesirable outcome), then it looks as if we toss "heads" (i.e., a positive, desirable outcome) far more often. In this way, many health professionals and patients alike are misled into believing that we should use ineffective or less effective treatments, simply because we are much more likely to see the "good" research results, and more rarely the "bad" outcomes that might call into question a therapy's universal benefit for everyone with a particular condition.

We often operate under the misconception that therapies that make it into the market or practice are tried and true, rigorously tested and evaluated interventions. Some certainly are, but Goldacre (2012) asserts than many are not. Tamiflu is a good illustration of these practices in recent years. Governments have spent billions of dollars stockpiling this drug, believing that it will reduce the rate of complications from influenza. But only about half of the trial results for Tamiflu have ever been published, and the manufacturer has stonewalled researchers trying to obtain the full clinical study reports. To critically assess the published Tamiflu findings, then, we might use our statistical imagination to place those results in their broader contexts, imagining what hidden forces (e.g., the failure to publish findings that show limited or no effect) might be shaping our interpretations of evidence that is presented. Doing so can help us reflexively assess many taken-for-granted notions in our work.

We must use a statistical imagination to provide context to the isolated bits of evidence that we are presented, in order to see them more clearly and honestly, particularly when so many behaviors and practices become institutionalized in a way that makes them seem natural or even inevitable. Welch and colleagues (2011) note, for example, that if we consider the number of diagnoses assigned per capita, Americans are by far the sickest population in the world. A reactionary interpretation might lead us to conclude that we need *more* health care in the United States. Welch and colleagues instead suggest that we might actually need *less*. How can this be? If we consider the broader context of these observations, then we see how trends in contemporary health care, biomedical research, reimbursement structures, law, and consumer demand actually drive a phenomenon called overdiagnosis in the United States. However, despite how dramatically different the diagnostic picture looks when we reconsider it with a statistical imagination, Welch and colleagues note that the responses to these shifts among many medical and allied health professions have, at least partly, created entrenched patterns of professional behavior that perpetuate this phenomenon, in turn contributing to rising health care costs, skyrocketing prescription drug use, unnecessary treatments, and often poorer patient outcomes. Calls in medical and allied health education for greater inclusion of epidemiology highlight the need to empower providers with a strong statistical imagination as part of responding to these trends.[1]

Finally, the statistical imagination imbues a strong sense of scientific skepticism, and a good scientist and thinker is always skeptical. When we observe a pattern or regularity, we never first assume that it is coincidental; rather, we approach it as something we need to explain using the rules of science. Many often fall back into the entrenched position that things are the way they are because they've always been that way. In other words, that is just the way that it is, but that doesn't cut it as a valid scientific explanation, despite the fact that we often believe this or that justification as truth. In short, a skeptical approach quickly unravels such claims.

As scientists we are also trained to tolerate a nearly constant degree of uncertainty in only cautiously drawing conclusions, because we can very rarely (if ever) be 100% confident that research results are valid. In fact, the only way to reach absolute certainty is to observe every single instance of an occurrence in an entire population. Let's put that into perspective by calling into question two simple, but generally, accepted claims: the uniqueness of fingerprints and snowflakes. Validating the claim that each fingerprint or snowflake is unique requires that we analyze the fingerprints of every single human being that has ever lived, or to closely examine every single snowflake that has ever fallen. If we understand scientific error and empirical uncertainty—including the fact that most claims based on evidence are based on analysis of small sets of a larger universe—then we can begin to discern

---

[1] There are other influential social forces that foster these trends as well (e.g., the practice of defensive medicine in the context of litigation risk, financial reimbursement structures, etc.).

the complexity of things that we might previously have taken for granted. We can also extend these ideas to critically evaluating other claims germane to clinical presentation, diagnosis, health care delivery, or treatment. In short, things are rarely what they at first seem and the rules of science help us critically and systematically assess the evidence presented in research.

What Is Science?

The word *science* is derived from the Latin word *scire*, which means "to know," but science is a term, and a concept, that is frequently misunderstood. To many, science refers to a prestigious and well-funded field of study (i.e., the health *sciences*), or a body of knowledge itself (i.e., the *science* of biochemistry), or equates with the term truth (i.e., these facts are *scientific* and are thus irrefutable). As a result, we often confuse the *content* of science with its *methods*. At its core, though, to say something is scientific simply means that it originates with scientific methodologies. So *science* itself simply refers to methodology that guides the discovery and production of knowledge that is grounded in the rules of reason (i.e., logical validity) and experience (i.e., empirical verifiability). In short, science refers to a systematic method of explaining empirical (or observable) phenomena (Ritchey 2007:8), or the study of phenomena through strict observation, evaluation, and theoretical explanation (Privitera 2012:7). In both these definitions, we can see the primary significance being placed upon methodologies of *logical inference* (i.e., drawing conclusions based on evidence), *falsifiability* (i.e., testability), *replicability* (i.e., reproducibility), and *generalizability* (applicability to larger contexts), which constitute the bedrock of scientific research. And because science is limited to directly *observable* phenomena, many ideas or objects must be measured indirectly (like motivations or attitudes, or even very small subatomic particles) or cannot be measured at all (e.g., the existence of God, or an afterlife).

The main goal of science, then, is to explain things that can be observed and measured (i.e., empirical phenomena), and a scientific explanation is generated based on the methods of science. These products of scientific inquiry are called *theories* and they help us achieve one of the principal objectives of science, which is to explain the observable world around us. Often, people think of theories as the untested ideas that are confirmed or disconfirmed as factual by scientific methods. However, this is a misconception. Because research results are always probabilistic (i.e., they are highly likely, but almost never absolutely certain), there is always a gap between the data itself and our assertions about what is actually happening in the world. Crossing this gap requires sound reasoning and interpretation. Theories, then, are sets of very specific statements, generally grounded in previous empirical research, which are continually tested against new observations. Over time, theories are gradually altered and refined in a way that ideally helps them explain things more effectively (typically a very slow process).

An acceptable theory typically accomplishes at least two things: (1) it provides an explanation, which helps us understand some phenomenon of interest, and (2) it allows us to make predictions about what should happen in the future, based on that explanation. In other words, we should be able to predict what will happen when changes in one *variable* (i.e., any observation that changes over time, or from

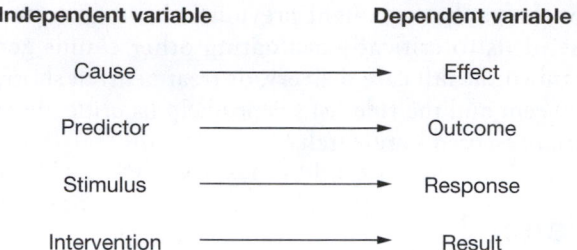

FIG. 3.1 Independent and dependent variables.

Source: Adapted from Ritchey, Ferris. (2007). *The Statistical Imagination.* New York: McGraw-Hill.

place to place, or among individuals) affect changes in some other variable. We call variables that help us make these predictions *independent* variables, and the variables that change as a result, *dependent* variables (Ritchey 2007) Figure 3.1. We measure these variables quantitatively (i.e., they can be represented with a number) to produce either *descriptive statistics* or *inferential statistics*. The former describes the frequency of an occurrence or general trends in the data, whereas we use the latter to develop cause-and-effect explanations. For example, based on existing explanations (i.e., current theories) of disease epidemiology, we might hypothesize that as the percentage of vaccinated persons in the Nashville, Tennessee, metropolitan area decreases (an independent variable), the incidence of measles in that area will increase (a dependent variable). Alternatively, based on theories related to health care policy, we might hypothesize that as access to preventative health care in Nashville increases (an independent variable), total health care costs in that area will decrease (a dependent variable). Because the geographic area (Nashville) in both of these examples does not vary, it is called a *constant*.

The Scientific Method

The various sciences (biology, physics, sociology, psychology, etc.) are united not by their subject matters, but by their methods and assumptions. Indeed, this is what distinguishes scientific approaches from other modes of seeking knowledge. A scientific *methodology* is simply a system of rules and procedures that provides the guidelines for conducting research and evaluating claims. We should also note that these procedures are neither static nor infallible. There are many different techniques and they are continually being developed or reformulated. But what various methodological approaches have in common are the goals of logical inference and generalizability. *Logical inference* refers to drawing careful conclusions on the basis of observation and analysis, while *generalizability* (also known as *external validity*) refers to applying results and conclusions from smaller-scale analyses to larger populations of similar phenomena. The methods that we describe below define the rules of the game for researchers and scientists to follow—the paradigm of scientific inquiry (Frankfort-Nachmias & Nachmias 2000). While different texts will conceptualize the process in slightly different ways, and some methodological approaches intentionally vary from certain procedures, the research process involves seven basic steps.

1. *Specify a research question.* The researcher must first define a question of interest for investigation. This research question should be something both important and innovative. For example, we might ask: *Does underwater treadmill training (UTT) improve physical function among persons with incomplete spinal cord injury (ICSI), over and above standard therapies already in use?* This question addresses a significant clinical health issue with far-reaching implications and the potential to improve many people's lives. So this is something that we would definitely want to explain.

2. *Review the extant literature.* After defining a research question, the researcher searches the existing body of scientific knowledge for information and other studies that in some way inform the proposed research. This step serves a dual purpose. First, no one wants to waste time and money designing and conducting research that someone else has already carried out; after all, research is often very expensive and time-consuming. Second, related previous studies might inform the new study in a number of ways (e.g., what independent variables should be considered, potential ways to measure phenomena, etc.). At this point, the goal is to locate the cutting edge of existing knowledge, and then build upon it. For our aforementioned research question about the effects of UTT on physical function of patients with ICSI, we might look to fields like physical and occupational therapy, medicine, nursing, or others to inform our research.

3. *Propose a theory and develop hypotheses.* Existing research should coalesce around a number of independent variables that likely predict variation in the chosen dependent variable (those that the researcher envisions, as well as those suggested by the existing research), such that the researcher can begin to assemble a theoretical framework to explain precisely *how* these variables work to produce specific outcomes. From that theory we derive at least one *hypothesis*, which is simply a predictive statement concerning the relationship between two variables, where changes in one variable correspond with changes in a second variable. In this way, hypotheses are derived from larger theories, and predict what observed outcomes might be expected under certain conditions. If we reproduce those outcomes, we corroborate the theory; if we observe something other than what was predicted, we might modify previous explanations in some way. Our research question above seeks to investigate the effects of one very specific independent variable (UTT), which should predict variation in our dependent variables, where physical function would be specifically measured by, for example, (a) *Activities of Daily Living,* or *ADL,* and (b) *motor coordination.* So to keep things somewhat simple, we might propose the following hypotheses:

   H_1: Those persons with ICSI undergoing UTT (independent variable) will exhibit fewer problems performing activities of daily living (dependent variable 1).
   H_2: Those persons with ICSI undergoing UTT (independent variable) will exhibit greater motor coordination (dependent variable 2).

Hypotheses generally constitute a restatement of a research question, but in more precise terms such that each variable is specified in a way that can be measured. As a result, another key element of this process concerns the careful *conceptualization* (i.e., definition or specification) and *operationalization* (i.e., measurement) of variables.

4. *Select an appropriate research design.* This step in the research process outlines how variables will be measured and how data will be collected. There are many options for how to conduct a study, including but not limited to experimental design, quasi-experimental approaches, surveys, personal interviews, and case studies. Think of these various approaches as simply tools in the researcher's toolbox. The tool one uses should correspond to the job at hand, meaning that it is up to the scientist to select the most appropriate research design and data collection methodology to address the questions under study. There is no "one size fits all" approach, just as you wouldn't want to use a screwdriver to hammer a nail. Selecting the appropriate design often involves balancing a variety of methodological, practical, and ethical considerations. We will discuss these concerns in more detail below.

5. *Collect data.* Here the researcher actually implements the planned research design to comprise a data set. Depending on the research design, this may involve testing, completing interviews, making repeated observations, administering surveys, and so on.

6. *Analyze data and draw conclusions.* This step involves analysis of collected data in a way that permits the researcher to compare observations to the predictions of the hypotheses made earlier. We either find support for our hypotheses, or we refute them. Either way, the researcher employs data analysis to gain a better understanding of the phenomenon under study. For example, we might find support for both of our hypotheses about UTT, support for neither, or support for one and not the other. In short, at this point in the research process, we seek to answer our research question via the data, by way of the hypotheses.

7. *Disseminate results.* In this final step of the scientific method, researchers share their findings and conclusions with two general audiences: the public at large and the scientific community. For public audiences, we might distribute reports or give presentations to emphasize the conclusions and practical significance of the research. Reaching scientific audiences typically means distributing your methods and results in a peer-reviewed journal or a conference presentation.

Importantly, scientific methods engender a cyclical process. The final step of the scientific method involves integrating results and conclusions into the existing body of scientific or professional knowledge, while the first step involves grounding your research question(s) in that very same ocean of extant literature. This is important because it explains how the accumulation of knowledge proceeds in a maturing scientific field. Further, this connects the individual researcher to the larger community of scientists in a particular discipline or area of investigation, with each study representing only a very small part of the intellectual force pushing a field forward. So what does one piece of research actually mean within this larger context? Well, even a well-designed and carefully conducted study with valid results may not mean very much on its own. Remember, the statistical imagination involves placing a single set of findings into the broader context of similar studies, developing a nuanced understanding of the often complex phenomena that we investigate, and

TABLE 3.1 **The Logical Model of Causality**

Covariation	When two or more phenomena (or variables) change together.
Nonspuriousness	The effects of other relevant variables are controlled, and the relation between variables is maintained.
Time Order	The presumed cause (or independent variable) occurs first and prior to the presumed effect (or dependent variable).

Source: Adapted from Frankfort-Nachmias, Chava & David Nachmias. (2000). *Research Methods in the Social Sciences.* New York: Worth.

critically assessing both the role of probability in a research design and the results in lieu of their practical applications and generalizability to real-world populations. To become part of the scientific canon in any discipline, a study's findings should be replicated in similar populations and under similar conditions (Benestad & Laake 2007). Many studies do not pass these tests for any number of reasons (some of which we will discuss below), and it will then be left to you to make sense of what they mean for your own practice. As noted, each research design possesses not only strengths but also weaknesses. Researchers typically strive to maximize the former while minimizing the latter, but critically evaluating research requires an understanding of each. As scientists we all strive to meet the burdens of causality, validity, reliability, and generalizability, but it is not always possible, feasible, or ethical to do so. In the next several sections we address these issues.

In Pursuit of Causality

The desire to explain is one of the core pursuits of science, and the issue of *causality* lies at the heart of most scientific explanations. For a causal relationship to exist, we would expect that changes in a study's independent variable (what we call *variation*) correspond with some observed changes in a dependent variable. However, this is not a sufficient condition to determine causality. That is, even in the presence of such *covariation*, we cannot conclude that we have identified a causal relationship. As a result, causality can be an elusive thing to determine empirically. This means that we must take great care in designing research and using appropriate logic when doing so. In practice, demonstrating causality involves three distinct steps (Frankfort-Nachmias & Nachmias 2000; Singleton & Straits 1999): *covariation, eliminating spurious relationships,* and *time order.* Understanding these three criteria is tremendously important to critical assessing research and proposed explanations. Many claims in the area of health and medicine that appear to be supported by evidence actually fall apart when subjected to these tests of causality.

Covariation

As noted above, the criterion of covariation means that two or more concepts, variables, or sets of observations change together. In other words, a positive or negative change in one or more independent variables (IVs) is associated with positive or negative fluctuations in one or more dependent variables (DVs). For instance, Rossi and colleagues (2012) reviewed studies investigating the impact of physical activity on mortality in patients with hypertension (i.e., high blood pressure). In this example, we might observe that, as the frequency of aerobic exercise increases (i.e., a single IV), blood pressure (DV_1) is expected to decrease, as is mortality (DV_2). As you might imagine, the independent and dependent variables change together systematically; that is, as frequency of aerobic exercise increases, blood pressure decreases. Therefore, the criterion of covariation is met, and we may say that the variables are *correlated* with one another. However, as the old adage goes, *correlation alone does not equal causation*. While causation requires correlation, the latter is not sufficient to claim the former.

We can also choose to specify more information regarding covariates, including *direction*, *strength*, *symmetry*, and *linearity* (Shi 2008). Direction and strength are probably most important for our audience, but the other attributes are arguably worth mentioning briefly as well. For example, in addressing direction we might describe a positive (or direct) relationship for variables that covary (i.e., they increase or decrease together). Alternatively, a negative (or inverse) correlation describes a situation when as one variable increases the other systematically decreases, or vice versa. In the example above, as frequency of aerobic exercise increased, blood pressure decreased. This means they were *negatively correlated*. Second, the *strength* of a relationship describes how tightly the variables are correlated with one another, something that can be quantitatively assessed.

Third, a relationship may be described as symmetrical or asymmetrical. A symmetrical relationship is bidirectional, where a change in either of two variables is accompanied by a change in the other (i.e., $X \leftrightarrow Y$). An asymmetrical relation, on the other hand, refers to a situation when change in one variable is associated with change in another, but not vice versa (i.e., $X \rightarrow Y$). Our study on frequency of aerobic exercise is a good example of an asymmetrical relationship if we can reasonably say that increases in the frequency of exercise are associated with decreases in blood pressure, but cannot reasonably say the opposite (it doesn't make much sense to say that as blood pressure decreases, frequency of aerobic exercise increases).

Finally, linearity concerns whether two variables change at the same rate regardless of whether the values of those variables are relatively low, moderate, or high (see examples in Figures 3.2a and 3.2b). The number of cigarettes smoked over time (measured in pack-years) and the chance of lung cancer might be described as linear, because the probabilities of disease increase as one smokes more and more. But the association between, for example, rates of Cesarean section (C-section) and maternal mortality is described as nonlinear (Volpe 2011). This is because when rates of C-section are very low, more women suffer complications that lead to death while giving birth. However, the benefit of C-section for maternal mortality eventually levels off. When rates of C-section are greater than about 12% there appear to be, on the whole, no additional decrease in mortality.

Eliminating Spuriousness

Eliminating spuriousness refers to the researcher's ability to demonstrate that covariation between two variables of interest cannot be explained, in whole or in part, by a

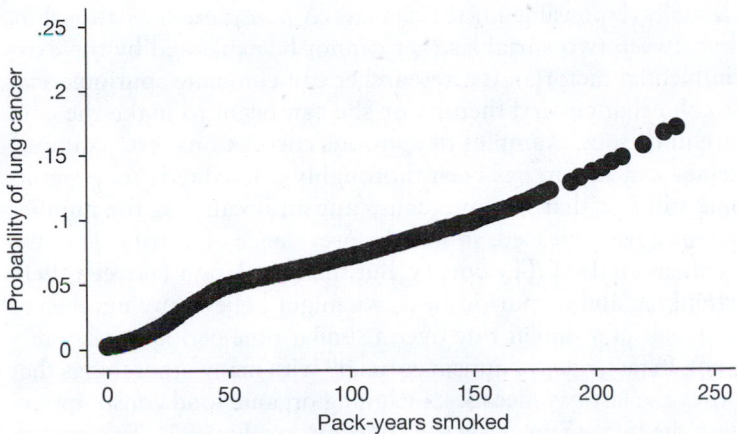

FIG. 3.2 (A) Example of a linear relationship (pack-years smoked by probability of developing lung cancer).

Source: Tammemagi, C. Martin, Paul F. Pinsky, Neil E. Caporaso, Paul A. Kvale, William G. Hocking, Timothy R. Church, et al. (2011). "Lung Cancer Risk Prediction: Prostate, Lung, Colorectal and Ovarian Cancer Screening Trial Models and Validation." *Journal of the National Cancer Institute* 103(13), 1058–68.

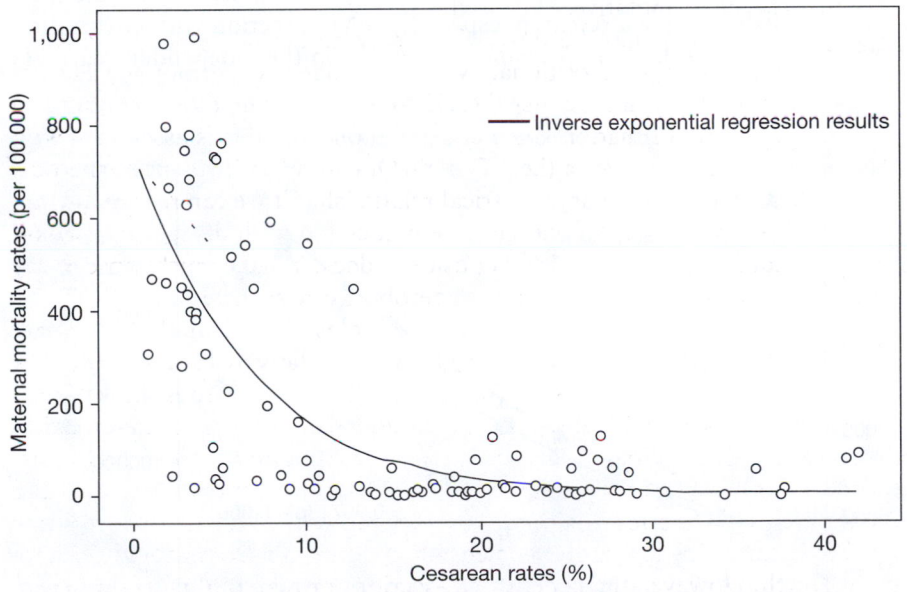

FIG. 3.2 (B) Example of a nonlinear relationship (maternal mortality rate-by-rate of Cesarean section).

Source: Volpe, Fernando M. (2011). "Correlation of Cesarean Rates to Maternal and Infant Mortality Rates: An Ecologic Study of Official International Data." *Pan American Journal of Public Health (Revista Panamericana de Salud Pública)* 29(5), 303–08.

third variable that is actually responsible for the changes. A *nonspurious* relationship, then, is a relationship between two variables that cannot be explained by the existence of some other influential factor(s). If a researcher can eliminate spurious relations amidst two variables that covary, then he or she can begin to make the case for causality. There are numerous examples of spurious correlations. For example, the link between vaccines and autism has been thoroughly discredited. Yet a significant number of people still fear that vaccines cause autism because as the number of childhood vaccinations have increased, so has the prevalence of autism. The two therefore appear related, and indeed they covary. But the correlation between them is spurious. Without thinking about spuriousness, we might believe any number of things that happen to change at a similar rate over a similar time period are *causally* related when they are not. In fact, rates of autism correlate with many other things that have been increasing over the last two decades, including organic food consumption. The correlation between the two, again, is clearly spurious (see Fig. 3.3). To establish causality, we need to rule out other things that may explain why our DV is changing.

Time Order

The third criterion for establishing causality is relatively straightforward: a hypothesized cause must precede the observed effect. That is, predictors must come before outcomes, or independent variables must precede dependent variables, for a causal relationship to exist. This makes intuitive sense, of course, but is sometimes difficult to establish in applied research, especially in conjunction with covariation and nonspuriousness. In the examples above, changes in the independent variable

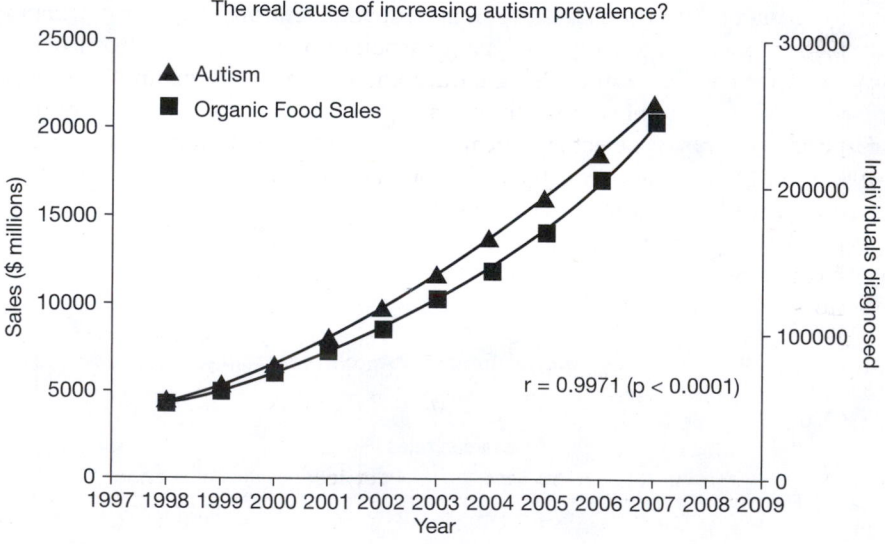

FIG. 3.3 The real cause of increasing autism prevalence?

Sources: Organic Trade Association, 2011 Organic Industry Survey, U.S. Department of Education, Office of Special Education Programs, Data Analysis Systems (DANS), OMB# 1820-0043. "Children with Disabilities Receiving Special Education under Part B of the Individuals with Disabilities Education Act"

This was created by a Redditor: http://imgur.com/1WZ6h

(physical activity) must precede changes to the dependent variables (blood pressure and mortality rate) in order to meet the criterion of time order. If all three of these requirements—covariation, nonspuriousness, and time order—are established, then a causal relationship may be supported.

As mentioned, there are many different types of research designs and each has strengths and weaknesses. Often the strength or weakness of a design centers on its ability to help us meet the three criteria for establishing causality. We begin our discussion of research design with *classic experimental design* because understanding the logic of the experiment helps us understand how the criteria of causality are demonstrated in applied research and how other methodologies attempt to meet those same requirements in alternative ways.

Classic Experimental Design

Empirical research in the biomedical sciences is typically quantitative, which means that it involves statistical analysis of numerical data, and we can categorize most of these studies as either *experimental* or *observational*. The goal of all studies is to generate *valid* (accurate) and *reliable* (reproducible) results that may be generalized to larger populations of interest. These goals are achieved through careful planning in both research design and data analysis strategies. The experimental method (or experimental design) is one of the most common and straightforward approaches to establishing causality between an independent variable and a dependent variable, specifically by meeting the three criteria of covariation, nonspuriousness, and time order. Figure 3.4 will serve as an illustration of the classic experiment as we discuss the ways by which these requirements are demonstrated.

An experiment typically focuses upon a single intervention (e.g., a drug, a therapy, or a condition), while carefully analyzing associations (i.e., covariation) between a single predictor variable and a single outcome between two groups of subjects. This logic serves as the basis for clinical and laboratory trials in the biomedical sciences, and attempts to detect significant differences between a *control group* and an *experimental group*, over time (i.e., time order) while ensuring that other possible causes of observed associations (i.e., nonspuriousness) are minimized or eliminated. In Figure 3.4 then, X signifies the independent variable, O_1–O_4 represent measurements of the dependent variable, and d_e and d_c denote the difference between the pretest and posttest in each group. To conduct an experiment, the researcher must purposefully control the conditions under which observations are recorded in order to isolate causal relationships involving the independent and dependent variables. This is accomplished by making the experimental and control groups as identical

Group	Pre-test	Post-test	Difference
Experimental	$O_1 \longrightarrow X \longrightarrow O_2$		$O_2 - O_1 = d_e$
Control	$O_3 \longrightarrow \hspace{2em} O_4$		$O_4 - O_3 = d_c$

FIG 3.4 Experimental design model.

Source: Adapted from Frankfort-Nachmias, Chava & David Nachmias. (2000). *Research Methods in the Social Sciences.* New York: Worth.

TABLE 3.2 Components of Classic Research Design

Comparison	The operation that determines whether two variables covary, or are correlated.
Manipulation	The operation that controls the assignment to the experimental and control groups, so that the researcher can determine the time sequence to ensure that the independent variable changes prior to changes in the dependent variable.
Control	The operation that enables the researcher to rule out rival explanations for observed effects, including intrinsic and extrinsic factors.
Generalizability	The extent to which findings can be generalized to larger populations and applied to different settings or environments.

Source: Adapted from Frankfort-Nachmias, Chava & David Nachmias. (2000). *Research Methods in the Social Sciences.* New York: Worth.

as possible in every way except the intervention itself. The researcher measures the dependent variable at two points within each group: before introducing the independent variable (*pretest*) and again following exposure (*posttest*). The differences in measurements of the dependent variable between the pretest and posttest are then assessed for both groups, and if these differences in the experimental group are significantly larger than the differences for the control group, the researcher may infer that the predictor is causally related to the outcome. This design, if carried out properly, ensures that the requirements of causality are met within a specific population of interest, and this is achieved through *comparison, manipulation, control,* and *generalizability* (Frankfort-Nachmias& Nachmias 2000).

Identifying a relationship between two variables depends first and foremost upon the process of *comparison*, whereby the researcher compares groups of individuals that differ on the basis of one variable (in the example above, exercise therapy) to examine variation on the basis of some other variable (e.g., blood pressure). In the classic experimental design, we must compare those subjects who completed the prescribed exercise (the experimental group) with those who did not (the control group). Second, to foster an ability to compare groups based on the key variable of interest, we often *manipulate* the conditions of interest. That is, we take two groups that are the same on virtually all accounts and intentionally do something different to one of them to see if it produces different outcomes between the two groups on the basis of our dependent variable.

Control is the third component of the classic experimental design and requires the researcher to eliminate all other factors that could represent competing explanations for the observed associations between the independent and dependent variables. This issue is called the problem of *internal validity* and there are both *extrinsic* and *intrinsic factors* that can compromise it. Extrinsic factors exist prior to the study. For example, if the subjects in the control and experimental group were different in some relevant ways to the outcome of the study, we would say an extrinsic factor (that difference between them) compromised the internal validity of the study. This is a common limitation of studies where subjects cannot be randomly assigned to control and experimental groups for logistical or ethical reasons (often called *selection bias*). Intrinsic factors, on the other hand, occur during the study (or observational) period and typically involve changes in the research subjects (e.g., history, maturation, or experimental mortality), changes in the measurement instrument (e.g., reliability), or the effects of observation itself. For example, if during a study of the effects of a drug, the subjects in the experimental group see their physicians twice as often as those in the control group, this could compromise the validity of the study, particularly if frequency of doctor visits ends up being related to the study outcomes (e.g., if those people become more health-conscious and begin to eat healthier foods because they receive that advice from their physician at each visit).

There exist a number of options with which to address intrinsic and extrinsic factors. Controlling intrinsic factors can be achieved by ensuring that the control and experimental groups experience identical study conditions, with the exception of the independent variable (in the example above, we might ensure the control and experimental groups see the physician with the same frequency). Researchers typically control extrinsic factors with either *matching* or *randomization*. Matching pairs subjects in control and experimental groups on the basis of known variables predictably related to a research hypothesis. For example, for each subject with several extrinsic characteristics of interest (e.g., sex, age, body mass index, education, and health status) in the experimental group, the researcher must also match an individual with those same characteristics in the control group. As you can imagine, it can be difficult to recruit two people who are identical in all of the potentially relevant ways, and it becomes more difficult as the number of factors that we are trying to match increases. Additionally, we don't always know all of the factors posing a threat to a study's internal validity. It is more suitable in this case to assign subjects randomly to control and experimental groups. This means that each subject has an equal probability of inclusion in either group. As long as the groups are large enough, the rules of probability ensure that various extrinsic factors in a population are spread uniformly across the study groups.

In addition to the critical concern of internal validity, researchers are also concerned with the extent to which a study's findings (which are based on samples) can be applied to larger populations of interest in the real world. This is called generalizability (or *external validity*). Generalizability is particularly important because research ultimately aims to uncover associations that actually matter in the real world. The key to generalizability is sample representativeness and a *representative sample* is one that most closely reflects the population of interest in as many ways as possible. In short, such a sample accurately *represents*, in a smaller form, the larger population of subjects. Take for example the study above concerning the frequency of exercise on blood pressure. If the average age of a person with high blood pressure is 57, and you recruit a sample with an average age of 35, we will have difficulty saying for sure if exercise indeed lowers blood pressure in all patients with hypertension, or whether this effect is limited to younger people (those around 35 years of age). Here again, a *random sample* is likely to produce a representative sample, because according to the rules of probability it is most likely to look like the larger population with respect to the potentially related factors (such as age).

Our review of experimental design demonstrates that, by randomizing subjects into multiple control and experimental groups, the researcher may observe the effects of an independent variable on a selected dependent variable, because the groups under observation should be similar with the exception of the predictor variable of interest. Experiments therefore simplify statistical analysis in many respects because only the differences between the groups need to be assessed (see Figure 3.4 above). If the difference measured (e.g., decrease in blood pressure) in the experimental group is *significantly* larger than the difference in the control group, then a relationship has been identified. How much of a difference indicates a *significant* difference is a question that we tackle in the section below on research translation.

Clinical Trials

As noted above, experimental design is generally considered the "gold standard" of research designs, provided it is feasible and ethical to carry out. One of the most common biomedical applications of such designs is the randomized clinical trial, typically conducted in evaluating medical treatments. The randomized trial was developed by epidemiologists in the 1940s, but unfortunately was slow to catch on. In fact, some (Welch et al. 2011) claim that we still don't use it enough, despite the fact that it is the most reliable way to determine what works in clinical practice. Clinical trials typically go through four phases. Phase 1 studies are typically conducted on relatively small samples of healthy volunteers in order to assess safety, toxicity, and side effects, along with data on how the drug is metabolized and excreted. After toxicity in human populations is determined to be acceptably low, Phase 2 studies generate preliminary data on the drug's effectiveness using persons with the targeted disease or condition. If Phase 2 studies establish a high enough degree of effectiveness with respect to treating the targeted condition, a Phase 3 investigation follows, evaluating different drug dosages using comparatively larger samples from various populations. Phase 4 testing (sometimes called *postmarketing*) then follows after the drug is marketed, examining its effectiveness and rate of adverse events in the general patient population, and to further refine safety and dosage guidelines (fda.gov; Skovlund & Vatn 2007).

The influential hypertension studies by the Department of Veterans Affairs (VA) illustrate how the principles of experimental design manifest in clinical trials (see also Welch et al. 2011). Before the VA hypertension studies, paying close attention to controlling blood pressure was not standard clinical practice, despite our ability to measure it reliably. Even as late as the 1950s, some experts believed that high blood pressure was essential to support organs and somatic systems. So these studies represented groundbreaking efforts to uncover cardiac health risks (and ultimately treatments) well before patients developed more serious complications. In Chapter 7, we critically evaluate how the results of these trials have been *utilized* in some questionable ways, but they nonetheless demonstrate our focus here on the value of well-designed experimental research for improving patient care.

In short, the original VA study was a true experiment. Participants with what we consider today severe diastolic hypertension were randomly divided into two groups. The experimental group received treatment for hypertension (hydrochlorothiazide combined with either reserpine or hydralazine), while the control group received placebos (i.e., inert sugar pills). Just like the classic experimental design described above, members of the two groups were alike in as many ways as possible

TABLE 3.3 Outcomes in the VA Randomized Trial of Treatment for Severe Hypertension

Outcome	No Treatment (Control Group)	Treatment (Experimental Group)
Death	4	0
Stroke	4	1
Heart failure	4	0
Heart attack	2	0
Kidney failure	3	0
Eye hemorrhage	7	0
Hospitalized for hypertension	3	0
Treatment complication	0	1
Total	**27**	**2**

Source: Welch, H. Gilbert, Lisa Schwartz, & Steven Woloshin. (2011). *Overdiagnosed: Making People Sick in the Pursuit of Health.* Boston, MA: Beacon Press.

(avoiding or minimizing *systematic bias* through randomization), so that any differences after the study period could only be attributable to the drug therapy (i.e., the independent variable). The original VA trial was not very large by today's standards (about seventy per group) and it was not a very long follow-up period (about eighteen months as opposed to several years or even decades). But the results were nonetheless powerful; Table 3.3 shows a summary of bad health events observed during the study's follow-up period.

The difference in the control and experimental groups at the end of the study were stark—twenty-seven bad outcomes in the control group, with only two in the experimental group. If treatment made little or no difference in a study like this one, we would expect the bad events (twenty-nine of them) to be roughly evenly split between both study groups, according to probability. Another way to think about the odds of getting a 27/2 split of negative outcomes between these groups simply by chance (i.e., if the medication had no real effect) is to think about flipping a coin. What would you say if you flipped a fair coin twenty-nine times and observed "tails" twenty-seven times and "heads" only twice? The odds of this happening are much less than one in a million. We point this out because such an event (whether coin tosses or distributions of bad events) is not likely due to chance. Rather, within the logic of the randomized controlled clinical trial, we can infer that the differences in these observations are likely due to the treatment itself. When we appropriately control for potential confounding factors, and we see differences in our outcomes (e.g., the rates of bad events between control and experimental groups) that are so large that they are very unlikely due to chance, we can say with a high level of confidence that the treatment is *causing* the outcome. While experimental models involve conditions that help us determine causality in this way, the ability to make this claim is the goal of all research designs.

Other Research Designs

Researchers typically aim to observe the effects of an intervention in an experimental design of randomly assigned subjects in treatment and control groups, so that investigators can maximize internal validity according to the principles that we outlined above. Such an arrangement is desirable if it is both *feasible* and *ethical*. Key ethical considerations include that (1) all competing treatments under study are expected to benefit the participants or at least are harmless; (2) the best treatment is unknown; and (3) subjects consent to random assignment (these issues are elaborated in Chapter 11). For the research to be feasible, the researcher must be able to control the assignment and delivery of treatments. If these cannot be met, the researcher may choose to employ *observational methods*. In short, researchers use these methods when the objective is still to uncover explanations of some phenomenon, but when direct comparison, manipulation, and control are not all possible or ethical. As noted, differences in study outcomes sometimes can result from initial differences in the groups themselves. These pretreatment differences (also called *selection biases*) generally take two forms: *overt biases*, which have been identified and can be accurately measured, and *hidden biases*, which have not been identified and measured, but are suspected to exist (Rosenbaum 2005). These are central issues in any discussion of observational studies because they can compromise the validity and reliability of empirical research.

In this section we very briefly describe several categories of observational design in which researchers attempt to recreate some aspects of the classic experiment by using any number of analytical adjustments that simulate its conditions. Remember that all research designs have strengths and weaknesses. We first introduced the classic experiment, considered the gold standard, to help you discern how other designs differ in their attempts to maximize internal validity and attributions of causality (see Frankfort-Nachmias & Nachmias 2000; Privitera 2012). Because these methods are commonly used to generate evidence in health and medicine, it is important to understand the strengths and weaknesses of each.

Quasi-Experimental Methods

Using the classic experiment as a model, scientists have developed several *quasi-experimental designs*, which are often employed when randomization, manipulation, or comparison cannot be achieved. These designs are considerably weaker than experiments in terms of internal validity, particularly because researchers frequently use statistical manipulations as a method of control. Quasi-experimental designs often allow for the selection of random samples from a population, but they do not require or permit random assignment of participants to comparison groups. This is typically because the independent variables are *quasi-independent*, meaning that characteristics of the participants themselves, like *sex* (male/female) or *race* (white/non-white), serve to differentiate the groups or conditions under comparison, thereby preventing direct comparison among identical groups of subjects. In other words, we could not design a study and randomly assign the characteristics of male/female, or white/non-white; we would instead just use that attribute as a way to classify comparison groups. These designs are generally superior to cross-sectional or correlational methods (described below) because they usually involve studying more than one sample, and often over an extended time period. A study may also be called quasi-experimental if only one group is observed (i.e., no comparison group). Examples of these methods include *contrasted-groups*, *planned variation*, and *panel* and *time-series* designs. All seek to achieve, in some way, the model of logical validity established in the classic experiment. For example, a quasi-experimental approach to the VA hypertension design above might seek to examine treatment benefit among males and females in different test groups. The variable *sex* is a preexisting attribute (also called a *categoric group*) that makes random assignment or matching unfeasible. Or we might choose to use age or race as a variable to predict hypertension. These are preexisting attributes that would prevent use of randomization in the classic experimental design. Ascribed characteristics that are relevant to the study question—such as whether race is related to hypertension—can't be assigned to each subject (i.e., it cannot be manipulated as we might a treatment in the classic experiment).

Correlational and Cross-Sectional Methods

While methodologies that attempt to recreate the attributes of experimental design are arguably more common in the biomedical sciences, correlational and cross-sectional methods are often employed in the social sciences, particularly survey research. In these approaches, researchers typically ask questions of random samples of populations and then statistically analyze pairs or sets of scores for individuals within the sample(s). This method is suitable for detecting relationships between variables (i.e., covariation), but falls far short in establishing causality, primarily because these designs are essentially a snapshot of measurements at one point in time and cannot meet the criterion of time order. Therefore, in most cases researchers are attempting to simply describe a pattern of relationships between variables. No variables are manipulated to create and observe different conditions, and there are no groups to which subjects are randomly assigned, thereby making adequate control over competing explanations and assessment of directionality problematic. While these factors limit internal validity, these methods enable investigators to study situations where random assignment to control and experimental groups is not possible or ethical. For example, suppose we want to study the relationship between poverty and attitudes toward seeking health care. It would be unethical and impossible for us to select people randomly and induce poverty (the independent variable) in one group to determine how their attitudes toward health care changed over time as a result. In this case, we may instead collect a broad sample of people from various socioeconomic positions and measure both their socioeconomic status and their attitudes toward health care to determine if they covary at one point in time (note that if we collect data over time, we would categorize our study as *quasi-experimental*). While we cannot control for both overt and hidden biases as with randomization in the classic experimental design, we can specify statistical controls (variables we believe might interfere with the outcome), to begin to address nonspuriousness. Additionally, we can use various probability sampling strategies (collecting a sample that more closely resembles the larger population) to maximize the external validity (i.e., generalizability) of the results.

Preexperimental Methods

Preexperimental designs are unsuited to experimental manipulation and do not permit randomization. Most do not include a comparison group at all, participants are not selected from larger populations of interest, and data analysis is not substituted for experimental control. Therefore, these are the weakest type of design from the perspectives of internal and external validity. There is a very high degree of potential error in drawing conclusions based on preexperimental designs, and they are probably most useful for empirically evaluating early hypotheses for later use in more sophisticated and focused research. A common example is the *case study*, which involves observation of a single group or individual patient at a single point in time, often after some phenomenon or event that allegedly produced an effect. This group of designs can permit investigators to collect data when no other design can be employed, or to show that further research or lines of inquiry are warranted, but they are very weak on validity and do not permit any logical attribution of causality.

Qualitative Methods

Most of our discussion thus far (and below) focuses primarily on *quantitative*, rather than *qualitative*, analysis and methods. The former rely on the numerical measurement of observable phenomena and the subsequent statistical analysis of those data. The latter category is vast, and enables researchers to gather information about all sorts of social and cultural phenomena through dozens of different methodological tools and orientations. These include participant observation, focus groups, interviews, ethnographies, content analyses, among others. We spend greater time on quantitative discussions in this chapter because for a number of reasons these are more common in the biomedical sciences and health professions, and you are thus more likely to encounter them in your work. Moreover, quantitative experimental and quasi-experimental designs aim to illuminate cause-and-effect relationships. As such, they seek to inform health and medicine by suggesting changing some particular practice will have an outcome for patients. Qualitative methodologies typically aim to provide a rich description of a multidimensional phenomenon that is not so easily captured with standardized numerical measures (e.g., things such as cultural values or ways of thinking). Because a full treatment of these methods is beyond the scope of this chapter, we will provide two examples to illustrate the usefulness of qualitative approaches in health research.

Qualitative methods generate data on individual and group experiences, perceptions, thoughts, notions, actions, and/or feelings, and are principally concerned with uncovering how people interpret and experience the world around them. As you can imagine, such data are not easily quantified, or it may be pointless or meaningless to quantify them at all. For example, communication with patients is clearly a core function of health care practice. After all, much of the diagnostic and treatment process relies on information solicited from patients, and the successful management of their health relies heavily on communicating treatment plans clearly. Moreover, good communication is not strictly a function of momentary dialogue, but is built upon a foundation of rapport and trust. So clearly it is important to understand how particular groups of patients understand their health, bodies, and relationships with health care providers and institutions through the lens of their own experience, including their cultural and religious values. In order to comprehend such things, it is necessary to explore how people perceive, experience, evaluate, and interpret the world around them, because in the real world these phenomena most often guide behavior over and above abstract logic and rational decision-making. If we wish, for example, to understand end-of-life decision-making among member of a particular religious community, we may choose to use a qualitative approach. This is because quantifying something as dynamic and multidimensional as cultural and religious belief is not only challenging, the standardization required of doing so means we have to force something multifactorial like cultural values into a single scale that is equivalent across all subjects. It is not always helpful or useful to handle data in this way, and qualitative methods help us study phenomena without requiring us to do so. These aspects of understanding may be critical elements of research in areas like health lifestyles, interprofessional dynamics, patient–provider communication, illness experience, and other areas of health care delivery and policy.

As a second example, Grimen and Ingstad (2007) describe the study of smoking behavior. There is a well-established causal relationship between smoking and lung cancer. Yet many people continue to smoke and new people continually initiate smoking—behaviors that go against rational thought in the face of over-whelming research evidence. So there must be some other explanation or set of explanations that help explain this phenomenon. To make sense of the simplified (and standardized) observations required of quantitative work, we might seek to uncover the diverse perspectives and interpretations of the world among smokers (or nonsmokers, for that matter), or their values or identities—objectives for which qualitative methods are well suited.

All research designs have their specific strengths and weaknesses—a fact that you will discover as you explore the world of scientific inquiry—and it might be tempting to orient qualitative methods in opposition to quantitative approaches. We discourage this and instead (as noted in our discussion of the scientific method above) urge you to consider the various methods that fall beneath these broad classifications as tools in your research design toolbox—like a hammer or screwdriver—that are appropriate for some situations and inappropriate for others. Rather than focusing on a particular methodological approach, as many researchers do in their profes-sional lives, we encourage you to examine the research question, the different ways in which we can operationalize its components, what we gain and lose by doing so, and then pursue the best methodology to uncover what it is that you want to know.

Research Translation: From Findings to Practice

Now that we have briefly outlined the structure of a few common research designs, we can specify key ways that you can critically evaluate them particularly as you make sense of their utility in practice (or lack thereof). We leave more extended practical discussions of applied research to other resources (see, e.g., Greenhalgh 1997a–i, 2014; Reinar & Bradley 2007), but nonetheless offer some tools with which to critically assess the research that you come across in your work. In this section, we have organized the concepts above into a series of questions that you should consider when evaluating the quality of research.

Does the Study Add to Our Understanding?

Very few studies yield completely new and groundbreaking results, but most work adds some small, but novel, piece of information to a larger and more complex picture. Think of a jigsaw puzzle: each piece contributes in a very specific and important way, but is less meaningful in isolation. Moreover, when assembling a puzzle, we might choose to move any single piece or group of pieces around until we discern where it best fits (i.e., where the overall picture becomes clearest). A body of research works in much the same way. Still, even current studies should further past work in specific ways. For instance, a follow-up period for a new study might be longer in duration than previous studies; it might have a larger sample size, which may improve our confidence in the results or our ability to generalize the results; the methods may be more rigorous or appropriate; or the study population might be slightly different in a way that informs how a particular treatment might be used or avoided.

Who Is Being Studied?

At first glance, this question seems to deal with the samples or the larger study population, but there are additional important issues at hand. For example, it is important to examine how subjects were recruited, who was included (or excluded), and how participants were actually observed. These are common sources of bias. For instance, if research aims to assess patient satisfaction and recruits survey respondents from a print advertisement in a newspaper, the sampling methodology is likely biased toward those likely to read newspapers (and these people may be on average older, for example, since younger people are more likely use digital media). We might also hypothesize that former patients with higher levels of dissatisfaction might be more likely to respond to such advertisements.

Also consider the fact that many studies limit their samples to just men or women, veterans (as in the VA studies mentioned above), individuals with a specific condition (e.g., hypertension), or some specified degree of a condition (e.g., mild hypertension). So if a study suggests that treatment X appears effective in men with moderate to severe heart failure, then its findings may say little about patients with milder forms of the condition, or for women. This again speaks to the issue of generalizability. We commonly hear a recent groundbreaking study's findings reported in the media, but upon closer scrutiny we often discover that findings cannot be applied to the general population. Frakt (2015) notes that this is often one of the chief limitations of randomized trials, many of which focus on very narrow populations and exclude older patients or children due to ethical or safety concerns. This can pose real problems for generalizability, like clinical trials for drugs known as proton pump inhibitors (PPIs) conducted on *adults*, which prompted a sevenfold increase in prescriptions for these drugs between 1999 and 2004 (and a sixteenfold increase for one "child-friendly" liquid form of PPIs) to *infants* with gastroesophageal reflux disease. Later study of infants revealed that these drugs caused adverse events in this population, with no more benefit than a placebo administered in randomized clinical trials (Carroll 2014).

Finally, are subjects observed in experimental or real-life surroundings? Were they provided detailed expectations of a treatment's potential benefits or side effects? These factors and others can significantly impact the behavior of research subjects and how they report treatment effects. For example, telling them a medication might improve their energy levels may actually increase their energy levels psychosomatically or make them more sensitive to mild increases in energy such that they are more likely to report them. And while these considerations might not completely invalidate a study's findings, they at the very least complicate their interpretation and practitioners must evaluate them accordingly.

Is the Research Design Appropriate?

While many research methods textbooks can be quite complicated, a great deal of research evaluation comes down to critical thinking and common sense. Are the variables measured in a way that makes sense (i.e., are they *valid*?) and are they reproducible (i.e., are they *reliable*?). This is particularly important when it comes to principal variables of interest. Some variables are notoriously difficult to measure at all. Study authors themselves commonly overestimate the suitability of this or that measurement or design so it is useful to apply the design components discussed above (comparison, manipulation, control, and generalizability), as well as the criteria involved in the logic of causality (covariation, time order, and nonspuriousness) and internal validity in evaluating specific studies. In short, do measurements and overall design appear suitable to the research question at hand, and do conclusions logically follow from the way that data are collected and analyzed?

Is Systematic Bias Avoided or Minimized?

Systematic bias refers to anything that erroneously influences a study's conclusions and distorts comparisons. For instance, when they are used, comparison groups should be as similar to one another as possible except for the variable under observation and analysis. Groups should receive the same explanations, the same contact with the researchers or health professionals, and the same amount of time and number of observations. Researchers should address bias in different ways for different research designs. Even methods with a very strong reputation for internal validity and causality are fraught with potential bias, as Figure 3.5 shows below (Greenhalgh 1997b:306–07).

Blind assessment is one key way that bias can be minimized. Quite simply, reporting and observation can be affected by knowledge of the study groups' membership. A *single-blind* study refers to a situation where patients do not know whether they are members of the control or experimental/treatment group, while a *double-blind* study refers to where both researchers (i.e., those observing and recording measurements) and subjects are unaware of group membership. Having no knowledge of group assignment is another important way to minimize or eliminate bias. When researchers expect to find certain outcomes, particularly when there is a degree of subjectivity in coding the data (e.g., determining whether a patient's reported energy levels are highly elevated, moderately elevated, or mildly elevated), the bias that we all have as humans in concert with the researcher's expectation of a result can compromise data and, in turn, the conclusions.

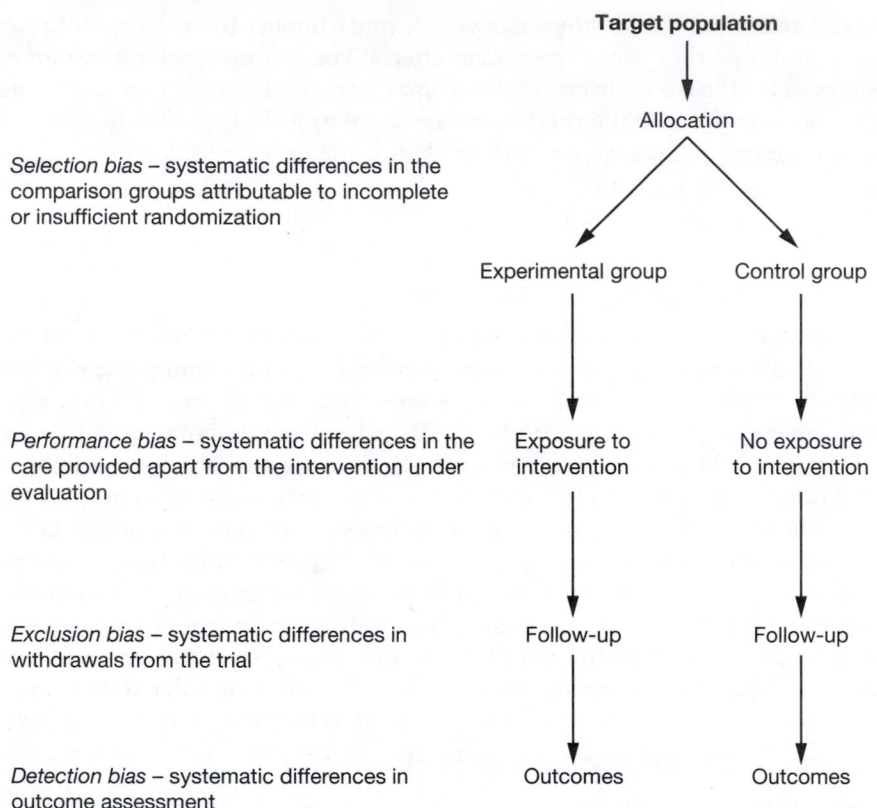

Selection bias – systematic differences in the comparison groups attributable to incomplete or insufficient randomization

Performance bias – systematic differences in the care provided apart from the intervention under evaluation

Exclusion bias – systematic differences in withdrawals from the trial

Detection bias – systematic differences in outcome assessment

FIG. 3.5 Sources of potential bias in a randomized controlled trial.

Source: Adapted from Greenhalgh, Trisha. (2014). *How to Read a Paper: The Basics of Evidence-Based Medicine.* Oxford: John Wiley & Sons.

Still other information that is important to assess involves the duration and completeness of follow-up during the study period. That is, a study must last long enough to detect anticipated changes in the dependent variable. A study period of two to seven days might be appropriate for assessing the effectiveness of a drug on postoperative pain, while many years or decades would be more appropriate for evaluating the long-term effects of vitamin or nutritional supplements administered during childhood or adolescence. Study periods were a key consideration in the VA hypertension analyses mentioned above, because over time, group differences became more pronounced with five- and ten-year follow-up periods. After five years the chance of a bad event was 80% for the control group and 8% for the treatment group. After ten years, 95% (control) versus 15% (treatment), and after fifteen years, 99% (control) versus 21% (treatment). There are also many reasons why subjects might drop out of (or withdraw from) a study, including adverse drug reactions, loss of motivation, comorbidities of clinical significance, moving out of the area, or even death. Our point here is that omitting all cases lost to follow up in analyzing data introduces bias into the research process, and tends to bias in the direction of the intervention or treatment under study. In the vast majority of cases, all data should be analyzed, and if/when it does take place, omission of *outliers* or withdrawals should be carefully and convincingly justified.

Statistical Considerations

We also need to consider the p-value (we use the letter p to symbolize the concept of *probability*) and the notion of *statistical significance*. In any inferential statistical test, computer programs will typically provide a p-value to accompany other sets of descriptive statistics, coefficients, group comparisons, and test values. It is the p-value, however, that is used to determine whether or not a finding is *statistically significant*. In technical terms, statistical significance means that the probability of getting the observed effect is less than a specified threshold of significance (also called *alpha*, α). *Alpha* corresponds to the amount of uncertainty that we are willing to tolerate in making a decision on statistical significance. The alpha value is set prior to analysis based on how much *confidence* we require of our results. Alpha values typically include the likely familiar thresholds of .05, .01, and .001, where *Level of Confidence (LOC)* = (1 − α). The decision of statistical significance revolves around comparing two values: the p-value (p) and *alpha* (α). If $p \leq \alpha$, then we say that the finding is statistically significant. For example, if we have a study finding where p = .02 and we have set α at .05, what this really means is that we have greater than 95% certainty that any observed effects are due to real effects in the population from which samples were drawn, rather than a product of random chance. If $p \leq .05$, we can be 95% confident in our results (where α = .05, and LOC = (1 − α), or (1 − .05) = .95, or 95%). Similarly, if $p \leq .01$, we can be 99% confident, and by the same logic, if $p \leq .001$, we can be 99.9% confident. If however, $p > \alpha$, then the result is not statistically significant, indicating that there is a sufficiently high probability that observed effects are due to random variation associated with sampling error—by *chance* alone. That is, if we set alpha (α) at .05, and $p > \alpha$, there is at least a 5% likelihood that random chance is the cause of any differences between the statistics we observe and what we would expect if there were no effects.

Notice that we used the term *likely* to indicate that our conclusions are probably what's actually happening in the population. The only way that we can be 100% sure of our conclusions, remember, is if we observe every single unit of the population under study, which we can rarely, if ever, do. But if we are not absolutely sure about conclusions, how do we know if our results are correct? The short answer: we don't. Uncertainty, as we noted above, is a ubiquitous element of applied research, and an awareness of this uncertainty and what it means is an integral part of the statistical imagination. In short, researchers carefully choose *alpha* (or *level of significance*) based upon how much error or uncertainty they are willing to tolerate in conclusions, and this decision is often guided by practical or clinical concerns (i.e., is 95% confidence good enough?).

Let's consider what a p-value symbolizes: it is *the probability (p) of the observed measurement differences occurring entirely by chance, if no relationship exists between variables under study.* Recall the VA hypertension study above where the observed difference following intervention was twenty-seven bad events in the control versus only two bad events in the treatment group. As we noted earlier, that's a large difference, even to the casual observer. But we can be even clearer and more precise about it. From a statistical standpoint, this difference is so large that it would correspond to a p-value somewhere around 7.56×10^{-7}, or .000000756. That is, there is only a .0000756% probability that we would observe such stark group differences by random chance alone. We would therefore conclude that those differences are likely due to real effects of the intervention itself, with 99.9% confidence (because $p < .001$). Understanding p-values and statistical significance in this way enables you to interpret all sorts of statistical findings, regardless of which tests are used.

A final consideration in evaluating research studies concerns the difference between statistical significance as we have just described, and practical significance. Sample sizes should be large enough to have a sufficiently high probability of detecting (as statistically significant) a sizable effect if one indeed exists. This allows us to be reasonably sure that no treatment benefit exists if it is not detected in the study (i.e., avoiding something called Type II error, which refers to failing to detect an effect when one actually exists, the statistical equivalent of a "false negative" – in contrast to a "false positive"). However, in selecting sample size, the researcher must also consider beforehand how much difference between the study groups would represent a *clinically significant* effect. This very well may be different from a *statistically significant* effect. If a new drug lowered experimental subjects' blood pressure by 10 mm Hg, the effect might easily represent a statistically significant ($p < .05$) reduction in the chances of stroke. However, if subjects exhibited symptoms of mild hypertension and reported few symptoms and no other risk factors for stroke, this effect could still be very small in reality, perhaps only preventing one stroke for every 850 patients treated (see Greenhalgh 2014). This statistically significant finding is not clinically significant precisely because the outcomes expected would not be worth patients taking the drugs in the first place (due to cost, side effects, hassle, etc.). Still, practitioners sometimes make treatment decisions based on statistical significance instead of clinical significance. This highlights the need to consider not just whether sample sizes are too small to generate confidence in the results, but also whether they are so large that their statistical significance is dramatically mismatched to their clinical significance. After all, results can be statistically significant even when the measured effect is very small if a very large sample size is analyzed. The result of confusing statistical and clinical significance with respect to the hypertension study described above is near-epidemic overdiagnosis and overtreatment of mild hypertension (see Welch et al. 2011; see Chapter 7).

Research Ethics

In Chapter 11, we discuss bioethics in general and the ethical requirements of human subjects research, in particular. It is important that research, just like clinical practice, meet key standards of morality, particularly where patients should be fully informed, give their consent for participation, and not be subject to undue risk. As the history of medical experimentation unfortunately demonstrates, many of these principles crystallized around ethical travesties in both research and clinical practice. However, because we later provide a more comprehensive treatment of bioethics, in this section we discuss the ethical obligations that researchers assume with regard to scientific integrity and fiduciary responsibility to the public, who depends on well-designed research and truthful reporting of results for the improvement of public health. Of course, researchers are expected, and in some cases required, to disclose potential conflicts of interest in the form of personal relationships, funding, income, investments, and any other situations that could call into question the objectivity of their results. Yet problems persist.

While it is likely that the vast majority of researchers do indeed disclose potential conflicts if they exist, even the appearance of potential bias or ethical compromise can be sufficient for some to call into question the conclusions of empirical research. We find a good example of this principle in the Goldacre (2012) work on health care research cited above. If there is no national or international registry within which all clinical trials are recorded, then there is at least the appearance that patients, practitioners, educators, and policymakers do not have uncompromised access to all results pertaining to a particular treatment or intervention. Add to this picture the fact that a majority of all biomedical research in the United States (see Dorsey et al. 2010) is funded by industry (i.e., pharmaceutical, biotechnology, and medical device firms), and we have significant potential for bias and conflicts of interest. This is not to say that all such research is unreliable; after all, someone has to fund that research, in addition to federal, state, and local governments, and private not-for-profits. Still, research is full of ethical quandaries that you should not only be able to recognize, but also spend some time thinking about as you assess its claims.

Another current example of potential ethical conflicts for researchers involves industry funding for research with the potential to shape public opinion as well as policymaking. Take, for example, the ongoing debate over the roles of caloric intake and exercise in obesity. O'Connor (2015) describes the large sums of money that Coca-Cola provides to influential researchers to advance the message that America's obesity crisis is due much *more* to the lack of adequate physical activity and much *less* about caloric intake. This message arguably is intended to direct consumer and policy attention away from sugary drinks and other sources of additional calorie consumption and their roles in obesity and type 2 diabetes. This also, and probably not by coincidence, comes at a time of increasing efforts to tax sugary drinks, remove them from schools, and stop companies from marketing directly to children. It's nothing new for the food and beverage industry to fund research (and this situation is not unique to just Coca-Cola). But if funded research consistently endorses a particular set of conclusions involving complex public health issues like this one, and especially when those conclusions are at odds with other valid research findings, some perceive these tactics as unethical. For instance, one recent analysis of beverage studies points out that research funded by Coca-Cola, PespiCo, the American Beverage Association, and the sugar industry were five times more likely to find no link between sugary drinks and weight gain, when compared to studies whose authors reported no financial conflicts, even when the best large randomized trials support a direct association between sugar-sweetened beverages and weight gain or obesity (Bes-Rastrollo et al. 2013). The point here is that in evaluating evidence for various claims, just as you need to be critical and even skeptical of confounding factors inherent to the research, one might be similarly critical and skeptical of external forces that can compromise the analysis of the data.

Conclusion: Evidence-Based Medicine and the Statistical Imagination

Evidence-based practice (or evidence-based health care) is a decision-making approach that seeks to synthesize research, practical circumstances, provider experience, and patient preferences. In other words, evidenced-based clinical expertise incorporates the wishes and circumstances of the patient along with the results of relevant research to generate optimal diagnostic and treatment decisions (Reinar & Bradley 2007). Only through combining the various dimensions above can practitioners effectively apply research-based knowledge in clinical practice, health care delivery, or policy making. Evidence-based practice requires critical appraisal of the evidence generated through the research process, implementing useful findings, and reflecting upon and evaluating that implementation.

We have outlined the various aspects of scientific inquiry up to this point in order to help you hone your abilities to critically evaluate information that you encounter. This means assessing causality and the logical, internal, and external validity of research, as well as evaluating the clinical relevance, quality, and applicability of conclusions emerging from that research. It is important to remember the distinction between statistical and clinical (or practical) significance in carrying out this process, and to carefully consider whether new knowledge can help you take better care of patients and/or to carry out your work more effectively and purposefully. Much of the ability to do this comes from experience, perhaps especially when it comes to the final step of evidence-based practice mentioned above—reflexivity. Reflexivity involves the continuous reflection and re-reflection upon your own critical appraisal and clinical decision-making processes and choices in a way that consciously facilitates your ability to become a better professional.

One particularly important way in which clinicians need to be reflexive about evidence concerns the interpretation of statistical results based on population-level groups. This is because applying such findings to any single individual could constitute a *reductionist fallacy*. Group (or *aggregate-level*) results apply to just that—the group (Wasserman and Hinote 2012). This is not to say that these have no relation to the individuals that make up the collective; it just means that within that group there is considerable variation (in statistical term it is called *error*) pertaining to each individual. The application of diagnostic criteria and laboratory findings is fraught with the potential for such reductionism. The example of hemoglobin A1C—a test that gives a three-month weighted average of glycated hemoglobin—illustrates these problematics, although we argue that many diagnostic thresholds are susceptible to this fallacy (see Welch et al. 2011 for discussion of various logical flaws in diagnostic and screening procedures). In particular, there is considerable variation in hemoglobin glycation based on race and age, such that interpreting the *clinical significance* of a patient's A1C levels requires not only determining where their values fall with respect to a general threshold, but also interpreting the data in light of various confounding factors and individual patient characteristics (Bloomgarden 2009). In short, instruments that employ summary statistical measures like averages should be cautiously applied to individuals because of common variations around social factors such as age, sex, race, and so on.

Being a good evidence-based practitioner requires an understanding of the core assumptions and features of applied research methodology and a flexible statistical imagination with which to evaluate research claims and findings. This involves the ability to think through complex practical and research scenarios, and a sound understanding of probability and the cyclical nature of scientific inquiry. Translating research to practice also means providing appropriate context to sometimes fragmented and often contradictory research findings. All of this represents a logical, common-sense approach intended to help you recognize both the strengths and limitations of empirical investigation and to determine what the large-scale tendencies of groups tell us about the particular afflictions of an individual patient. Simply put, being a good clinician requires a solid statistical (and sociological) imagination.

CHAPTER 3 ACTIVITY

Thinking Critically about Research

1. You are a researcher who wants to study how single mothers cope with stress. You decide to do an online survey. Describe the various ways that this research design might be problematic.

2. You are reading an online article and are directed to a peer-reviewed journal article on the relationship between height and professional achievement. The article found a strong association between being taller and making more money. The authors note that the mean height of individuals in the sample was 67.5 inches (5 ft. 7 in.) and did not collect data on any other variables. Discuss various potential confounding factors that could call into question these results.

3. A colleague approaches you about conducting a study on pain relief for low back pain following transcutaneous electrical nerve stimulation (TENS). The American Academy of Neurology (AAN) has said TENS is not effective for chronic back pain, but your colleague has used TENS in his physical therapy practice for years and says he has seen firsthand how it has been helpful as part of a therapy protocol involving a number of treatments. How would you design a study to examine whether your colleague is correct? (Think not only about

conditions for which to control, but also different ways to sample the population of patients, and the pros and cons of each approach).

4. One of your patients is extremely afraid of doctors. She told you that she read a "report" that claimed that the more doctors there were in a particular area, the higher the number of people who died in that same area. Using your statistical imagination, how might you respond to her concerns?

5. A study of 10 million people, half of whom are taking the (fictitious) drug Rendynizone and half that are not, shows that those on the drug have a BMI that is 0.7 kg/m^2 lower than those not on the drug, which is statistically significant ($p<.001$). Will this affect your prescribing habits as a practitioner? Why or why not?

6. You are a practitioner working in an intensive care unit in an area with a large population of Somali refugees, many of whom you frequently see as patients. You decide that you want to learn more about their cultural tendencies and values, how they tend to understand illness and view death and dying. Explain how would you design a research project to better understand these phenomena?

PART II

Social Epidemiology and Determinants of Health

CHAPTER 4

Social Class and Health

LEARNING OBJECTIVES

After reading this chapter, students should be able to

- Describe the important roles played by social determinants of health and disease in human populations, especially following the epidemiological transition.

- Define the concept of socioeconomic status (or social class) and articulate how it operates as a fundamental cause of health and/or disease.

- Describe how socioeconomic status and life chances shape the way we perceive and define the world around us, thereby shaping behavior.

- Discuss the association between socioeconomic status and health outcomes and the mechanisms that create the health–wealth gradient.

- Identify and discuss the various ways that neighborhood, community, and other place-based contexts shape behavior, and thereby health outcomes.

- Articulate the ways that social causation explanations compel us to rethink various elements of contemporary health care delivery.

The pervasive links between socioeconomic status (SES) and a range of health and disease outcomes will not come as any great surprise to most clinicians. After all, their experiences tend to illustrate that individuals and groups with more and better resources (e.g., money, education, etc.) tend to experience fewer severe disease episodes, fare better when they get sick, and are better able to adhere to professional advice. But beyond the relatively straightforward and rarely disputed insight that higher socioeconomic rankings are associated with a variety of good health outcomes, it is important to unravel precisely how good or bad health profiles emerge from these complex, multifaceted relationships. To do this, we need to delve deeper into the social determinants of health. More importantly, we must explore precisely what these insights mean for the work of clinicians and other professionals who not only routinely confront illness and disease, but are increasingly called on to promote health, which is a much more complicated prospect.

To be clear, unraveling social determinants of health, even in a cursory way, is difficult because factors such as social class, gender, race/ethnicity, and others are inextricably interconnected. Additionally, these mechanisms change over time and vary from group to group as populations and disease profiles continually shift and evolve in response to biomedical, environmental, and socioeconomic changes. Hence the rise of social epidemiology, a vast and complex field of study. Despite this complexity, issues surrounding the social determinants of health converge upon a handful of important insights pertinent to clinical work in the health professions. These ideas constitute Part II of this book because understanding the etiology and epidemiology of disease today is especially important to how health professionals organize and conduct their work. As we note in Chapter 2, this is particularly significant following recent epidemiological transitions that spawned many of the challenges we encounter today in clinical practice, health policy, education, and the like. These are challenges that we discuss in coming chapters. As a result, we will spend time in this chapter specifically highlighting the roles of socioeconomic factors. In Chapter 5 we will discuss the much larger matrix of health inequalities including race/ethnicity, gender, age, and culture, while in Chapter 6 we will examine the significance of health behavior and lifestyles.

In this chapter, we will first introduce the group of variables known as the social determinants of health before moving on to a more specific discussion of SES. Because SES and other related factors are such powerful and ubiquitous predictors of health and well-being, we will describe them as *fundamental social causes* of health and disease as we explore the role they play in shaping individual and population health profiles. As we will see, the effects of SES stretch well beyond an individual's social position or ability to afford health care; as a result, they span multiple levels of analysis and experience. These insights directly inform the work of health professionals, so we conclude by exploring their clinical implications to emphasize their significance for patient care over and above population health in the aggregate. In other words, we will begin to unpack exactly what the broad social patterns at the nexus of social class and health mean for health practitioners.

The Social Determinants of Health

In conceptualizing the social determinants of health, think for a moment about two questions. *First, if we could somehow cure all sick people in our society right now, would this solve the problem of poor health? Why or why not?* For the second question, imagine yourself on the banks of a river enjoying a picnic when, coming around a bend of the river, you see a person in obvious distress, struggling against the current. Possessed of empathy and compassion, with a touch of courage, self-sacrifice, and proficient swimming skills, you leap into the river and pull this person to safety. Now if you have ever pulled another person from a body of water, you will know that this is an exhausting task. Just as you are catching your breath, another person comes around that same bend in the river, struggling mightily against the current, and again you dive into the water and rescue the person. By now you are a hero and perhaps feel pretty good about your efforts. Then you look again to see three more people fighting for their lives coming down that river. Even though you want to, you are doubtful that you will be able to save all three. This brings us to our *second* question: *What do you do in this situation?*

The first question is one posed by social epidemiologist Leonard Syme to illustrate the basic insight that public health concerns more than curing disease. Even if we could "fix" everyone suffering from disease or poor health *at any given time*, countless individuals and groups would manifest the very same disease states that we cured, precisely because factors external to the individual actually cause disease in the first place. Put another way, there are factors that create circumstances and conditions in which we are statistically more likely to become ill and perhaps even die prematurely. Why? Because health and disease are inextricably intertwined with factors beyond us as individuals, and if those go unaddressed, they will continuously push at-risk individuals into the ranks of the sick and disabled (see Adelman 2008; Hinote 2014b). But let's consider the second question and scenario. Many might be willing to heroically dive back into that river with knowledge that they cannot save everyone, and just do the best that they can. They might even be willing to sacrifice themselves to save as many people as possible. This is certainly laudable, well intentioned, and can produce a good result, at least for some people. But it might be wise and potentially more effective to travel upstream to see why so many people are falling into that river in the first place (see also Weiss & Lonnquist 2015).

Both scenarios metaphorically illustrate important ways to begin to think about the social determinants of health and disease. The first highlights that social factors and institutional arrangements, coupled with the ways that we relate to these influences and how they shape our thoughts and behavior, always impinge upon us in ways that have great potential to promote good or bad life outcomes, including good or bad health. Put simply, we can keep curing sick individuals, but more sick individuals will inevitably come behind them, leaving the underlying social causes of disease unaffected. Acknowledging this reality brings the implications of our second scenario into better focus. Those in the river represent the sick and the suffering. Clinicians and practitioners can rescue some, but not all, of those people. If, however, we more closely consider the broader social and cultural influences from which these people emerge, the social influences that create sickness and suffering in the first place (i.e., the *upstream* factors), perhaps we can think more deeply and critically about our approaches to disease. Within the context of the social determinants of health, we assert that contemplating and understanding these broader influences will deepen your understanding of patients' experiences, the character of their illnesses, and engender a more humanistic kind of care that takes account of not just how disease presents in the clinic, but how it is nested in larger, influential social arrangements. Doing so will facilitate your recognition of at-risk patients and allow you to intervene before problems arise, or to consider treatment recommendations that take account of the various challenges faced by patients in their social environments. After all, once patients leave the clinic, where do they go? Most return to the social contexts in which they face all of the various dimensions of life that very well could have brought them to the clinic in the first place.

The term *social determinants of health* refers to conditions into which we are born, and in which we grow, work, live, and age, along with the wider set of forces and systems that shape the conditions of everyday life and thereby, health (see CSDH 2008; who.org). This definition is noticeably broad and encompasses more examples than we can include here. But it also seems to describe two important and interconnected domains—*social conditions* and *social forces*—that link individuals together into the environments, communities, collectivities, and societies in which they live (recall the reflexive model of social reality from Chapter 1). While these influences are increasingly popular in research and policy discussions, knowledge of these factors has existed for centuries, even since ancient times. Most experts widely recognize the roles that social factors like poverty, stress, unhealthy environments, and poor lifestyles play in making people sick. However, many frame these health-related social forces as secondary in importance to actual pathogenic (i.e., disease-promoting) mechanisms. That is, while nearly all agree that social factors exercise a great deal of influence in constraining or enabling health (Cockerham 2005), the majority of attention, both research and clinical, continues to focus somewhat narrowly on the physiological factors involved in disease. In fact, there was relatively little research on the *social causation of health and illness* (discussed below) until very recently.

Few would dispute that those occupying positions toward the bottom of social hierarchies (e.g., those who are poorer, for example) tend to exhibit greater morbidity and mortality than those occupying positions toward the top of those hierarchies. As we will see, distributions of disease are much more subtly complex than this. The first error that many people make is in thinking about socioeconomic disadvantage as only a secondary (distal) factor that exposes individuals to other primary (proximal) influences that eventually make them sick. For example, one might posit that poverty leads to stress, which leads to poor diet and lack of exercise, and ultimately results in diabetes. This view emphasizes diabetes not as a direct result of poverty per se, but of those more proximal health behaviors. Similarly, one might assert that socioeconomic disadvantage leads to lack of health care coverage, which prevents early detection of chronic disease or immediate treatment for other conditions, which leads to poorer health status and potentially premature mortality. These are plausible models of how social factors shape disease. But the simple, linear way in which disease causation is portrayed in them makes it easy to disregard the causal role of social factors, especially when it appears that those more proximal factors (i.e., exercise habits) fully explain the emergence of disease. Put another way, it is equally plausible to argue that the *true* cause is farther back in the causal chain—upstream, as opposed to downstream, factors. The reality is that many factors and probabilities coalesce to cause disease, and each is therefore important for clinicians to understand and consider.

The contours of disease in advanced industrial nations today are so strongly affected by social factors and conditions that without these elements, diseases may not develop at all. These social determinants are not like biological pathogens, but overlooking or minimizing their critical roles in pathogenesis disregards an integral element of how specific diseases emerge and persist in particular populations, whereas those same illnesses might scarcely affect other groups. The hypothetical examples above illustrate this point: if a social determinant yields exposure, then it can be considered causal. And the available epidemiological data support this conclusion as well. Figures 4.1 and 4.2 depict respondent-reported prevalence data for heart disease and stroke in the United States (two of the top three causes of mortality in the United States) over the past two decades. On the horizontal axis you will see clusters of time period data corresponding to population groups organized by the percentage of the federal poverty level (FPL). The percentage of American adults

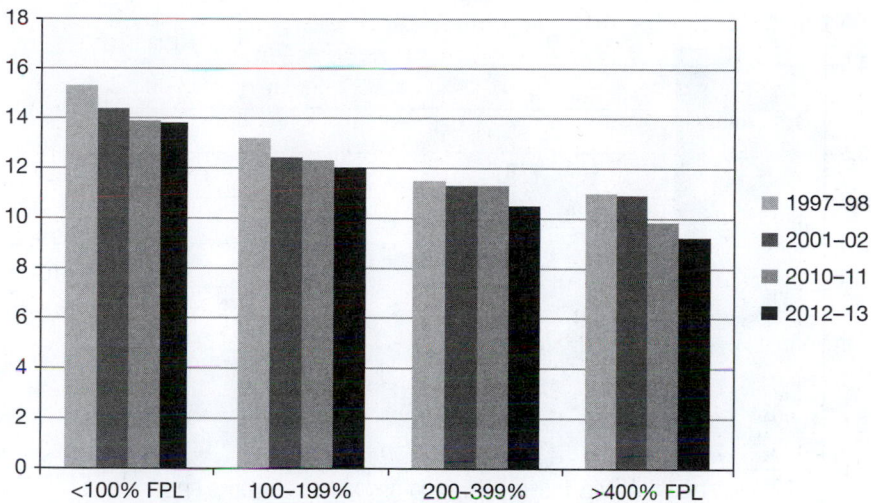

FIG. 4.1 Respondent-reported prevalence of heart disease among adults aged 18 and over, United States, 1997–98 through 2012–13.

Source: Data adapted from National Center for Health Statistics (NCHS). (2015). *Health, United States, 2014: With Special Feature on Adults Aged 55-64.* Hyattsville, MD: U.S. Department of Health & Human Services, Centers for Disease Control & Prevention.

(age 18 and over) is plotted on the vertical axis. There are distinct patterns that you will immediately recognize in these graphs. Here, we will focus on the prevalence of these conditions *among* the socioeconomic groups depicted (i.e., the four clusters of data), and then the change in prevalence over time *within* each cluster.

Both conditions are more prevalent in the lowest socioeconomic stratum reported (<100% FPL). For example, this subgroup exhibits more than twice the percentage of stroke when compared to the highest socioeconomic category (Fig. 4.2). Across both conditions, the prevalence tends to trend downward as we ascend the socio-economic hierarchy. The changes within each cluster across these time periods also reveal valuable information. For heart disease, we see generally declining prevalence for all subgroups, but declines were greater for the >400% FPL subgroup when compared with all others, especially the lowest subgroups. Stroke is a different story. Rate of stroke actually *increased* in prevalence over time among the three lower SES groups, while again, the highest exhibited declines. Remember from Chapter 3 that when we as researchers see relatively clear and obvious data patterns, we predict that there is something that is likely shaping those patterns; that is, they are not random. We can similarly say with relative certainty (with vast research) that underlying influ-ences are shaping these data, because there is an infinitesimally small chance that such an obvious trend would appear by random chance (especially in these very large samples and across multiple conditions, only two of which are depicted here).

In light of the data in Figures 4.1 and 4.2, we might explore whether or not there is something about membership in one of these socioeconomic categories that puts people at higher risk for cardiovascular disease or stroke. We know that the leading modifiable risk factors for heart disease and stroke include hypertension, high cholesterol, cigarette smoking, diabetes, poor diet, physical inactivity, overweight,

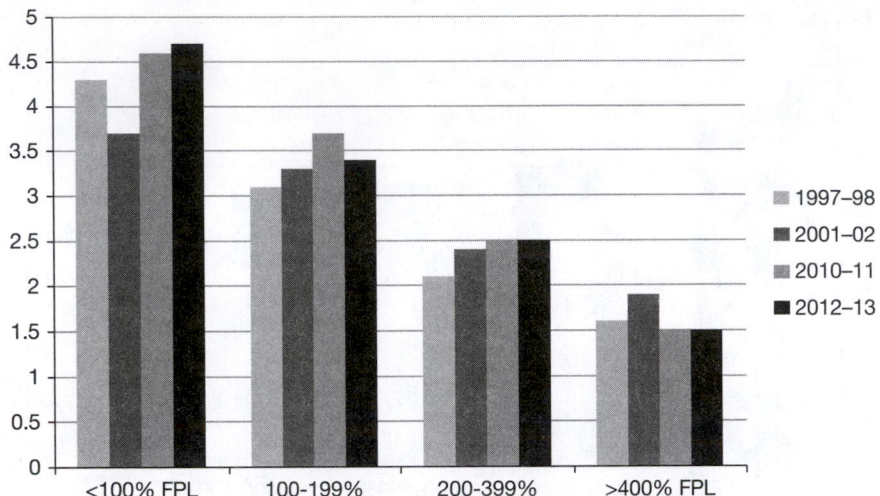

FIG. 4.2 Respondent-reported prevalence of stroke among adults aged 18 and over, United States, 1997–98 through 2012–13.

Source: Data adapted from National Center for Health Statistics (NCHS). (2015). *Health, United States, 2014: With Special Feature on Adults Aged 55-64.* Hyattsville, MD: U.S. Department of Health & Human Services, Centers for Disease Control & Prevention.

and obesity (Lloyd-Jones et al. 2010). So in investigating the shape of the data, our question might now be: Are these risk factors, and the ability to successfully modify them, somehow directly related to socioeconomic factors? If a higher prevalence of these modifiable risk factors can be demonstrated empirically, then we could argue for an important causal role for SES in the prevalence of heart disease and/or stroke. In the next sections of this chapter, we will begin to unravel the underlying mechanisms involved in these associations. Doing so can become quite a complex and burdensome task, because the etiologies of the most common diseases (especially chronic diseases, but others as well) are very complex, especially when compared to infectious diseases or injury, which were the leading causes of mortality in earlier historical periods (see Chapter 2). We now find ourselves at a point in history where biomedicine, coupled with tremendous advances in technology, has created the capacity for humans to avoid diseases and premature mortality, and all of this makes social influences and conditions dramatically more important in matters of both individual and population health (Link 2008), as well as health care delivery and clinical practice (Wasserman & Hinote 2012).

Socioeconomic Status

SES, also sometimes called *social class*, is one of the most important and powerful influences among the class of factors called the social determinants of health. This is because SES not only is an influential element of our lives, but is also so closely associated with many other important causal factors. Beyond the confines of health and medicine, SES shapes how we see ourselves and the world around us in all sorts of ways. It thereby exerts a strong influence on human behavior generally. First, however, we must understand how to define the concept. Empirically, researchers from multiple disciplines measure SES by using one or more assessments of income, education, occupational prestige, and wealth. Importantly, this is a largely sociological operationalization that reflects an individual's or group's ranked position in a particular social hierarchy. But if SES were only a position in a hierarchy, its effects would not be nearly so pervasive across so many domains of life and health. In reality, SES is also very closely associated with the variety of opportunities to which an individual may or may not have access—a concept called *life chances* that will be key to understanding the social epidemiology of health and disease, and to which we will return in Chapters 5 and 6 (Dahrendorf 1979; Weber [1922] 1978).

The term *life chances* essentially refers to the probabilities of finding the good things in life. In short, those in more privileged positions enjoy more favorable life chances, while those living in less advantaged circumstances enjoy less favorable life chances. This might seem to go against the American ethos of individualism and meritocracy, but data clearly demonstrate that those born at or nearer the top of American society, for example, possess greater odds of success than those born nearer the bottom. This is why the structures and hierarchies of society tend to remain relatively stable over time and across generations. McNamee and Miller (2013), for example, use the metaphor of a relay race to describe the pursuit of success in the United States. Largely due to the resources ascribed to us by virtue of being born into a particular class, some of us begin at the starting line, while others start one-quarter, one-half, or three-fifths of the way around the track, much closer to the finish line. This doesn't mean that people born into disadvantage don't or can't have success. It does mean that they typically must work harder to overcome more obstacles to achieve success compared to those who start with greater and more accessible socioeconomic resources. Moreover, in a relay race, each runner hands a baton off to another runner and they complete the race as a team. In the example above, the runners who are positioned closer to the starting line pass that advantage on to the next runner. Thinking about social class from an intergenerational standpoint, the advantages enjoyed by one generation are passed on, and they accumulate over time. This is a good way to think about how life chances work not only generally, but also when it comes to health. In short, those with less favorable life chances must overcome many more barriers to good health.

Dahrendorf (1979:73) describes life chances as the "probability of finding satisfaction for interests, wants and needs," along with the chances of good events taking place to help bring about that satisfaction. In fact, we can think about society as a broad, layered (or stratified) structure of social groups, organized from top to bottom with varying compositions of life chances. When it comes to health outcomes, then, the higher the status of a particular socioeconomic bracket, the better their life chances, and the greater the probability of enjoying more health-promoting (and less disease-promoting) aspects of life. On the other hand, in relatively lower strata, probabilities are flipped. Applying the analogy of the relay race above to Dahrendorf's (1979) probabilistic definition of life chances, this means that over time, those with more resources will, as a group, accrue more successes than those with fewer resources. That is, those with a head start on the racetrack will tend to win the race a disproportionately high number of times (though perhaps not always).

It is important to remember that SES as a social factor, from the perspective of any one individual, *shapes* or *influences*, rather than *determines*, our health outcomes. But SES is a social *determinant* of health where it determines the shape and contours of health through the simple accrual of probabilities among various groups. That is, while individuals may vary widely, even within socioeconomic brackets, the laws of probability tell us that, over time and with large enough numbers, the comparatively limited chances for health (e.g., to purchase healthy food, live in healthy neighborhoods, to receive preventative care, etc.) among low-SES groups will manifest in predictably worse health for those groups in the long run. This is not to lose sight of the role of individual choice in all of these processes (discussed further in Chapter 6), but from a broad socioeconomic perspective, SES is firmly connected to life chances and the material and nonmaterial resources that can either facilitate or impede good health (Hinote 2014a).

So far it might seem that we are referring to SES and related processes as a set of mysterious *external* forces swirling around us that shape our lives, experiences, and choices, but SES also profoundly affects processes that are *internal* to the individual. The socioeconomic conditions around us affect the ways that we perceive and react to the world. They influence our behaviors and responses to particular situations or life events and even how our bodies respond physiologically to external stimuli. One of the most important mechanisms responsible for this is called *socialization*, or the process through which individuals learn the norms, roles, structures, and ideologies of the social group(s) to which they belong, from their family groups all the way up to the levels of culture and society. These processes first take place within the family, who is responsible for transforming us from helpless infant into a (hopefully) functioning adult and productive member of society, and continues into other settings like school, church, sports, work, and so on. (i.e., virtually every other social institution in which we participate). We will talk about these important processes in greater detail in Chapter 6, but just as we learn what is appropriate behavior for a mommy or daddy, boy or girl, doctor or nurse, we also learn group-approved behavior in many other situations. The social class circumstances in which we are raised are no different. We are socialized within specific socioeconomic contexts, and the attendant behaviors, dispositions, beliefs, and values attached to those influences become part of the way that we see and interpret the world (Bourdieu 1984; Cockerham 2013; Mead 1934).

Social class influences within socialization processes unfold in a number of ways. They show up in broad social structures and institutions, face-to-face interactions, and the ways that we perceive the world around us. Fiske and Markus summarize the extensive research emerging from various disciplines to note that, "social class shapes social interactions in every domain of life," reporting:

> that doctors, middle class by virtue of their occupation, prescribe simpler treatment regimes for their working-class than for their middle-class patients; that middle-class jurors tend to be more assertive than jurors from the working class; that working-class parents are more likely than their middle-class counterparts to defer to teachers' views of their children; that, relative to middle-class adults, working-class adults are more attuned to the emotions of others and relatively more concerned with helping and giving back to their communities; that working-class or

first-generation college students can be disadvantaged by the university focus on self-expression and choice; and that middle- and working-class Americans together perpetuate a broad and deep stereotype of middle-class competence. (2012:1)

Importantly, social class represents a powerful influence on not just how we are ranked in large groups, but also how we develop a sense of self-identity. It turns out that, whether we are aware of it or not, we are constantly aware of our ranking in a social group. Fiske and Markus go on to note the psychological implications of these processes, where:

those with higher rank have a sense of themselves as independent from others and as influencing and controlling social interactions. Those with a lower rank experience themselves as relatively interdependent with others and as adjusting and deferring to others in interaction. The self in a high-status position is likely to focus on expressing and promoting one's own interests, choices, and goals. The self in a lower-status position is more likely to be relatively socially responsive and to focus on avoiding threat or harm and tuning into others' goals, emotions, and needs. (2012:2)

Despite the evident power of SES, discussion has been scant in the United States, especially when compared with other advanced industrial countries. For example, social class is far less institutionalized in the United States than, say, gender or race/ethnicity. Statistical agencies commonly collect and publish data comparing men with women, African Americans with whites, and Hispanics with non-Hispanics. And though the U.S. Census Bureau publishes data by educational attainment or income, it never specifically categorizes data by social class or SES (DiMaggio 2012). This seems somewhat odd, especially when public health agencies in several European nations routinely collect and report data comparisons including social class and SES, generally ranking individuals and groups according to occupational hierarchies reflecting meaningful differences in social standing. In the United Kingdom and France, for example, such data have been available for nearly a century. At least five socioeconomic groups are regularly reported in the United Kingdom, while other nations report as many as six or more such categories. Indeed, these data are invaluable public health tools, precisely because SES group membership is so tightly correlated with health outcomes and epidemiological trends. On the other hand, data on health differences across socioeconomic groups, especially analyses that go beyond relatively simple differences based on education and income, are less common in the United States (Braveman et al. 2010). Still, measurement and data limitations have not prevented American scholars from studying these important differences.

Even though these classifications are not typically tracked in the United States as they are in other nations, the effects of social class are just as pervasive. In fact, inequality and stratification on the basis of SES in the United States is much larger than most Americans think (Kiatpongsan & Norton 2014; Norton & Ariely 2011), and is among the highest in the industrialized world (see Murtin & d'Ercole 2015; Organisation for Economic Co-operation & Development 2014). In the United States, just as in other countries, the association between SES and health is so strong that it forms a gradient, meaning that not only are there differences between highly disparate groups (e.g., upper and lower classes), but there are significant differences between proximal groups as well (e.g., upper and upper-middle class). The higher in the hierarchy, the better the health of the individuals comprising that socioeconomic group. The group at the top of the hierarchy tends to exhibit the best health and greatest longevity, while the group immediately below the top is slightly worse, and on and on down the social ladder. This is a pattern first uncovered in the Whitehall studies performed several decades ago in the United Kingdom. But when researchers began looking for similar patterns in the United States, they showed up for virtually every condition as well as overall mortality and within many different groups. While other social determinants of health (see Chapter 5) demonstrate less consistent patterns with respect to shaping health and mortality, the effects of SES are incredibly robust and pervasive. In fact, along with strong associations with virtually all health outcomes, social class meets other criteria (discussed in Chapter 3) to substantiate an even stronger claim: Social class is not only *correlated* with health outcomes, but it is a fundamental *cause* of health and disease as well.

Social Class as a Fundamental Cause of Health and Disease

As we have described, the rise of increasingly complex diseases following the epidemiological transition compelled many to reconsider the individualist (or *reductionist*) approaches to health and disease causation. The parameters characteristic of purely biomedical approaches to health and disease, which tend to focus more narrowly on germs infecting tissues, thereby expanded to include physical and social environments. Put another way, treating disease by focusing only on the individual (e.g., their individual choices, genetic makeup, etc.) becomes less and less effective when the conditions most likely to make us sick emerge from the seemingly infinite number of micro-decisions that we make over the life course, all of which are constrained or enabled by our life chances. For example, people don't "catch" diabetes or heart disease like they might with the common cold. Rather, these conditions emerge over relatively long periods of time as we live out our lives within social environments that strongly influence our behaviors (including our health behaviors). The ascendency of chronic illness as the most significant mortality threats in developed countries compels us to critically reexamine the traditional risk factors for disease, the ways that we treat it, and the groups who tend to be affected to a greater or lesser degree. The origins of disease are so closely tied to the social influences and conditions surrounding the individual patient that they complicate and sometimes confound the typical diagnostic and treatment paradigms of modernity (i.e., the cause-and-effect assumptions that characterized infectious disease etiology). Today, many scholars explain the variety of causal processes involved in a way that can help clinicians and policymakers develop better methods with which to approach patient care and public health. The fundamental cause explanation is particularly influential and informative for clinicians on the front lines of treating diseases that emerge from complex social environments (e.g., Link 2008; Link & Phelan 1995, 2000; Phelan et al. 2004).

There are two key things to consider as we move beyond a more traditional focus on disease causation. First, the more proximal, individual risk factors for disease (e.g., diet, exercise, etc.) are poorly understood unless we properly contextualize them within larger sets of social conditions. In other words, we must look to the social conditions that put people *at risk* for those more proximal risk factors. Second, some social conditions (like SES) are likely fundamental causes of disease themselves, because they embody access to important resources, affect multiple diseases through multiple mechanisms, and maintain an association with disease even when intervening variables/mechanisms (i.e., risk and protective profiles) change over time. More specifically, there are four criteria needed to say that social factors *cause* disease. A fundamental social cause must (1) influence multiple diseases; (2) affect disease through multiple risk pathways; (3) be reproduced over time; and (4) involve access to resources that can facilitate avoiding risk, embracing protection, or minimizing the consequences of disease if it appears (see Link & Phelan 1995, 2000; Phelan et al. 2004). Thinking about the social causes helps us to better focus on those upstream factors that shape health, why they are important, and how the insights gleaned from this line of research can inform the work of clinical health professionals (Cockerham 2013).

While the particular mechanisms involved may change over time, the association between SES and health has existed for centuries. Its validity extends to multiple diseases through multiple pathways, and involves resources that permit individuals to navigate risks and protection. As a result, SES is considered a fundamental cause of disease. This is important because, *SES embodies resources that permit some individuals (and deny others) the ability to successfully navigate risk and protective factors in a way that health threats can be minimized or avoided altogether.* In other words, nearly all known health-promoting (i.e., salutogenic) or disease-promoting (i.e., pathogenic) social factors are associated with SES, so that those with higher SES have a higher likelihood of embracing the protective effects and simultaneously avoiding the risks associated with those very same factors or conditions. Regardless of the health threats facing the population as a whole, higher-SES groups and individuals are most likely to have and utilize resources that can protect their health (Glymour et al. 2014).

There are so many pathways in the association between SES and health that it is impossible for us to list all of them here. In fact, existing research probably has not yet uncovered all of them, but the most important to date probably include neighborhood advantage, living and working conditions, health lifestyles, stress, social support, sense of control, and self-efficacy (see Fig. 4.3). Figure 4.3 shows a basic model whereby SES corresponds to a variety of specific conditions that can be advantageous or disadvantageous for any number of resulting health outcomes. Examine the relationships between SES and health that runs through neighborhood advantage, for example. SES affects what kinds and qualities of neighborhoods one can afford to live in. Those in higher-SES groups can afford to live in environments free of hazardous chemicals, mold, and other health risks, and in neighborhoods that promote health and well-being. This includes areas with safe parks, well-maintained playgrounds, and other areas encouraging leisure-time exercise, in addition to places to purchase fresh fruits and vegetables. Neighborhood advantage also extends to the positive relationships and other social connections, like the quality of interaction with neighbors, visitors, or law enforcement. Living in a desirable, high-resource, aesthetically pleasing area is also positive for self-esteem and sense of security,

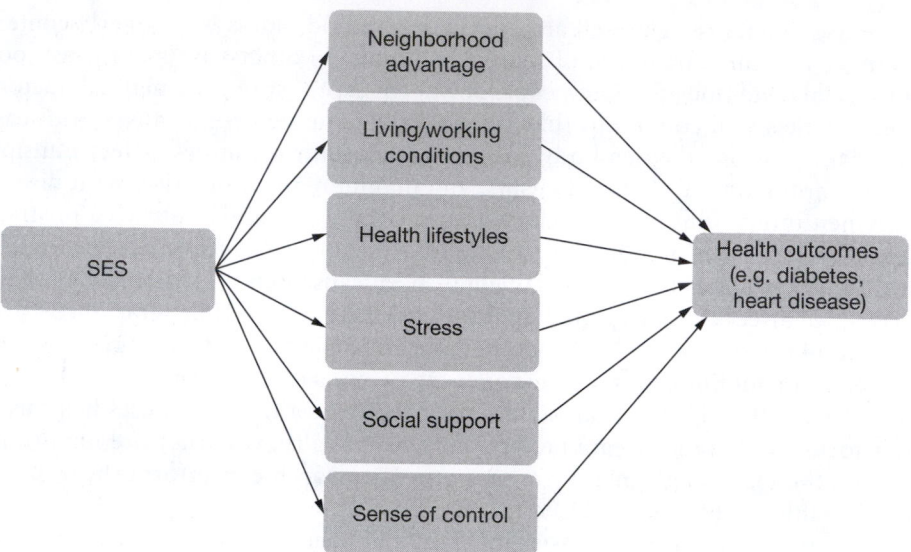

FIG. 4.3 Basic model of SES as social cause of disease through multiple pathways.

and these same neighborhood conditions tend to attract business and capital that fills tax coffers and supports local merchants that contribute to the area. All of these neighborhood advantages are a function of SES and all of them affect health because they increase the likelihood of healthy diet, exercise, exposure to clean air, and a range of other individual health-related factors.

Another major SES-related factor concerns stress. While no one is free from the stress of social life, SES position is also associated with how much stress we encounter, how continuous or intermittent it might be, and the manner that we respond to stressful stimuli, both behaviorally and physiologically. Chronic stress may influence us to engage in sets of behaviors that might be good (e.g., exercise, meditation, etc.) or bad (e.g., alcohol/drug use, risk taking, etc.) for our health. Or chronic stressful conditions stemming from disadvantage can cause physiological responses where, for example, an individual's endocrine system produces sustained, elevated levels of cortisol. This can affect metabolism, the immune response, and promote serious long-term physiological effects like heart disease (see Whitworth et al. 2005). Cognitive orientations like having sense of control over one's life (also conceptualized as internal locus of control, or self-mastery), as opposed to a sense of fatalism (external locus of control, or powerlessness), are strongly associated with SES and play critical roles in how we manage stress and distress (see Fig. 4.3). Social support and positive relationship networks offer even more protection when it comes to stress, and are similarly associated with SES (see discussion of the stress process model in Chapter 8).

Across the life course, SES and the resources emanating from it can affect brain development, dietary and nutrition preferences, intelligence, self-efficacy, and other outcomes associated with physical, emotional, psychological, and social development and well-being. The effects of disadvantage may even be observed in utero, and related to premature birth and low birth weight (see Margerison-Zilko et al. 2015), or physiologically, where conditions of disadvantage might even cause our bodies to age more rapidly at the chromosomal level (see Needham et al. 2013). The fundamental cause explanation illustrates how social conditions like SES help us avoid or minimize risk to our health, thus leading to more positive health outcomes, lower morbidity, greater longevity, better survivability following disease onset, and greater quality of life across the life course. Without understanding the larger context of disease causation, it is difficult to make sense of why certain groups have disproportionately high rates of diseases such as heart disease, diabetes, and the like. In short, individual risk factors (i.e., individual behavior and genetics) alone are insufficient in explaining these strikingly stable patterns, while social factors are better able to explain population-level epidemiological trends and give us new insights about the origins of disease. Most importantly for clinical practitioners, the social determinants of health begin to illuminate how we might intervene within these processes, along with how we might reconceptualize the methods through which we deliver health care, and the ways that we interact, assess, and advise patients. In the next section we further elaborate on neighborhood disadvantage (as only one example illustrating the nature of fundamental social causes), but shift our focus toward ways in which clinical practitioners can utilize this knowledge to improve patient care.

Neighborhood Disadvantage and the Role of Clinical Practice

The places in which we live and work produce some of the strongest and most important SES-related effects on health and well-being. In the preceding section, we briefly discussed how neighborhood advantages or disadvantages affect health. Neighborhoods are sources of exposure to healthy or unhealthy environments, and SES drives the ability to live in areas with more of the former and less of the latter. Moreover, people are socialized within neighborhood environments (among other contexts) such that they internalize the health habits and patterns to which they are exposed. In this section, we introduce a more detailed framework to help you visualize the various ways that place-based effects on health manifest over time, in particular populations, and in specific locales. We believe that this approach is useful to think about the health effects of place and neighborhood and to help us visualize the ways that environments can shape or even delimit individual choices and behaviors. In turn, these can inform clinical practice in multiple ways as well. Macintyre and colleagues (2002:131) describe five features of local areas that influence health in positive or negative ways:

1. *Physical Features.* These include characteristics shared by all residents in a specific area, including air and water quality, pollution, and the general character and appearance of the community or neighborhood. Research demonstrates that lower-SES neighborhoods are more likely to be in close proximity to pollutants, highways, airports, or waste disposal facilities (Fitzpatrick & LaGory 2013). Individuals with higher SES can afford to avoid the inconveniences of living near these types of facilities (noise, heavy equipment traffic, etc.). But this also represents a health advantage, where they simultaneously avoid the physical health threats of these areas.

2. *Availability of Healthy Environments at Home, Work, and Play.* These attributes don't affect everyone living or working in an area in the same way that

broad, physical features do, but nonetheless represent phenomena that tend to cluster around neighborhoods in which we live and work, and thereby affect health. These include things like safe housing, steady employment, and nonhazardous work conditions, whose relationship to health is fairly obvious, but also very consequential. For example, children from low-SES families also tend to live in older housing structures, which are also more susceptible to leaks and resulting mold. As a result, these children are more likely to develop asthma and its more severe forms (Chen et al. 2006). Other key elements of healthy environments include safe areas for children to play, and for everyone to engage in leisure-time physical activity. These also confer significant health advantages.

3. *Services Provided to Support People in Daily Life.* These resources include quality schools and other educational opportunities, street cleaning and lighting, public transportation, waste removal, policing, and health and welfare services. These various features affect community life in a variety of ways related to health. The physical condition of streets and sidewalks, for example, is associated with outdoor physical activity in neighborhoods, which, of course, has a variety of positive physical and mental health outcomes, including risk of obesity (Lovasi et al. 2009). When municipalities maintain neighborhood infrastructures, it has positive effects on the health of residents, but poorer neighborhoods often do not receive sufficient service and maintenance.

4. *Sociocultural Features.* These characteristics refer to the political, economic, ethnic, and religious fabric of a community or neighborhood, including norms and values, social integration and interaction, crime and other threats to personal safety, and networks of social and community support (remember the Roseto study from Chapter 1). The connectedness of a community represents an important health resource. Socializing with others not only confers psychological benefits like stress reduction and a sense of trust and belonging, but also represents access to resources that other people in a social network can provide in times of need (Cohen et al. 2000).

5. *Reputation.* This refers to how both residents and nonresidents of a particular area (including business investors, community/economic planners, etc.) evaluate and perceive a community. These are groups with the potential to influence or even transform the infrastructure and resources of an area, along with the self-esteem and morale of residents, as well as who tends to move into or out of that space. The morale of residents is no small feature with respect to health. How neighborhood residents feel about their neighborhoods, and whether they feel discriminated against or isolated from others, affects the degree to which they are fatalistic about life in general and their health in particular (Pampel et al. 2010). Such attitudes directly affect health behaviors, including risk-taking behaviors such as smoking, unprotected sex, and the like.

A variety of neighborhood factors coalesce to promote or impede health. The number of opportunities to purchase healthy foods, engage in physical activity, avoid pollution and crime, and embrace feelings of safety and social cohesion all contribute to the overall health profile of a particular population. When we measure the combined effects of all of these features, the exposure to which is highly dependent on SES, we rank neighborhoods on how healthy they are. For example, a study by Wasserman et al. (2014) illustrated that body mass index (BMI) among elementary school children largely depended on a variety of neighborhood features, including the average SES of the neighborhood, number of fitness centers and parks, and the rate of population increase or decline (something reflective of reputation insofar as it measures whether people want to live in that neighborhood or not). These researchers uncovered a 25-point difference in BMI percentile across all race/ethnic and gender groups among a very large sample. That is, on average, children in the most unhealthy neighborhoods had an average BMI percentile rank falling between the 75th and 85th percentiles, whereas for those in the most healthy environments it fell between the 47th and 57th percentiles. These represent huge differences in the predictable health outcomes of children in the most "obesogenic" environments (i.e., those with the fewest parks and fitness facilities, along with lowest SES, etc.).

While they offer an important set of factors with which to assess neighborhood and community attributes, Macintyre and colleagues (2002) also point toward a useful crossover into how these structures also affect the psychology and future prospects of the individuals living within them, using the work of Abraham Maslow ([1962] 2014) and his widely known *hierarchy of needs*. This hierarchy emphasizes the various needs that should be met on the way to self-actualization, or realizing our true potential as human beings. Importantly, this also represents for clinical practitioners an important bridge between their patients' social environments and their individual attitudes, behaviors, and health outcomes. Clinicians may be able to offer little in the way of "fixing" the larger-scale problems of social environments through which patients acquire and manage their illnesses. However, they can make themselves aware of these influences and thereby address not only the actual health outcomes that emerge from them, but also the cognitive orientations that patients acquire within them.

As a psychologist, Maslow notes that place (particularly where one lives and works) occupies a central role in health matters because health is largely dependent on environments. Individuals typically adapt to the situations in which they find themselves, but they do so in more or less healthy ways. For example, one might respond to stress by increasing their physical activity (healthy) or smoking (unhealthy). Importantly, this means they alter their choices and behavior in ways that accord with social contexts (or how they perceive those social contexts). In turn, once basic environmental needs of individuals are fulfilled, they will expand their perceived sets of choices, and their sense of their own ability to make choices that matter (i.e., self-efficacy). In other words, in healthier environments, individuals can turn to other concerns, like their "potentialities and capacities, their talents, their latent resources, their creative impulses, their needs to know themselves and to become more and more integrated and unified, more and more aware of what they really are, of what they really want, of what their call or vocation or fate is to be" (Maslow [1962] 2014:24). For Maslow, meeting these essential needs also means "relative independence of adverse external circumstances, such as ill fortune, hard knocks, tragedy, stress, [and] deprivation" ([1962] 2014:24). In short, immediate environmental contexts are key to flourishing as humans. Interestingly, the baseline of Maslow's hierarchy begins with requisites like unpolluted air, clean water, availability of nutritious food, and safe and secure housing, before moving into relationships and social integration—all closely related or directly associated with the neighborhoods and communities in which we live.

To highlight the clinical implications of the ways that SES affects health through neighborhood mechanisms, let's return to the example of childhood asthma. SES is strongly associated with the types and characteristics of neighborhoods in which people can afford to live. Those with higher SES can afford safer, healthier neighborhoods. Conversely, those with fewer SES resources tend to live in less safe neighborhoods, with more pollution, more incivilities (e.g., vandalism, graffiti, and litter), less access to healthy foods, less access (both real and perceived) to opportunities for physical activity (e.g., safe parks and other facilities), and lower quality infrastructure when parks and playgrounds are present (Pampel et al. 2010; Suminski et al. 2012, 2013, 2014). SES amplifies or attenuates the degree to which people experience these healthy or unhealthy material/physical features of neighborhoods (see Fig. 4.3), and the resulting multifaceted health consequences. For instance, children from low-SES families live in neighborhoods that expose them to physical environments that promote greater rates of asthma (in older, dilapidated housing). This is exacerbated where lack of physical activity opportunities decreases the prevalence of physical activity. But the internalization of unsafe environments with greater degrees of incivility, lower social cohesion, and the like also promotes significantly higher levels of stress among these children, and stress also exacerbates asthma (Chen et al. 2006). So the pathway between SES and childhood asthma is complex and multifactorial, precisely because SES works through neighborhood to shape living and working environments, which affect health behaviors like diet and physical activity, as well as social psychological processes like stress and coping. All of these are intricately interconnected and ultimately affect the rates and severity of asthma among low-SES children.

Understanding the multiple pathways through which SES can affect health is critical for practitioners, because it highlights the various ways they might feasibly intervene in these processes. For example, a clinician seeing a child (from a low-SES family) presenting with asthma may need much more than a steroid inhalant. We might also spend greater time inquiring about the physical environment of the home, gleaning important information with which to develop recommendations accounting for those insights. The clinician might consider referring the family to nonprofit mold remediation programs that exist in some cities, or emphasizing pro bono legal resources to force landlords into providing safe rental housing, or assessing the feasibility of relocating. We might also spend greater time inquiring about stress and giving the patient and their families stress-reduction tools,[1] or discussing ways to enhance one's sense of perceived control over situations, or perhaps talk about ways to draw from existing networks of social support or coping resources. The key point is that while clinicians may not be able to remediate economic disparities or rebuild decaying neighborhoods, they can account for the multiple ways in which social structures like SES operate through various pathways to affect individual health outcomes. Without an awareness of these pathways, clinicians miss the opportunity to provide better and more effective treatment that accounts for the social and environmental factors that cause or exacerbate illness. An individualist approach might suggest the child with

---

[1] For example, there are numerous studies showing the benefits for patients incorporating mindfulness-based stress reduction (MBSR) as a "nonpharmacologic clinical tool" (Williams et al. 2015).

asthma needs a particular medication, but adding a social scientific approach compels us to ask what upstream factors (like neighborhood and housing conditions, and stress) might also require attention to best care for the patient.

Conclusion

The complexity and multidimensionality of social determinants of health make them particularly perplexing for many practitioners today because they contradict several important principles of modernist health care (see Chapter 2). For example, the notion of social factors as causal elements of disease challenges several of the core ideas of biomedicine, especially that disease is a condition of the individual that can be successfully treated by eradicating an invading pathogen (i.e., a germ, virus, etc.) through the use of chemotherapeutic or prophylactic interventions. This way of thinking rose to dominance after great success in treating infectious diseases before the epidemiological transition. Unfortunately, purely biomedical explanations also displaced other important ways of thinking about health and illness (several examples of which we provided in Chapter 1). The social determinants of health are initially perplexing for many professionals because we often oversimplify very complex disease processes by reducing them to microbes, foreign invaders, or solely individual-level (often genetic) malformations, guided by the principles of biomedicine (Hinote 2014b).

Thinking about social determinants also appears to invalidate the idea that the clinic is where treatments and cures are produced. As an important element of biomedicine, the clinic is historically the practitioner's quarantine, where he or she may isolate the sick person from outside influences in order to diagnose, treat, and cure the patient. As a result, training to practice within the confines of the clinic conditions many practitioners to view social causes of disease as beyond their scope of expertise or intervention. Many clinicians therefore are trained, perhaps unintentionally, to ignore or minimize the effects of social determinants, despite the fact that few would deny their true significance.

Despite these and other contradictions, understanding the logic of social determinants of health, and developing strategies to apply the insights gleaned from that logic, is an important part of training for health professionals. Moreover, framing social determinants of health in opposition to the biomedical features of disease is a false dichotomy. After all, the logic of social determinants does not invalidate the principles of biomedicine any more than the biomedical model eliminates all possibility of social causes of disease. In fact, these two ways of thinking complement one another, so much so that integrative training in both has the potential to help you become a well-rounded professional grounded in the tenets of biomedicine, but with the ability to integrate the insights that come from understanding the social nature of disease epidemiology and the humanistic elements of patient care. The structures of professional training, clinical practice, diagnosis/treatment, health care delivery, and health policy have shifted dramatically in the past, and as we have already noted, they are in the midst of transforming yet again. When the leading disease threats are chronic in nature, and they emerge from conditions and behaviors so firmly connected to social factors like the ones we discuss in this and the following chapters, understanding the social dimensions of epidemiology becomes imperative for those working on the front lines of health care delivery.

CHAPTER 4 ACTIVITY

The Flint Water Crisis: The Many Dimensions of Class and Health

On September 24, 2015, Dr. Mona Hanna-Attisha, a pediatrician at Hurley Medical Center in Flint, Michigan, went public with the results of her study of lead levels in Flint children. She found that the percentage of children with lead poisoning had more than doubled since April 25, 2014, when the city switched its municipal water source from the Detroit water system to the Flint River.

While much of the discourse surrounding the Flint water crisis date the origins of the problem to the day when the water source was switched (see Lurie 2016a for a detailed timeline of events), it is important to consider the larger context in which these events unfolded. Flint is a paradigmatic example of postindustrial economic decline. A manufacturing city built around automobile production, declines in the manufacturing sector decimated Flint (its economic decline and the resulting social problems are catalogued among other places in Young (2013) and Michael Moore's film *Roger and Me*). These economic declines, in concert with accusations that local officials had mismanaged the city's finances, led to the appointment of Darnell Earley as "Emergency Manager," empowered by Michigan Governor Rick Snyder to make decisions on the premise of restoring fiscal solvency to the city.

It was Earley who spearheaded the switch to using the Flint River as the water source. By the summer of that year, residents were complaining about discolored and foul-tasting water, and *Escherichia coli* was detected, prompting a warning to residents to boil tap water before drinking it. Perhaps more startling, automobile manufacturer General Motors announced in October 2015 that it would stop using the water after it became apparent that the water was corroding engine parts in its Flint factory. By January 2016 Flint issued a warning that chemicals in the water may be unsafe for older and medically fragile residents, but claimed it was still safe for other groups. At the same time, increasing numbers of Flint residents were complaining

not just about flavor and color of the water, but a range of symptoms they were experiencing. While a variety of state and local agencies continued to insist that the water was safe, a state government building in Flint began purchasing water coolers of purified water for its employees. When the city of Detroit offered to switch Flint back to its own water system, Earley rejected the offer.

By the spring of 2016, investigators were finally detecting high lead levels in the water. After noticing rashes, severe abdominal pain, and seemingly stunted growth in her children, LeeAnne Walters successfully insisted that the City test her water (Lurie 2016b). Across multiple tests, they found lead levels between ten and twenty-seven times higher than the EPA limit. However, the City contends that these lead levels resulted from the home's internal plumbing, and shortly thereafter the new Emergency Manager for Flint, Jerry Ambrose, unilaterally nixed a City Council vote to switch back to the Detroit water system. A few months later, independent researchers from Virginia Tech found that water from the Flint River was nearly twenty times more corrosive than the water from Detroit. It appears that the corrosive nature of the water caused the older, already dilapidated water infrastructure in the Flint Water Plant to leach lead into the water supply. The corrosive nature of the water also damaged the pipes of homes in Flint, particularly those in the older and more disadvantaged sectors of the city. As in other places in the country, lead exposure affected Flint's poorest children the most.

Yet when Dr. Hanna-Attisha released her results, which made clear that lead toxicity increases since the switch constituted a public health crisis, state and local public health agencies lined up to dispute her data. It would be several months before environmental health leaders in the area would acknowledge that the problem was real. In the wake of this event, it is estimated that 5% of children in Flint have toxic levels of lead in their blood, and the water is implicated in an outbreak of Legionnaires' disease that had killed twelve people by April 2016.

Discussion Questions

1. Identify the multiple ways in which social class may have played a role in how the Flint Water Crisis unfolded.

   Helpful Hint: Explore the role of poverty in setting the social and political stage in which the events unfolded, but also in terms of residents' exposure to lead, and investigate how poverty might amplify the negative consequences of exposure.

2. How do you think the Flint Water Crisis will affect issues of class and health going forward?

   Helpful Hint: Think about economic development at the city and regional levels, but also the challenges of economic and academic achievement facing the children of Flint. Think about social and physiological pathways to achievement.

3. What is the role of a clinical practitioner in promoting health, not just among his or her patients but also among the public in general?

4. Discuss ways that the Flint Water Crisis could have been prevented.

CHAPTER 5

A Matrix of Health Inequalities

LEARNING OBJECTIVES

After reading this chapter, students should be able to

- Articulate the significance of social determinants in the contemporary landscape of health and illness.

- Describe how the cohort effects of age affect health outcomes, clinical presentation, and the health care system.

- Explain the ways that gender shapes individual- and population-level health.

- Clarify the ways that race and ethnicity influence health.

- Explain how culture constitutes a significant context within which health unfolds.

- Describe the intersectionality of various social determinants of health and how these constitute a matrix of inequality.

In the preceding chapter we introduced socioeconomic status (SES, or social class) as one of the most powerful social determinants of health today. Because it affects multiple diseases through multiple pathways, reproduces their effects over time, and involves access to resources germane to disease risk and/or protection, SES constitutes a fundamental cause of health and disease (Link 2008; Link & Phelan 1995). But it is easy to focus on a single factor like SES, which alone wields considerable influence over disease outcomes, while ignoring other dimensions of inequality and difference. If we focused solely on SES, for instance, we would slip into a similar fallacy as those focusing solely on the most proximal causes of disease, without considering the various causes further *downstream* (recall the analogy from Chapter 4). That is, we may overlook other health-related aspects of social life that put people at risk of various risks. Social determinants of health include many other conditions into which we are born, and in which we grow, work, live, and age, along with the wider set of forces and systems that shape the conditions of everyday life (CSDH 2008; who.org). There are at least two important insights to acknowledge in this definition.

First, social determinants stretch across all areas of our experience and environments, including but not limited to age, gender, race/ethnicity, and culture. As a result, we must account for many other influences over and above SES; even this very powerful concept does not fully explain all health disparities. Second, these influences never affect us singularly (i.e., as SES *alone*). Rather, the additive and multiplicative effects of *multiple* factors and conditions continuously exert influence on us throughout our everyday lives and experiences. The ubiquitous and multidimensional nature of social determinants of health makes unraveling their impacts a quite complicated endeavor, like analyzing multiple moving targets simultaneously. For one, today the concepts of health and disease are more ambiguous than in the past. Chronic diseases, for instance, often constitute evolving, long-term, and dynamic states of managed dysfunction. As a result, what it means to be sick or well is in many regards variable and subjective. Moreover, the meanings attached to phenomena like gender, race/ethnicity, and culture are largely socially constructed, which means that individuals and groups experience and respond to them in different ways. Add to all of this the fact that primary sources of morbidity and mortality today operate through causal and risk pathways that are far more *individuated* (or unique to each patient) when compared to earlier historical periods, which were largely dominated by comparatively simpler infectious ailments that were more discretely observable and temporary (Wasserman & Hinote 2011).

For example, someone with syphilis is infected with an organism that needs to be eliminated from their body, a process clearly delineating when they are *sick* and the moment they return to *health*. Chronic illnesses, on the other hand, are far more complicated. Sometimes they have no obvious symptoms at all (hypertension, perhaps) and often move very slowly over time through different degrees of dysfunction. Additionally, when one is living *with* a chronic disease, their definitions of how sick they are tend to revolve around the extent to which the illness impacts their daily functions (see Chapter 8), which is very different for different individuals. However, greater complexity does not mean that diseases are chaotic and disorganized. Rather, it means that health professionals must approach the clinical encounter with the ability to make sense of the complexity emanating from the various conditions in which individual patients live, work, and age, all situated within broader social contexts like class, gender, race/ethnicity, and culture. This is no small task for practitioners, but is necessary to understand how and why people become sick and how well positioned they are to manage their illness. In this chapter we explore how various social factors beyond SES influence health and give rise to inequalities in disease epidemiology and illness management. We conclude by exploring how these social factors intersect as a *matrix of inequalities*.

Age

The variables that we discuss in the coming pages are characteristic of all people in one way or another, but they also constitute important connections between us because they reflect the many groups or *collectivities* to which we belong. More importantly, however, membership in these collectivities is associated with different levels of access to broader sets of resources, power, and advantage. When talking about age, we usually think about chronological age (i.e., how many years an individual has been alive). This is certainly important, since as we age we typically experience physical and mental declines. But the concept of age is also much larger than these individual experiences, because age also connects us to broader groups of people like us, called *age cohorts*.

Age cohorts exhibit both life course and historical dimensions. The *life course* dimension describes how groups of people move through the life course together, sharing similar life events, roles, and experiences along way. For example, they go to school together and get married, have children, and retire around the same time. In other words, they shared similar roles in their pasts, they occupy many similar roles in the present, and are likely to share much of the same into the future. As they move through the life course, they give way to successive cohorts, while at the same time replacing preceding cohorts, and so forth. Because individuals share similar trajectories across the life course, these processes, called *cohort flow*, can produce similar perspectives, attitudes, and interests within cohorts. As such, these experiences shape expectations of health, attitudes toward health care providers, interpersonal demeanor, and so on (Cockerham 2013; Riley 1987).

The *historical* dimension emphasizes how cohort members experience distinct historical periods together, including major events, from their unique perspective. Put another way, all of us share many culturally significant events, but we frame those events within very different outlooks and experiences, which are shaped by our cohort membership. Take for instance, the September 11, 2001 attacks, the HIV/AIDS epidemic, and the advent and proliferation of the Internet, each representing a culturally significant development in the United States. While shared by an entire population, individuals experience events somewhat differently in terms of their impact and meaning. Membership in a particular age cohort is one context that shapes the ways that we perceive, define, and evaluate those phenomena. Older cohorts might see terrorism as another threat to American security, similar to the attacks at Pearl Harbor, to be overcome with the same tools that led to victory in World War II (another major event experienced by this cohort). Younger cohorts who did not experience those same key events might perceive the 9/11 attacks quite differently, perhaps necessitating a fundamental shift in American foreign policy, international partnerships, society building, and homeland security. Older cohorts may view HIV/AIDS as a disease of deviance and of stigmatized groups that engage in unacceptable behaviors. Younger cohorts might frame this epidemic as a disease affecting many of their friends, as very serious but not indicative of some deeper moral shortcoming. Older cohorts may perceive the Internet as a convenient curiosity, while middle cohorts recognize the way that it continues to fundamentally transform virtually every aspect of our lives. And the youngest cohorts of our society never remember a time when things like the global war on terror, HIV/AIDS, and the Internet did not exist. Age, particularly through cohort membership, matters a great deal in terms of shaping how we view and interpret the world around us (just like the influences surrounding SES discussed in the previous chapter). As such, cohorts and cohort flow can influence individual health outcomes and significantly impact the health care system and the broader society.

The annual report, *Health, United States*, compiled and published by the National Center for Health Statistics (NCHS) includes data on mortality, morbidity, disability, risk factors, prevention, health insurance, health care access and utilization, health care costs, and more. The 2014 report explores in detail the age cohort born between 1950 and 1959, individuals who were between 55 and 64 years old at the time data were collected (NCHS 2015). This group was born during the Cold War, raised in the turbulent 1960s, and at the time of the report were approaching retirement. They occupy the heart of the "baby boom" generation,[1] and are significant for a number of reasons. The first concerns its size and diversity. Between 2000 and 2013, the size of the age 55–64 cohort increased substantially, constituting 8.6% of the total U.S. population in 2000, to 12.4% by 2013 (see Table 5.1). Projections suggest that by 2030 this cohort will contract to about 10.8% as the baby boomers move through cohort flow, eventually swelling the older cohorts greater than 65 years of age. A closer look at Table 5.1 indicates that older (≥65 years) cohorts are already increasing significantly and have been for a long time, especially among women. While nearly all age cohorts grew, signifying overall increases in the population, the oldest cohort (≥85 years) grew more than tenfold from 1950 to 2013. As the baby boomers move through the population structure, we can expect these trends to accelerate as the number of very old adults increases even more dramatically.

The age 55–64 cohort is also more racially and ethnically diverse than its predecessors, with non-Hispanic white adults decreasing from around 79% of the population to just below 74% across the 2002–03 and 2012–13 cohorts, while non-Hispanic black adults increased from 9.5% to 10.9% and Hispanic adults aged 55–64 increased from 7.5% to about 10% (see Table 5.2). Educational attainment increased within this cohort, but so did the percentage living below the poverty line. Fewer adults report retirement in the 2012–13 group, while those unemployed due to disability increased from 11.5% to 12.7%. Those within the age 55–64 cohort in 2012–13 were less likely to be married and more likely to report cohabiting, than their 2002–03 counterparts (NCHS 2015). Again, these are noteworthy shifts, with real implications for clinicians and patient care, as well as the burden of disease within our health care system. While the changes might seem small when measured in percentages, the absolute numbers involved become quite large when applied to the total U.S. population of more than 300 million people.

Understanding the sociodemographic profile of the baby boomers is important in providing context to their epidemiological experience. While chronic conditions may develop at any age, the odds increase around midlife and accelerate as we get older. In fact, about one-third of the age 55–64 group in 2013 report two or three chronic health conditions, with nearly one in ten reporting four or more. In addition, cancer and heart disease accounted for more than half of deaths within this age group in 2013. This is noteworthy because today managing such conditions is a complex process that typically involves the patient and family caregivers (see Chapter 8), multiple health care providers (and coordination among them), several drug therapies, many diagnostic tests and retests, and more. As more Americans enter age ranges characterized by increasing disease risks, cohorts exert substantial pressure on the health care system in terms of costs, quality of care, patient demand, and service utilization.

The attributes of the age 55–64 cohort are not altogether gloomy. In comparing the 2002–03 and 2012–13 cohorts, the latter smoke less and engage in more leisure-time exercise, although these are not equally distributed across various socioeconomic subgroups. Nonetheless, those aged 55–64 in 2012–13 also report

[1] This cohort comprises individuals born between 1946 and 1964, a time of very high rates of childbirth driven by a booming economy and the fact that many couples had delayed having children during the preceding Great Depression and WWII.

TABLE 5.1 Resident Population by Age and Sex, United States, Selected Years, 1950–2013

Sex, Race, Hispanic Origin, and Year	Total Resident Population	Under 1 year	1-4 years	5-14 years	15-24 years	25-34 years	35-44 years	45-54 years	55-64 years	65-74 years	75-84 years	85 years and Over
							Number, in Thousands					
All persons												
1950	1,50,697	3,147	13,017	24,319	22,098	23,759	21,450	17,343	13,370	8,340	3,278	577
1960	1,79,323	4,112	16,209	35,465	24,020	22,818	24,081	20,485	15,572	10,997	4,633	929
1970	2,03,212	3,485	13,669	40,746	35,441	24,907	23,088	23,220	18,590	12,435	6,119	1,511
1980	2,26,546	3,534	12,815	34,942	42,487	37,082	25,635	22,800	21,703	15,581	7,729	2,240
1990	2,48,710	3,946	14,812	35,095	37,013	43,161	37,435	25,057	21,113	18,045	10,012	3,021
2000	2,81,422	3,806	15,370	41,078	39,184	39,892	45,149	37,678	24,275	18,391	12,361	4,240
2010	3,08,746	3,944	16,257	41,026	43,626	41,064	41,071	45,007	36,483	21,713	13,061	5,493
2011	3,11,592	3,997	16,166	41,039	43,798	41,790	40,628	44,718	38,062	22,482	13,175	5,737
2012	3,13,914	3,943	16,056	41,145	43,944	42,309	40,516	44,269	38,586	23,985	13,273	5,887
2013	3,16,129	3,945	15,926	41,221	43,954	42,845	40,453	43,768	39,316	25,217	13,447	6,041
Male												
1950	74,833	1,602	6,634	12,375	10,918	11,597	10,588	8,655	6,697	4,024	1,507	237
1960	88,331	2,090	8,240	18,029	11,906	11,179	11,755	10,093	7,537	5,116	2,025	362
1970	98,912	1,778	6,968	20,759	17,551	12,217	11,231	11,199	8,793	5,437	2,436	542
1980	1,10,053	1,806	6,556	17,855	21,419	18,382	12,570	11,009	10,152	6,757	2,867	682
1990	1,21,239	2,018	7,581	17,971	18,915	21,564	18,510	12,232	9,955	7,907	3,745	841
2000	1,38,054	1,949	7,862	21,043	20,079	20,121	22,448	18,497	11,645	8,303	4,879	1,227
2010	1,51,781	2,014	8,305	20,970	22,318	20,632	20,436	22,142	17,601	10,097	5,477	1,790
2011	1,53,291	2,044	8,256	20,971	22,432	21,044	20,223	22,019	18,358	10,476	5,573	1,894
2012	1,54,492	2,017	8,199	21,026	22,512	21,339	20,174	21,807	18,603	11,203	5,648	1,964
2013	1,55,652	2,017	8,136	21,061	22,525	21,641	20,145	21,569	18,957	11,798	5,761	2,042

Continued

TABLE 5.1 Continued

Sex, Race, Hispanic Origin, and Year	Total Resident Population	Age										
		Under 1 year	1-4 years	5-14 years	15-24 years	25-34 years	35-44 years	45-54 years	55-64 years	65-74 years	75-84 years	85 years and Over
Female												
1950	75,864	1,545	6,383	11,944	11,181	12,162	10,863	8,688	6,672	4,316	1,771	340
1960	90,992	2,022	7,969	17,437	12,114	11,639	12,326	10,393	8,036	5,881	2,609	567
1970	1,04,300	1,707	6,701	19,986	17,890	12,690	11,857	12,021	9,797	6,998	3,683	969
1980	1,16,493	1,727	6,259	17,087	21,068	18,700	13,065	11,791	11,551	8,824	4,862	1,559
1990	1,27,471	1,928	7,231	17,124	18,098	21,596	18,925	12,824	11,158	10,139	6,267	2,180
2000	1,43,368	1,857	7,508	20,034	19,105	19,771	22,701	19,181	12,629	10,088	7,482	3,013
2010	1,56,964	1,930	7,952	20,056	21,309	20,432	20,635	22,864	18,882	11,617	7,584	3,704
2011	1,58,301	1,953	7,910	20,068	21,366	20,746	20,404	22,699	19,704	12,005	7,602	3,843
2012	1,59,422	1,926	7,857	20,118	21,432	20,971	20,343	22,462	19,983	12,783	7,624	3,923
2013	1,60,477	1,925	7,791	20,160	21,429	21,203	20,307	22,198	20,360	13,419	7,686	3,999

Source: National Center for Health Statistics (NCHS). (2015). *Health, United States, 2014: With Special Feature on Adults Aged 55-64*. Hyattsville, MD: U.S. Department of Health & Human Services, Centers for Disease Control & Prevention.

TABLE 5.2 **Health, United States, 2014 Profile of the Age 55–64 Cohort, 2002–03 and 2012–13**

Characteristics	2002-03		2012-13	
	Percent Distribution	SE	Percent Distribution	SE
Sex				
Men	48.0	0.3	48.0	0.3
Women	52.0	0.3	52.0	0.3
Race/Ethnicity				
Hispanic	7.5	0.3	9.6	0.3
Not Hispanic				
White only	78.9	0.5	73.6	0.5
Black only	9.5	0.4	10.9	0.5
Education				
Less than high school diploma	16.1	0.4	11.7	0.3
High school diploma or GED	31.8	0.5	27.4	0.4
Some college	25.0	0.4	29.6	0.4
Bachelor's degree or higher	27.1	0.5	31.3	0.5
Percent of Poverty Level				
Below 100%	9.3	0.3	10.0	0.3
100%-199%	13.7	0.4	14.7	0.4
200%-399%	27.9	0.5	28.1	0.4
400% or more	49.1	0.6	47.2	0.6
Employment Status in Past Week				
Employed	60.0	0.5	61.4	0.4
Not employed due to retirement	17.0	0.4	14.6	0.3
Not employed due to disability	11.5	0.3	12.7	0.3
Other	11.5	0.3	11.3	0.3
Marital Status				
Married	71.7	0.5	67.6	0.4
Divorced or separated	14.6	0.3	16.5	0.3
Widowed	6.8	0.2	4.7	0.2
Never married	4.4	0.2	7.3	0.2
Cohabitating	2.5	0.2	3.9	0.2

Source: National Center for Health Statistics (NCHS). (2015). *Health, United States, 2014: With Special Feature on Adults Aged 55-64*. Hyattsville, MD: U.S. Department of Health & Human Services, Centers for Disease Control & Prevention.

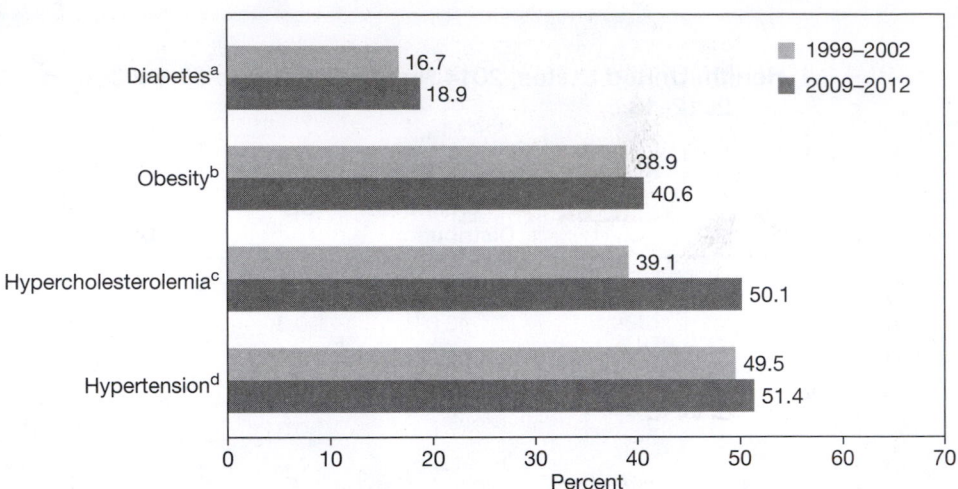

FIG. 5.1 Selected chronic conditions among adults aged 55–64, United States, 1999–2002 and 2009–12.

[a]Defined as respondent report of physician-diagnosed diabetes, or undiagnosed diabetes (measured fasting plasma glucose of at least 126 mg/dL or a hemoglobin A1c of at least 6.5%.

[b]Defined as body mass index greater than or equal to 30.

[c]Defined as reporting taking cholesterol-lowering medication or having a measured serum total cholesterol level of at least 240 mg/dL.

[d]Defined as reporting taking antihypertensive medication or having a measured systolic blood pressure of at least 140 mm Hg or a measured diastolic blood pressure of at least 90 mm Hg.

Source: National Center for Health Statistics (NCHS). (2015). *Health, United States, 2014: With Special Feature on Adults Aged 55-64.* CDC/NCHS, National Health and Nutrition Examination Survey. Hyattsville, MD: U.S. Department of Health & Human Services, Centers for Disease Control & Prevention.

higher levels of mild to moderate psychological distress and exhibit higher rates of several chronic conditions than previous cohorts did at the same age (NCHS 2015). Figure 5.1 depicts the prevalence of conditions like diabetes, obesity, high cholesterol, and hypertension between the 1999–2002 and 2012–13 cohorts of 55–64-year-olds in the United States. These trends are noteworthy because increasingly large cohorts of citizens are entering the age brackets where chronic conditions are more prevalent. Put these data together with the data from Table 5.1 on population growth and one can begin to sense the magnitude of the issue. For example, the prevalence of high cholesterol increased about 11% among the age 55–64 groups between 1999–2001 and 2009–12. But the number of individuals aged 55–64 increased by almost 12 million during that same time period. Without considering other influential risk factors, if half of them (50.1%) have high cholesterol, it translates into about 6 million more people. If we similarly analyze other disease categories, and include even older cohorts, the seismic nature of the problem comes into sharp relief.

Unsurprisingly, as a result of the risk factors and chronic conditions just mentioned, the age 55–64 cohort is responsible for a large number of health care visits (see Figure 5.2; NCHS 2015). They require care for conditions that they have already developed, but they are a group that could substantially benefit from preventative care and screening as well. As such, maintaining a source of affordable, comprehensive health insurance is very important. Most of today's 55–64-year-olds benefit

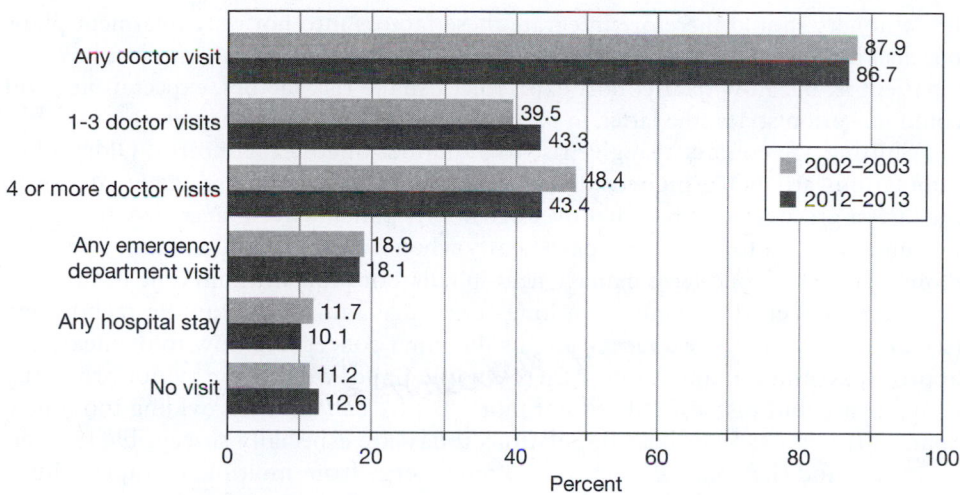

FIG. 5.2 Health care utilization in the past twelve months among adults aged 55–64, United States, 2002–03 and 2012–13.

Source: National Center for Health Statistics (NCHS). (2015). *Health, United States, 2014: With Special Feature on Adults Aged 55-64.* Hyattsville, MD: U.S. Department of Health & Human Services, Centers for Disease Control & Prevention.

from employer-sponsored private coverage, but that number is steadily decreasing. Additionally, many will not be able to maintain their coverage into retirement as employers increasingly scale back retiree insurance benefits, or eliminate them altogether. In coming years this cohort will exert tremendous pressure on providers, as well as insurance and reimbursement structures. Within a decade, Medicare, a system already under considerable pressure, will pay for nearly all of this cohort's care. Health providers, administrators, and policymakers, then, must face a variety of complex issues pertaining to access and treatment among this group, along with how their health care needs will affect various sectors of the workforce (see also Chapter 12).

Just like the age 55–64 group, each age cohort possesses collective attributes and each exerts profound influences upon its members. Not only do members of the same or similar cohorts tend to share perspectives and experiences, as a group they also share some similar health beliefs, practices, behaviors, lifestyles, and health risks. While it is easy to focus upon the elderly when thinking about health risks, each successive cohort in our society possesses its own set of perspectives and health experiences. As a result, we may observe cohort effects in younger age groups as well. Cockerham (2013) notes that cigarette smoking was quite prevalent among younger cohorts of both men and women in the 1940s, largely due to tobacco advertising in the media and shifting gender roles for women entering the American workforce. These behaviors created and sustained health risks culminating in elevated lung cancer mortality some decades later among members of this same cohort. From a clinical perspective this means it is important to understand and consider both cohort and aging processes. That is, providers should account for patients' life experiences as members of particular age cohorts, along with the fact that as they age they encounter new health challenges including dementia, falls, chronic sensory declines, and changes in cognition, in addition to other chronic conditions listed above.

Practitioners should therefore integrate these factors into not only treatment plans but also interpersonal interaction and communication, considering not just how old a patient is, but how their cohort experiences shape risk factors, expectations, and communication styles (the latter, in particular, is elaborated in Chapter 9).

Shifting age cohorts also give rise to a number of ethical concerns. Older adult populations are increasing worldwide, and among those who are age 60 and over, the fastest growing cohort is that over age 80. As patients live longer, new treatment dilemmas emerge for clinicians, particularly when chronic and degenerative diseases require complex, long-term management in collaboration with multiple health care providers. Given the advances in long-term care and life-sustaining technology (see also Chapter 11), we face a serious dilemma concerning how to delineate the appropriate amount and kind of care. On one hand, we can err by not providing enough care, but just as easily (if not more so), we can err by providing too much. Span (2015) notes that older populations today are especially susceptible to over-treatment and the complications that often emerge from multiple therapies aimed at treating many comorbidities. It is just this type of problem that is characteristic of clinical practice today, largely due to the complexity of health and disease in the chronic illness era. Graham (2014) describes the difficulty involved in merely calcu-lating the dosage for, say, a diabetes medication, for older adults, especially consid-ering complications associated with unpredictable diet, depression, dementia, vision loss, and other issues with self-care. As a result, Tseng and colleagues (2014:259) report that "among persons aged 65 years or older, hypoglycemic agents (sulfony-lureas and insulin) are the second most common medications associated with emer-gency department visits or hospitalizations and adverse drug events reported to the U.S. Food and Drug Administration, closely following warfarin."

Our health care system, which historically developed around treating acute conditions (see Chapter 2), is also ill equipped to meet many of the complex and chronic challenges associated with an aging population. The baby boomer cohort described above, for example, will move through a health care system (and a society) that is not likely to have the specialized personnel or facilities to care for such large numbers of older adults, especially considering recent declines in geriatric specialists (Wasserman 2015). This cohort will also continue to exert significant pressure on reimbursement systems like private insurance markets and Medicare. In sum, age is not only a very important determinant of patient health, but also poses substantial challenges for clinical practice and health care systems.

Gender

In social science disciplines, *sex* typically refers to a biological classification as male or female.[2] In contrast, the concept of *gender* refers to culturally specific ideas of what constitutes a man or woman. At the risk of oversimplification, we

---

[2] In the past this was determined by the physiological features of one's genitalia, but today is better described by chromosomal makeup of an individual (XX for female and XY for male). Recently, the United States Institute of Medicine (IOM) began to draw upon the definition advanced by the World Health Organization (WHO) and the style manual of the *Journal of the American Medical Association* (JAMA): "The classification of living things, generally as male or female, according to their reproduc-tive organs and functions assigned by chromosomal complement" (see Springer et al. 2012).

may conveniently define sex dichotomously, while gender exists along more of a continuum of ideas and expectations with masculinity at one pole and femininity at the other. As a result, when we talk about *sex differences*, we are talking about biology, while *gender differences* pertain to socially constructed notions of what it means to adhere to norms for men and women. Both are likely important in explaining gendered health disparities (Springer et al. 2012), which are complex and often appear inconsistent. For example, one of the most striking epidemiological findings of the past century involves the *gender paradox* in longevity (Bird & Lang 2014; Liu 2014). In the United States, in 2013, women could expect to live about 81.2 years on average, while men could expect to live about 76.4 years (NCHS 2015). But despite their advantage in longevity, women report poorer health, suffer significantly more comorbidities as they age, and use more health services than their counterparts. Even controlling for reproduction-related care, women experience more physical illness, sick days, and hospitalization than men. Hence the adage: *women get sicker, men die quicker*. In this section we explore the relationship between gender and health, largely through this paradox, because it emphasizes so many interesting and complicated features of that relationship.

A large part of the paradox of higher morbidity but lower mortality among women involves gender differences in the prevalence of fatal and nonfatal diseases and the types of chronic conditions affecting men and women. In most developed societies, men experience more life-threatening conditions at younger ages, while women exhibit a higher prevalence of chronic debilitating and nonfatal disorders. Men more likely develop serious conditions like cardiovascular disease and diabetes, and smoking-related diseases like lung cancer and chronic respiratory conditions. Women, on the other hand, tend to experience autoimmune and rheumatoid disorders, as well as less life-threatening but painful conditions such as arthritis and migraines, along with anemia and thyroid disease, compared with men of similar age. At the end of life, women tend to die of similar conditions as men, but at later ages. Women's longevity advantage shows up across multiple societies, but it is not universal, nor has it always existed. Bird and Lang (2014:602) note that, "it occurs almost exclusively in social and environmental contexts where average life expectancy is high for both men and women [and] appears to vary with environmental and behavioral risk and protective factors as well as with genetic, biological, and hormonal processes." But to simply say that men live shorter lives than women misses the complexity of gender as a determinant of health influenced by both biological and social factors.

Biological explanations tend to emphasize the role of physiological differences involving hormonal mechanisms and differential immune and stress responses (Bird & Rieker 2008), and biological differences tend to advantage women. Maklakov and Lummaa (2013:717) point out that greater female longevity is observable across many species, and explore two plausible hypotheses for male disadvantages in mortality: *unguarded* X, and the *mother's curse*.

> Early biological hypotheses that aimed to explain the sex differences in lifespan centered on the role of sex chromosomes and relied heavily on the fact that recessive deleterious mutations occurring on X (or Z) chromosome are not "guarded" by alleles on the second chromosome in the heterogametic sex resulting in increased mortality. Another commonly cited reason for increased male mortality

is maternal inheritance of mitochondrial DNA, which could lead to accumulation of male-specific deleterious mutations in the mitochondrial genome (so-called "mother's curse").

Emslie (2008) describes increased vulnerability for male embryos when compared with females, and greater morbidities linked to male sex chromosomes. Boys appear to be more susceptible to infection than girls, with estrogen potentially exerting a protective effect on women prior to menopause. Furman and colleagues (2014) also document the more robust immune responses among women, although mechanisms are not well understood, and observe greater antibody responses to influenza vaccination among females, with more elevated testosterone levels among men associated with the lowest antibody responses. But in reality, it is difficult to disaggregate sex and gender. Springer and colleagues (2012) acknowledge the neuroendocrine pathways between sex and cardiovascular disease, for example, but also make a compelling case for the many ways that sex and gender are "entangled," or "inextricably interwoven" with one another, thereby making investigation of one or the other, and the attribution of causality, problematic. "While the causal link between 'sex' and 'gender' is often thought to flow automatically from biological to social difference, recent research has forcefully demonstrated that the influence often operates in the other direction" as well (Springer et al. 2012:1818).

Stress response represents a good example of the interwoven biological and social pathways between gender and health. For both men and women stress appears to be linked to cardiovascular disease, but physiologically, men and women respond differently to stress and to different stressors (Steptoe & Kivimäki 2013).[3] In one study of middle school children, girls tended to have greater affective responses to stress, but they also utilize strategies of engagement versus disengagement to a greater degree to mitigate stressful situations (Sontag & Graber 2010). Together, this highlights the interactional nature of biological and social factors and the difficulty of disaggregating them. In this case, there may be physiological reactions to stress that tend to be stronger in a particular sex, but stress responses such as engagement (including talking to a person causing the stress, expressing one's feelings, etc.) may be more socially acceptable and socially encouraged among women compared to men, even beginning at early ages.

While a variety of physical health outcomes are differentially patterned among men and women, the supposed gap in mental health offers another opportunity for us to think more deeply and critically about the ways that gender shapes symptomology, case presentation, and health statistics. Liu (2014) points to the widely cited claim that women have higher rates of depression. Researchers in the 1970s (e.g., Bernard 1972; Gove & Tudor 1973) claimed that women were more depressed

---

[3]Interestingly, early stress research argued that women faced fewer stressors than men due to their relegation to the private sphere of home and family life, an element that protected them from the stress and strain of the masculine world of being a breadwinner. This work tended to focus on the socioeconomic stressors common to men's experience, while more recent research demonstrates that men and women both experience stress, but from a different range of stressors, and while drawing from different coping resources (Bird & Lang 2014). This example is an important case study showing the ways that social biases can affect health research, by shaping how we develop and operationalize variables of interest (see Chapter 3).

than men because of their less rewarding and more demanding marriage and family roles, a claim that many later studies supported. In response, however, Dohrenwend and Dohrenwend (1976) took a different approach, arguing that women did not necessarily exhibit greater psychological distress than men when different, *gendered* dimensions of mental well-being were considered, like personality disorders, substance abuse, and antisocial behavior. In other words, women appeared to report poorer psychological health largely because most research used depression as the primary proxy for mental well-being.

When other dimensions of mental well-being are considered, the results are substantially different. Men tend to externalize such experiences of distress through drinking alcohol, sometimes in excess, and through other substance abuse or conduct disorders. Women, on the other hand, tend to internalize, thereby manifesting symptoms of depression and/or anxiety (Cockerham 2013; Simon & Nath 2004). Liu (2014:631) summarizes the research:

> focusing on depression as the primary or sole measure of mental health more likely reflects women's psychological distress, but may not fully capture men's levels of distress. When both female and male prevalent measures of mental health (e.g., depression and alcohol consumption) are used, researchers find that gender differences in mental health may not be as large as expected.

For clinicians, this brief example highlights the ways that outward expressions of underlying social and psychological conditions may vary considerably across gender distinctions. Grasping this important insight is critical to providing effective patient-centered care attuned to the nuanced experiences of various social groups, and avoiding the tendency to retreat into mere stereotypes in the clinical encounter (i.e., women are emotional, distressed, and therefore depressed).

As some of the examples above highlight, *social explanations* for the gender gap emphasize the effects of social structure, stratification and inequalities, roles, and normative health behaviors (Bird & Lang 2014; Cockerham 2013; Courtenay 2000; Hinote & Webber 2012; Liu 2014). Just as with SES (see Chapter 4), patterns of mortality and morbidity are gendered in that they are shaped by access to resources and exposure to risks. Within industrialized nations, men historically worked in manual labor and other high-risk occupations, while women tended to work in service sectors or in desk jobs, often supporting the work of men. As a result, men enjoyed access to well-paid jobs in the twentieth century, but were also susceptible to higher odds of work-related injury or accidental death. While gender segregation has certainly decreased in recent decades, these trends continue to affect incomes in the United States, in part because, "the women's rights movement focused more on equal access to occupations than on income equality across occupations which has been the focus in much of Europe" (Bird & Lang 2014:604). Emslie and Hunt (2008:810) also point out that "men still occupy higher status, higher paid jobs and benefit from the gendered division of labour, and women may suffer more role conflict than men, given that many work a 'double shift' in the public and the domestic sphere." As a result, gendered divisions of labor persist today, and in part offset the increasing similarities between home and work roles for men and women. While many of these trends are still in flux, all exert direct and indirect effects on the health of both men and women.

Another compelling social explanation pertains to riskier and generally less healthy behavior and lifestyle patterns among men. Compared to women, men are more likely to smoke cigarettes, drink heavily, abuse illicit drugs, be involved in violence, and work in higher-risk occupations. All of these increase mortality risks from lung cancer, accidents, suicide, homicide, and so on. According to Courtenay (2000:1386):

> Many sociocultural factors are associated with and influence health-related behaviour. Gender is one of the most important of these factors. Women engage in far more health-promoting behaviours than men and have more health lifestyle patterns. Being a woman may, in fact, be the strongest predictor of preventive and health-promoting behaviour.

Of course, pervasive gender norms condition the propensity for men to engage in such risky behaviors and women's tendency to avoid them. Historical and cultural notions of masculinity and femininity shape what it means to be a man or a woman in any society, and how to behave accordingly. The greater social value placed on attractiveness in girls and women may result in greater attention to their bodies, which may in turn make them more aware of their symptoms and more generally concerned about their health than men. Women typically possess more knowledge of health and well-being, thereby offering more accurate reports of their self-rated health (Bird & Rieker 2008). Women also use a greater quantity of health services than their counterparts and do so more often. They are more than twice as likely to utilize outpatient mental health services and the number of women in a household is closely associated with the total number of physician visits for that household (Cockerham 2013). Of course, the fact that women actually have greater morbidity than men, as described above, may also explain their greater use of health services. But these differences may also be due to gendered attitudes and social norms, where women are more open to seeking help if it is needed and more likely to adopt the sick role. Men may be more likely to perceive such help-seeking behavior as weak and standing in contrast with often rigidly gendered stereotypes of masculinity.

Liu (2014) notes that many of the conditions responsible for excess male mortality are associated with specific health behaviors like smoking, which explains a substantial portion of the gender difference in mortality. Of course, historical notions of femininity have often been accompanied by repressive stereotypes that disadvantaged women in any number of ways. But they may have also, in some respects, served a protective function with regard to health. Today, for example, shifting gender norms could be responsible for shrinking differentials in risk factors like smoking, drinking, high-risk occupations, and other such behaviors among men and women, thereby attenuating the gender gap in life expectancy (NCHS 2015). That is, contemporary notions of femininity have promoted increased uptake of many risk factors related to smoking and binge drinking that, in earlier decades, were largely the behaviors of men who, in turn, suffered the associated health consequences. As a result of increased smoking, for example, the rate of lung cancer in women rose from about 5 per 100,000 in 1965 to more than 40 per 100,000 in the year 2011 (roughly equivalent to the rate among men in 1960; NCHS 2015;

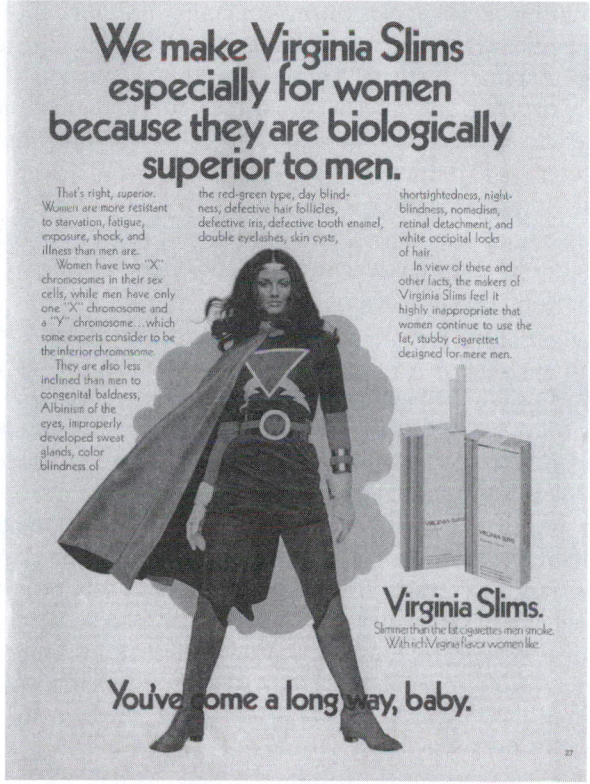

PHOTO 5.1 Cigarette advertisement targeting women.

Siegel et al. 2013). The Virginia Slims cigarette company even specifically marketed their product to the newly liberated woman of the 1960s and 1970s (see Photo 5.1), but since 2005 these trends have begun to reverse due to targeted antismoking campaigns. Nonetheless, they clearly illustrate that gender exerts powerful influences as a social determinant of health, and frequently intersects with age and other variables to shape health behavioral profiles, health care utilization, and morbidity and mortality.

Race and Ethnicity

Race and ethnicity are complicated and often problematic constructs. Traditionally, *race* refers to shared physical characteristics while *ethnicity* refers to shared national or cultural background. But of course, the two often overlap in common language usage and in some research and population data. Research studies often operationalize race in problematic ways, for example, by blending race and ethnic categories together when reporting data. Such data are often separated into five categories such as white (race), black or African American (race), Hispanic (ethnicity), Asian (race), and other. This may lead us to overlook important aspects of race or ethnicity, such as the experience of black Hispanics or multiracial/multiethnic individuals, because they are often forced to select one category, and because the categories themselves lack specificity (see Aspinall 2001 for a more elaborate discussion of such problems). Nonetheless, both systemic and interpersonal race/ethnic biases lead to a decidedly *racialized* experience, particularly for underrepresented minorities.[4] That is, one's race/ethnic characteristics, particularly those that are easily discerned by the public (like skin color or language), confer a set of advantages or disadvantages, and often trigger psychological, physiological, and behavioral responses that affect health. These phenomena are therefore relevant to practitioners seeking to treat patients in a racially and ethnically diverse society.

Race and ethnicity affect health through at least two general mechanisms. The first concerns the material advantages or disadvantages conferred by a racially stratified society. Marginalized groups may, for example, have less access to health care resources or they may be segregated in neighborhoods that are less conducive to health. The second mechanism concerns the internal group processes, behaviors, and patterns that develop between members of a race/ethnic group as they interact with each other within the confines of their shared social positions. Here too, these patterns of behavior (something which could be considered *cultural*, the social determinant discussed in its own right in the next section) can be healthy or unhealthy, but they emerge from interactions between people that are distinguished in social space by a shared race/ethnic identity. Before looking at broader data on race/ethnic health outcomes in the United States, however, we use the African American experience as a case study for how both of these mechanisms affect health patterns.

From slavery to segregation through the present day, the health of African Americans has been substantially influenced by their social position in a highly racialized society. For example, while slaves typically received medical care similar to that of the families who owned them, this was not out of benevolence, but rather was an effort to protect the family's investment, just as farmers provide veterinary care to livestock. In keeping with the state of medicine at the time, this care typically involved harsh treatments like bleeding and purging, and slaves were often punished for trying to avoid treatment through concealment or self-care using Caribbean or African traditions brought from their home cultures (Savitt 1978). Free blacks during this time were largely left to care for themselves, particularly because they tended to be too poor to afford care from a formally trained physician. This hindered their access to health care until the growth of hospital-affiliated medical schools began to provide care to the poor. Even then, however, that care doubled as a training opportunity for students, and black patients often feared such hospitals as places of wanton experimentation. Folklore about "night doctors" who would kidnap and kill blacks was widespread (Savitt 1982). Although there were no confirmed accounts of such night doctoring, instances of medical experimentation on black slaves left indelible marks on the collective conscience of African Americans that were later amplified by the exposure of unethical research programs (described below).

---

[4] Racialization is a term used to describe how social life is structured and influenced by race/ethnicity and how one's experiences are significantly affected by race status and social position.

After emancipation, freed blacks were largely marginalized within a segregated social system, including the nascent social institution of health care. Hospitals were largely segregated and, as with the educational system, those dedicated to caring for black patients were underfunded and substandard as a result. In some states, white nurses were prohibited from touching black patients, and nursing and orderly duties often fell to untrained black staff or the patients themselves (Wailoo 2001). A shortage of African American physicians exacerbated problems of access to medical care, particularly after the Flexner Report (see Chapter 2) of 1910 led to the closing of all but two African American medical schools (Howard University in Washington, DC and Meharry Medical College in Nashville, Tennessee). The American Medical Association (AMA) also affirmed the local chapters' rights to deny entry to women and minority physicians no less than twelve times from 1939 to 1968, and many local organizations, particularly in the South, availed themselves of that opportunity. Medical experimentation, including the Tuskegee Syphilis experiment, exacerbated an already established culture of distrust toward health care and medical professionals.

Today, race/ethnic health disparities in the United States reflect much of the legacy of slavery and segregation, and persist through the two mechanisms described above. On the one hand, African Americans are disproportionately less affluent and tend to live in racially segregated neighborhoods that confer a range of health disadvantages (see Chapter 4). They are more likely to be unemployed and less likely to have health insurance than their white counterparts (Kaiser Commission 2013). These factors therefore limit their access to health resources and health care itself. But a culture of marginalization is also a palpable result of this historical narrative. The lack of access to health care, coupled with an historical experience of mistreatment, has created extensive distrust of the health care system. Rates of certain types of complementary and alternative medicine, particularly when those include the use of prayer, are higher among African Americans, just as they were more than a hundred years ago (Barnes et al. 2004; Dubois 1899). African Americans also report higher levels of what we might call *spiritual fatalism*, the idea that one's fate is in God's hands (Abrums 2000; Wasserman et al. 2005).

While we provide a cursory account above, the African American example illustrates how physical or material alienation—laws and policies that segregated and marginalized them; economic factors that priced them out of health care; residential segregation that forced a group of similarly alienated citizens to form strong internal bonds with each other—resulted in particular group tendencies or "ways of being" with respect to medicine. Connecting this historical experience to current disparities, as well as health behavior and care-seeking trends, is an important function of the sociological imagination that may be transposed into a more robust understanding of other groups and other social factors. Moreover, understanding these tendencies is clinically relevant. While we should never assume that an individual blindly carries in some wholesale way the patterns of the groups to which they belong, we certainly want to remain sensitive to those trends and their origins when we do see them. For example, in Marion, Alabama, a small town of only 3,600 residents, a recent tuberculosis outbreak resulted in twenty-six people with active infection (and more than two dozen others infected but asymptomatic; Blinder 2016). This is a rate of infection that is dramatically higher than the rest of the state, actually resembling (or worse than) many developing nations. The overwhelming majority of these individuals were African American, and the high prevalence and rate of contagion have been linked to delayed care-seeking, which means greater contact with others while contagious, and the reticence of patients to give a full report of their contacts to public health authorities (Blinder 2016). Both of these are intimately tied to distrust of health care and governmental agencies among a population that resembles the victims of the Tuskegee study in many ways. Practitioners are on the front lines of detecting these types of epidemiological events and they need to be aware of the social factors that exacerbate the spread of disease.

Awareness of the relationship between race and health has clinical relevance in the treatment of chronic illnesses as well. Take one study examining compliance with prescribed hypertension management. The authors report that African Americans were less compliant in taking their medication, but a significant part of their explanation pertains to *temporal orientation* (Brown & Segal 1996). That is, those individuals who are future-oriented tended to be more compliant than those who are present-oriented. "Compared to more future-oriented respondents, present-oriented people perceived themselves to be less susceptible to the consequences of hypertension [and] believed more in the benefits of home remedies and negative aspects of prescribed medication" (Brown & Segal 1996:350). Importantly, however, African Americans were disproportionately overrepresented among the present-oriented group. Thinking about the history of marginalization from health and health care, it is not difficult to understand how an orientation might emerge as a tendency that undervalues the benefits of physician-prescribed medicines or overvalues home remedies. Across generations, the social influences to which we are resigned can often engender patterned ways of behaving that are handed down, much like other family traditions. Where historically, African Americans have been alternately alienated and abused by the medical system, there exists not only persistent marginalization, but a culture of reticence (if not resistance) that likely will take decades to change.

This reflects an important concept in the social science literature known as the *structural amplification* of disadvantage. Articulated by Ross and colleagues (2001:569), "Structural amplification exists when conditions undermine the personal attributes that otherwise would moderate the undesirable consequences of those conditions. The situation erodes resistance to its own ill effect." In this case, a history of systemic marginalization from health care has promoted, in various ways, poorer health outcomes, but also behavioral and cognitive tendencies that exacerbate rather than alleviate those issues. Importantly, we see the outcomes of this history in a number of interesting social patterns discernible in the mortality statistics for different race/ethnic groups (Table 5.3). Highlighting the ongoing health disparities discussed above, for example, African Americans have substantially higher mortality rates than whites (860.8 compared to 731.0 per 100,000 persons). To state these numbers in more consumable terms, they illustrate that, at 2013 rates, out of every 10,000 African Americans, 86 of them will die in a given year, while out of every 10,000 whites, 73 will die.

Other interesting patterns are worth briefly mentioning here as well. For example, despite having disproportionately high rates of mortality across most

TABLE 5.3 Age-Adjusted Death Rates by Sex and Race/Ethnicity, 2013

Cause of Death	All Persons	White	Black or African American	American Indian or Alaska Native	Asian or Pacific Islander	Hispanic or Latino
			Age-Adjusted Death Rate per 100,000 Population			
All causes............................	731.9	731.0	860.8	591.7	405.4	535.4
Diseases of heart.................	169.6	168.2	210.4	120.6	92.8	121.2
Cerebrovascular diseases......	36.2	34.9	49.0	24.6	29.4	29.6
Malignant neoplasms............	163.2	163.7	189.2	110.2	100.5	114.5
Chronic lower respiratory diseases........	42.1	44.8	29.5	30.8	13.6	18.7
Influenza and pneumonia........	15.9	15.8	16.7	15.0	15.0	13.2
Chronic liver disease and cirrhosis........	10.2	10.7	7.3	24.8	3.3	14.0
Diabetes mellitus..................	21.2	19.4	38.4	34.1	15.8	26.3
Alzheimer's disease...............	23.5	24.4	20.1	12.7	11.1	17.7
Human immunodeficiency virus (HIV)............	2.1	1.2	8.9	1.3	0.4	2.1
Unintentional injuries............	39.4	41.9	32.6	47.1	15.2	26.9
Nephritis, nephrotic syndrome, and nephrosis............	13.2	12.1	25.0	11.4	8.1	11.1
Suicide...............................	12.6	14.2	5.4	11.7	5.9	5.7
Homicide.............................	5.2	3.1	17.8	5.3	1.5	4.5

Source: National Center for Health Statistics (NCHS). (2015). *Health, United States, 2014: With Special Feature on Adults Aged 55–64.* Hyattsville, MD: U.S. Department of Health & Human Services, Centers for Disease Control & Prevention.

causes of death, African Americans have disproportionately low rates of death on other measures. Suicide rates among African Americans remain substantially lower than among whites (though they have risen among younger cohorts). While there are many explanations, two of the most convincing suggest that higher levels of spirituality and high levels of in-group social ties function as protective mechanisms (Willis et al. 2003). First, the same phenomenon of spiritual fatalism that works against actions that might have healthy consequences in the distant future may also promote a resignation, if not resilience, to psychological stress and strain. Second, while residential segregation limits access to health care resources, it simultaneously may promote greater development of *bonding* social capital,[5] the connections of social support within one's own social groups, including neighborhood (Gittell & Vidal 1998; Woolcock & Narayan, 2000). Thus, while African Americans may have limited access to some health resources, ironically they may also, by virtue of their collective disfranchisement, have strong ties to family and community, which represent important psychosocial supports that buffer against suicide. Both of these examples highlight the complex and multifactorial nature of the connection between race/ethnicity and health. The same phenomenon may be simultaneously healthy and unhealthy depending on the condition we are examining. Nowhere are these complex dynamics more clear than with the Hispanic paradox (Markides & Coreil 1986).

The Hispanic paradox refers to a phenomenon discernible in the mortality data in Table 5.3, where "Hispanics, as a group, have mortality (but not morbidity) outcomes equal or surprisingly better than non-Hispanics in the United States, even though they rank low in most socioeconomic indicators" (Franzini et al. 2002:280). That is, despite disadvantages like poverty, residential segregation, and a lack of other socioeconomic resources that would suggest mortality rates similar to those of African Americans, the data show that Hispanics, specifically those of Mexican American descent in the American Southwest, tend to fare better than whites (535.4 compared to 731.0 per 100,000 persons). Epidemiologically, this group fares better even than the non-Hispanic white population. But socioeconomically, they are closer to other less advantaged minority groups like African Americans. This is paradoxical because it defies the SES-health pattern on indicators like heart disease, stroke, and cancer (the three leading sources of mortality in the United States), as well as infant mortality and life expectancy.

There are a number of explanations for this phenomenon, each illuminating the various complex roles that race and ethnicity as social factors play in influencing health. There are two different migration-related theories for explaining the low mortality among Hispanics (Franzini et al. 2002). The *healthy migrant hypothesis* suggests that only the healthiest Hispanics are able to migrate to the United States in the first place. Alternatively, the *Salmon bias hypothesis* suggests that Hispanic migrants tend to return to their countries of origin as they approach death, thereby lowering the recorded mortality rate in the United States. There are data supporting both hypotheses, but these only partially explain the paradox. Notably, the Hispanic

[5]We can articulate two distinct forms of social capital: *bridging* and *bonding*. The former refers to the number and strength of social ties that one has toward individuals in groups other than one's own, while the latter refers to the number and strength of social ties that one has within one's own groups.

paradox also holds for *infant* mortality, which is roughly 10% lower among children born to Mexican immigrant women, suggesting that neither migration hypothesis tells the whole story (Hummer et al. 2007). Other explanations focus on culture and lifestyle, including low rates of smoking among women, strong family ties, and a well-developed cultural norm of helping others, including caring for elderly family members. Interestingly, however, once the protective effects of culture, lifestyles, social support, and group cohesion begin to break down with increasing *acculturation*,[6] the health advantages of this demographic group erode, especially among members of the next generation (Adelman 2008).

Clearly many of these patterns could be articulated as cultural phenomena instead of matters of race/ethnicity per se. The boundaries between the two are difficult to navigate, because the characteristics associated with race/ethnicity have significant social meanings and implications in a racialized society. Thus, what gives race/ethnicity its significance is that it results in shared experiences that confer widely shared sets of knowledge and understanding. What is clear, however, is that the propensity to divide ourselves socially and geographically along race/ethnic boundaries generates a number of health-related influences in the United States. These can be good or bad for health, and in fact, can be both at the same time. But importantly, clinicians should understand that the prominence of race/ethnicity in patients' lives and experiences, particularly those from underrepresented minority groups, is related to a host of social factors affecting relationships, resources, and expectations. While one should never assume that individual members of different race/ethnic groups necessarily represent all or even some of these dynamics, knowledge of the social determinants of health can sensitize practitioners, making them aware of important social but health-related information they otherwise might overlook.[7]

Culture

Culture is another powerful social determinant of health, and one that intersects virtually all others. While the meaning varies across disciplines and conceptual perspectives, in very simple terms we may define *culture* as a "shared understanding"—pertaining to everything around the individual in a particular time and place that holds meaning or significance. Note that cultural differences need not refer to vast geographical distances across countries and continents. Rather, analyses of culture and health also pertain to differences among subgroups of a community or country (e.g., North and South, or rural and urban). We can also distinguish *material* and *nonmaterial* culture. Cockerham (2013) illustrates this distinction by describing culture as knowledge and ways of living transmitted from one generation to the next, including abstract ideas, norms, habits, customs, and rituals (i.e., nonmaterial), as well as artifacts, food, dress, housing, art, music, automobiles, and so on (i.e., material). The shared understanding that constitutes culture affects health in numerous ways, shaping, for example, how cultural

---

[6]This term refers to "the process whereby one culture group adopts the beliefs and practices of another" (Guttman 1999:175).
[7]We will return to the notion of "sensitizing concepts" in the concluding chapter of this book.

groups think about the body, health, and disease, along with the practices that may be better or worse for health. As a result, health outcomes clearly reflect cultural patterns. Quah (2014:926) goes further to suggest that the role of culture in health matters is central:

> Practically all social science research on health and illness in the twenty-first century acknowledges the influence of culture on health-related behavior and attitudes. We have advanced from the early assumption that culture was one of several predictors of health behavior. Today we know that culture is not just one of many factors associated with health, but is the context within which health behavior unfolds.

Put another way, culture is so pervasive and influences so many factors that in turn affect health—residential patterns, social support, dietary practices, religious affiliations, spiritual practices, and so on—that it arguably underlies or intersects all other social determinants.

Drawing together work from a variety of sources, Quah (2014) summarizes the effects of culture across three categories of health-related behaviors: preventative behavior, illness behavior, and sick-role behavior. *Preventative health behavior* "refers to the actions of a person that believes he or she is healthy for the purpose of preventing illness" (Quah 2014:929; see also Kasl & Cobb 1966). A person's subjective evaluation of their own health will obviously affect their likelihood of adopting preventative health measures. Because the idea of "health" is so closely tied to values and norms, there are often significant cultural variations in the ways that people evaluate their own health status. Therefore, culture may strongly influence these types of health behaviors, because shared understandings about health and disease vary across cultural groups.

Next, *illness behavior* "refers to the actions of a person that feels ill, for the purpose of defining the illness and seeking a solution" (Quah 2014:930). What people tend to do when they start feeling sick; the way that they recognize, define, and respond to symptoms; and the meaning that they attach to them, all vary across culture. Two classic examples include Mark Zborowski's (1952) analysis of pain responses among Jewish, Italian, and "Old American" (i.e., white, American-born, and Protestant) patients in a New York City hospital, and Irving Zola's (1966) comparison of American patients at two Boston hospitals of Irish, Italian, and Anglo-Saxon descent in differentially expressing their symptoms (Cockerham 2013, 2016). Zborowski demonstrated significant variations in pain responses, with Jewish and Italian patients displaying greater sensitivity toward pain and a propensity to dramatize the experience of pain in the hospital setting when compared with Old Americans, despite similar ailments. This study also described how Jewish and Italian subjects diverged in the ways that they respond to and communicate pain in the home setting, and in attitudes toward pain and in doctor–patient interactions pertaining to their discomfort. Similarly, Zola found that Americans of Irish descent were likely to deny or minimize their symptoms, Italians tended to dramatize them, and Anglo-Saxons discussed their symptoms in a more calm and detached manner. In all, culture very clearly frames the ways that individuals define, respond to, and communicate their symptoms and discomfort with providers and others around them (Twaddle 1969).

Sick-role behavior refers to actions of people that view themselves as ill, for the purpose of getting well (Parsons 1951; Quah 2014; see also Chapter 7). Illness behavior typically comes before sick-role behavior, with the latter including elements of responding to symptoms as well as seeking what the individual deems "technically competent" help. Here, culture shapes who or what the sick person considers the most well-suited source of guidance, help, treatment, and so on (i.e., a certified health professional, a faith healer, a folk healer, etc.). In this way, culture influences the nature and structure of provider–patient interaction, including how the interaction is conducted and who is involved. Similarly, "just as cultural variations are observed among sick people searching for help from healing experts (whether traditional or modern), so the seeking of emotional and social support and the presence and quality of informal social support from family and friends also vary across cultures" (Quah 2014:931). As a result of such robust, consistent, and far-reaching research findings, there is a distinct need for health professionals to cultivate a sense of cultural competence in patient care and provider–patient interaction, not to mention interprofessional interaction and communication as well (these issues will be further elaborated in Chapters 9 and 10).

Two other examples also very clearly illustrate the effects of culture on health and disease. The first is the story of Roseto, where Bruhn and Wolf (1979) provide compelling evidence of a relationship between cardiovascular and mental health, on the one hand, and the culture of an Italian-American community in east-central Pennsylvania. Bruhn and Wolf confirmed a local physician's observation that the rate of heart attacks among Rosetans remained remarkably low when compared to rates among all Americans: 1 per 1,000 males and 0.6 per 1,000 females in Roseto versus 3.5 per 1,000 males and 2.09 per 1,000 females in the United States. Even the rates for two nearby communities (Bangor and Nazareth) were substantially higher, more closely approximating the national rates, even though those communities also included many Italians, and even relatives of Rosetans and many persons born in Roseto that moved away at an earlier age with their parents. In other words, it seemed as though there was something special about Roseto itself. The subsequent fifteen-year study by Bruhn and Wolf (1979) compared medical histories, physical examinations, and laboratory tests among Rosetans and members of the two neighboring communities to explain these vast differences, which persisted even amidst risk factors like greater obesity among Rosetans.

Further examination of dietary habits revealed that Rosetans ate at least as much animal fat as residents of Bangor and Nazareth, and the prevalence of hypertension and serum cholesterol concentration were similar in all three locales. There was also little divergence in smoking and exercise behaviors in the three towns, and the researchers were also able to eliminate genetic factors as valid explanations. In other words, the widely accepted risk factors for heart disease did not explain Roseto's dramatically reduced prevalence. As Bruhn and Wolf (1979:ix) note, "One striking feature did set Roseto apart from its neighbors, however, namely its culture, which reflected tenaciously held Old World values and customs." Among other differences, the researchers found that family and community relationships were stronger and more central to life in Roseto:

Our first sociological study of Roseto revealed that crises and problems were coped with jointly by family members with support from relatives and friends. Following a death in the family, interfamilial differences were forgotten, and the bereaved received food and money from relatives and friends, who at times temporarily assumed responsibility for the care of the children of the bereaved. When financial problems arose, relatives and friends rallied to the aid of the family, and in instances of abrupt, extreme financial loss the community itself assumed responsibility for helping the family. Personal and family problems were usually worked out with the help of other clan members and often the priest. The elderly were cared for in the homes of their kin and were usually institutionalized only when extreme physical and mental deterioration prohibited further home care. (Bruhn & Wolf 1979:42)

Bruhn and Wolf (1979:42–43) also identified other elements of community culture including the "maintenance of close family ties, the security derived from their religion, and the knowledge that the respected people in the community are on their side. These attitudes are considered essential in coping with family crises. 'When you have these things,' one woman said, 'then you can carry your cross.' " As another Rosetan explained (Bruhn & Wolf 1979:41), "People in other places live too fast. It's nice and quiet around here. People around here are friendly. I like the people all sociable and with a good heart, religious, like a big family all raised together. Where else can you go where your friends and relatives all help out in time of trouble? Everyone trusts everyone else."

Contrast this cultural milieu with contemporary life for most people in the United States, a fast-paced and highly mobile society where individuals are less likely to live close to family members, know their neighbors intimately, or socialize with groups nested in the communities where they actually live. Sociologist John Brueggemann (2010:3) goes so far as to equate contemporary American culture with Mount Everest's "death zone," the threshold beyond which human (and most other) life is unsustainable, and where if you try to go further when it is time to turn around and descend, or even stop to help a fellow climber, the consequences could be catastrophic:

Several aspects of the Death Zone make it a useful metaphor ... I am talking about unforgiving conditions in which sacrificing one's own interests for another is extremely costly, and split-second decisions have vital consequences. To reach our goals in such circumstances, we must be utterly committed, disciplined, and focused. To get "there," we need to block out all distractions along the way, even worthy ones like taking care of someone in need. Such a thin line separates winners from losers that we dare not gamble being on the wrong side ... For many, the risk and allure inspire total devotion. And for anyone who wants to be in the game tomorrow there is no space for altruism ... The frenzied pursuit of the next big achievement blinds us... We see the "Everest psychology" manifest in our daily attempts to not just keep up with but beat out the Joneses. If I can just get in to the right school, find the right mate, land the right job, buy the right house. The elusive summit is always within sight but just out of reach ... I may keep long hours at work with some awareness that I do not need the money or other rewards and my family does need me. I may grasp that my burning ambition and narrow focus are costing me friends, health, balance, and perspective ... nevertheless, I must proceed to the peak. Higher. Better. More.

Indeed, research suggests that the health consequences of such a culture are toxic, while slower-paced, noncompetitive, and slower-to-change environments appear to significantly promote longevity (see Adelman 2008; Cockerham et al. 2000).

The second example illustrating the effects of culture on health involves the prevalence of diabetes among American Indians, most notably the Pima tribe in the Southwestern United States. The 2013 mortality statistics presented in Table 5.3 illustrate a very high mortality rate from diabetes of 34.1 per 100,000 persons among American Indian/Alaskan Natives, a figure that actually represents a sizable decline from ten years earlier when the rate was over 50. But diabetes was almost nonexistent in the population before the nineteenth century when the Anglo population began to expand into the area, developing mining and agricultural operations (Smith-Morris 2004). Eventually the Gila River was dammed to supply these developments, cutting off irrigation to the Pima further downstream, who relied on subsistence farming supported by the Gila. The crops traditionally farmed were then replaced with government rations containing processed foods that were high in fat and carbohydrates.

Of course, agricultural collapse led to greater reliance on unhealthy foods for survival, and replacing the intensive labor of farming with a more sedentary lifestyle (Smith-Morris 2004). These shifts, in turn, promoted rising rates of diabetes. But perhaps more interesting are the cultural transformations that have exacerbated these developments. Driving through the Southwest today, you will likely see signs for Indian fried bread (usually drizzled with honey), something sold to tourists under the auspices of traditional Native American fare. But these "Indian Tacos," as they are sometimes called, have become traditional cultural emblems in the wake of the resource limitations pressed onto the culture, particularly where government rations contained flour, shortening, honey, and the like. Moreover, the prevalence of diabetes itself has created a widespread expectation among the group that diabetes is inevitable. In the documentary *Unnatural Causes* (2008), Dr. Don Warne, a physician who treats members of the Pima community, explains:

> When we have a population of people that feel disenfranchised or disconnected from tradition and from hope for a healthy future, that's going to have an impact on social behavior and whether or not people live in a healthy way. So not only is there unhealthy components of diabetes, there also is so much diabetes, that what we've seen is a culture of diabetes. And when people grow up in a community where their grandparents, their parents, aunts, uncles, siblings, even children have all gotten diabetes... if you have a non-community member who's a health care professional telling them that this is preventable, that might not be very believable ... In my own medical practice I've had quite a number of patients who say things like "I don't have diabetes *yet*." And what are they telling me? That they believe they are going to get diabetes. And when you think about things historically and things from a cultural perspective, really the culture of diabetes has created generations of people who believe it's inevitable.

This fatalism of course mitigates efforts to take up healthier lifestyles that might prevent diabetes. Thus, in the example of the Pima, we can see how sociopolitical forces create physical and material changes to social environments, which in turn worsen health. But more importantly, we can see how over time, as health behaviors become habituated, they can become part of cultural traditions and then self-perpetuate (we will return to this process in Chapter 6 in discussing the notion of *habitus*).

At an epidemiological and community level, we can see how culture clearly impacts health insofar as cultural perspectives include lifestyles and behavior that can be better or worse for health. But culture matters for health professionals at a clinical level as well, and cultural competence should be an integral element of training, particularly as a component of any patient-centered clinical encounter. It matters because communicating across cultural boundaries can be challenging, but a good first step entails recognizing that patients, by virtue of their cultural traditions and practices, may have radically different views about the body, health, and disease. Understanding these is a prerequisite to working with patients on health-related goals (see further discussion in Chapter 6 about health behavior and stages of change, as well as Chapter 9 concerning patient–provider communication). It is also important because treatment goals should allow space for, and attempt to align with, cultural traditions and practices. Prescribing significant lifestyle changes for individuals whose cultural habits might impede or prevent them from making those changes will not likely be effective. This certainly creates a challenge for clinicians. But remaining conscious of the various influences emanating from culture promotes the important recognition of what might underlie or exacerbate patient complaints, and can also inspire creative and well-targeted treatment plans that are feasible for patients to adopt, given their frameworks of understanding (i.e., their culture).

Conclusion: A Matrix of Inequalities

In this and the previous chapter, we outline a number of social factors that strongly influence health and well-being today, including SES, neighborhood disadvantage, age, gender, race, ethnicity, culture, and others. As mentioned above, social factors have always been important in health matters, but as modernization, public health, and health care delivery have slowly reigned in the widespread effects of many major infectious diseases, many of the same social factors have become critically important in the contemporary chronic disease era. After modern advances in public health, biomedicine, and technology enabled us to avoid or eradicate many diseases, along with a large proportion of premature mortality, social influences and conditions are now dramatically more important in matters of both individual and population health (Link 2008), as well as health care delivery and clinical practice (Wasserman & Hinote 2012).

We chose to deconstruct these various concepts over the last two chapters in order to fully unpack each in a way that emphasizes their true significance, as well as their potential health effects. Although a useful didactic exercise, it is somewhat misleading to think of these factors in isolation from one another. After all, humans are simultaneously affected by various factors like SES, living and working conditions, age, gender, race, ethnicity, and culture throughout their lives, relationships, interactions, and experiences. During the course of our discussions thus far, we have continually emphasized the significance of epidemiological changes toward greater *complexity* and *multidimensionality*, and what those shifts mean for health providers and patients. This also means that the ways that we conceptualize risk and vulnerability in patient populations must match that complex and multidimensional nature of health and disease today. As Hankivsky (2012:1713) explains, central to the notion of intersectionality is:

> the idea that human lives cannot be reduced to single characteristics; human experiences cannot be accurately understood by prioritizing any one single factor or constellation of factors; social categories such as race/ethnicity, gender, class, sexuality, and ability are socially constructed, fluid, and flexible; and social locations are inseparable and shaped by the interacting and mutually constituting social processes and structures that are influenced by both time and place.

What is needed, then, is a way to think about how these factors converge and intersect.

A more comprehensive understanding of health disparities, and the patients deeply affected by them, necessitates an intersectional perspective able to explain the interactions and overlap of many different human characteristics—one that is able to focus more clearly on the many relational contexts that shape both individual lives and the health of larger groups. *Intersectionality* refers to an approach that emphasizes the complex nature of social positions and experiences in understanding the needs and outcomes of vulnerable populations. While this approach is not entirely new in the social and behavioral sciences (Collins 1990), its application represents a somewhat novel approach within clinical and epidemiological contexts. Even though intersectional approaches to health and health care are in their early stages of development, they represent a way of thinking that is of great value to clinicians and health professionals (Hankivsky 2012). Such an intersectional approach to clinical practice rests upon a number of core ideas (Hankivsky & Cormier 2009:8–9):

- Individuals' social lives are complex and dimensions of social life cannot be delineated into separate measurable elements.
- It is important not to assume that all members of a single social group share similar experiences, perspectives, and needs.
- Social categories such as race, ethnicity, gender, class, geography, and so on are fluid and flexible.

Considering these factors enables practitioners to see how social conditions come together to create a specific matrix of risk within specific patient populations. In thinking this way, we might also see the social determinants of health as a *matrix of inequalities*, meaning that different conditions, including membership in different SES, age, gender, cultural, and race/ethnic groups, amplifies or attenuates health-related social influences not in isolation, but in tandem. For example, the disadvantages faced by African Americans might be attenuated, though not totally eclipsed, by the advantages associated with higher SES.

There are many research examples that illustrate intersectional approaches to health, demography, epidemiology, and the like. For example, some point to the clear intersection of SES, age, and race/ethnicity in the rising mortality rates among young and middle-aged white Americans, particularly those with lower educational attainment (Case & Deaton 2015; Kolata 2015; Kolata & Cohen 2016). This mortality is not the result of the leading causes of death in the United States (i.e., heart disease and cancer) or complications associated with the most common chronic conditions (i.e., diabetes, hypertension, overweight/obesity). Instead, it is an epidemic fueled by suicides and substance abuse, particularly alcoholic liver disease and overdoses of heroin and prescription opioids. This exemplifies how the social advantages associated with being white must be understood as always in tension with other factors that might confer any number of countervailing disadvantages.

Further, medical sociologists William Cockerham and Brian Hinote contextualize the study of health lifestyles amidst the many intersections of gender, SES, age, culture, and history in examining health trends and excess mortality in Eastern Europe and the countries of the former Soviet Union (Cockerham 1999; Cockerham et al. 2006a; Hinote & Webber 2012; Hinote et al. 2009a, 2009b). Their historical and quantitative analyses elucidate the ways that social factors and conditions converge to produce aggregate epidemiological trends, most closely linked to deeply embedded patterns of alcohol and tobacco use, and dietary practices. For example, there appear to be cumulative health disadvantages associated with being a working-class, middle-aged man in Russia and other Soviet and post-Soviet societies, such that the additive effects of membership in these categories and others often promote increasingly destructive lifestyle practices and dramatically lower longevity. The authors (Hinote et al. 2009b) extend this line of inquiry to health lifestyles among women amid these same intersectional conditions and contexts as definitions of gender have transformed following the collapse of the Soviet Union.

The recent American Heart Association (AHA) statement on Social Determinants of Risk and Outcomes for Cardiovascular Disease (CVD) offers one final example through which to emphasize the significance of intersectional approaches to engaging the social determinants of health. Havranek et al. highlight their general importance, writing:

> [A]lthough we have traditionally considered CVD the consequence of certain modifiable and nonmodifiable physiological, lifestyle, and genetic risk factors, we must now broaden the focus to incorporate a third arm of risk, the social determinants of health. Failure to demonstrate awareness of this third dynamic will result in a growing burden of CVD, especially in those with the least means to engage in the healthcare system. (2015:888)

The statement carefully outlines that the prevalence of heart disease is expected to increase by about 10% between 2010 and 2030 in the United States—a shift resulting from an aging population but also a dramatic increase in obesity, hypertension, diabetes, and physical activity over the past twenty-five years. The most likely explanations for these trends, the report asserts, include "changes in societal and environmental conditions that have led to changes in diet and physical activity" (Havranek et al. 2015:873), and "at present, the most significant opportunities for reducing death and disability from CVD in the United States lie with addressing the social determinants of cardiovascular outcomes" (Havranek et al. 2015:874). Perhaps most importantly, however, the AHA statement pointedly addresses the ways that social determinants of health "cluster at the *intersections* of social, economic, environmental, and interpersonal forces" (Havranek et al. 2015:874, emphasis added). Noting that population-level approaches are indeed valuable in addressing these factors and their ill effects, the AHA statement also endorses continued attempts to intervene at the individual-level as well. This includes the work of clinical practitioners, who can adopt an intersectional approach to providing effective, patient-centered care amidst the shifting tides of health and disease today.

CHAPTER 5 ACTIVITY

Historical Memory, Inherited Culture, and Distrust of Health Care: The Tuberculosis Outbreak in Marion, Alabama

The town of Marion is the county seat of Perry County, Alabama, and sits about an hour west of the state capital, Montgomery. Like many small rural towns, its population has declined nearly 25% over the last three decades, down from 4,600 to about 3,500 residents in 2013. Perry County is relatively poor, with a median household income of $25,528, compared to $53,482 for the United States generally. Only 69.6% of Perry County residents who are 25 and older have a high school degree and only about 9.1% have a college degree, whereas nationally, 86.3% of those 25 and older hold a high school degree and 29.3% have a college degree (United States Census Bureau 2016). Additionally, 22.6% of those under 65 in the county are disabled (compared to 8.5% nationally) and a 2014 survey showed more than 15% remained uninsured (compared to 12.0% nationally). About two-thirds of the residents of Marion are African American.

Early in 2014, physician and public health officials in Marion began to see cases of tuberculosis (TB), and within a year, more than twenty cases of active TB had been diagnosed in Marion, with six other cases in the state linked to the city. By that time, three Marion residents had died of the disease. Financial incentives for screening led to the identification of at least three more cases of active TB and by early February 2016, after more than 2,000 Marion residents had been screened, there were just over 150 residents who tested positive for TB exposure (though not the active disease).

The rate of active TB in Marion is about 253 per 100,000, which is greater than the rate of the disease in places such as Afghanistan, Cameroon, Ethiopia, and Vietnam (Brooks 2016; World Bank 2016). By comparison, the rate of active TB in the United States is about 3 per 100,000 persons.

But the story of the Marion tuberculosis outbreak does not begin with the residents who were infected. The social and historical contexts of the region significantly shaped the contours of this epidemiological event. In particular, a history of racial oppression against African Americans constitutes a significant part of the history of the city and the historical memory of its residents. Like many places in the South, many black slaves in and around Marion before the Civil War became its indentured sharecroppers afterward. The city also sits less than 80 miles from Montgomery, where the Freedom Riders were severely beaten at the Greyhound bus station in 1961 by a violent mob, and just over 100 miles from Tuskegee, where 399 black men with syphilis were intentionally not treated as part of a government study (see Chapter 11). Less than 30 miles from Selma, Marion occupies a prominent place in American civil rights history. The shooting death of Jimmie Lee Jackson, a civil rights activist and Marion resident, by Alabama State Trooper James Fowler served as a key impetus for the Selma to Montgomery march and Jackson was eulogized by Martin Luther King, whose wife, Coretta Scott King, was born and raised in Marion. In only one clear indication of how these historical events still hold significant meaning for the people of Marion, and Alabama generally, it was not until 2007 that Fowler was indicted for the killing. This is a community truly still reeling from its racial history.

So when there was an outbreak of TB in Marion, the social and cultural history of the area, combined with its relative poverty, created just the right conditions for rapid transmission. While African Americans comprised about two-thirds of the city's population in 2016, the Director of the Alabama Department of Public Health noted, "All the cases in Perry County involve black people" (Lucas 2016)." As Alan Blinder (2016) notes, "Many people in Marion, where about 63 percent of the residents are black, said they knew little about what had happened in Tuskegee, but they often said their wariness of medical professionals had been passed on through generations." In addition to the general wariness of getting medical care, the solicitations for testing by government agencies may particularly trigger concerns. Beyond getting screened and seeking care, both of which are necessary to stop the spread of an epidemic, individuals may be reluctant to disclose the names of others with whom they have had contact for a variety of reasons (Blinder 2016).

Discussion Questions

1. Discuss the various ways in which the social and cultural factors in Marion promoted its susceptibility to this epidemic.

   Helpful Hint: Along with the socioeconomic state of affairs and the racial history of the area, think about factors such as residential and social segregation.

2. How might other factors like age and gender amplify or attenuate the various factors related to TB contagion in Marion?

   Helpful Hint: Think about whether older people versus younger people or men versus women might be more or less at risk and the various reasons this might be the case.

3. While the financial incentives for getting screened appear to have been successful, what longer-term changes and interventions in the social dynamics of the area might prevent future epidemiological crises such as this?

4. As a practitioner in Marion, what might you do to facilitate trust and rapport among your patient population?

Health Behavior and Lifestyles

LEARNING OBJECTIVES

After reading this chapter, students should be able to

- Explain the various shifts underlying renewed interest in health behavior and lifestyles across multiple disciplines.

- Define health behavior and health lifestyles.

- Demonstrate the significance of health behaviors in terms of epidemiology, health care delivery and policy, and clinical practice.

- Discuss the significance of *habitus* in patient care and clinical decision-making.

As with other areas of health and illness, current considerations of health behavior largely revolve around (1) an evolving definition of health, (2) the epidemiological transition, and (3) the clinical challenges emerging from these important shifts. These transformations (emerging from the period called late modernity; see Chapter 2) compel us to rethink how we define health and therefore what constitutes health behavior. In the past, comparatively simpler, infectious diseases were primarily responsible for most morbidity and mortality. As a result, health was typically conceptualized in a binary way, where individuals were either sick or well. In that landscape, health behavior largely referred to activity undertaken by healthy people to prevent illness (see Kasl & Cobb 1966). Today, that conceptualization remains important, but has become outdated. Health today reflects more of a continuum of functionality and satisfaction across multiple domains of human experience, and contemporary disease threats are largely chronic (and certainly more complex). We must therefore reframe and expand the ways that we think about health behavior to match that complexity. Accordingly, the notion of health behavior today is a broader and more complicated definition, referring to activity undertaken by people for the purpose of maintaining or enhancing their health, preventing health problems, or achieving a positive body image (Cockerham 2012).

This definition opens up significantly the range of behaviors that deserve exploration in the next few sections. Indeed, the topic is so vast that we could make it the focus of its own book (and many have done so). But in this chapter, we first discuss the significance of contemporary health behavior, and explain how health behavior and lifestyles are among the strongest predictors of morbidity and premature mortality today. These phenomena are certainly a matter of concern for individual patients and the professionals working alongside them, but like other social determinants of health discussed in Chapters 4 and 5, they are also linked to broader resource and opportunity structures, group socialization and membership, and ways of perceiving the world and our choices within it. As a result, understanding how health behavior and lifestyle patterns emerge necessitates accounting for both individual choice (a *micro*-approach) as well as the surrounding influences always impinging in one way or another upon those choices (a *macro*-approach). We therefore integrate individualist approaches to understanding health behavior with more contemporary structural explanations of health lifestyles, both of which help us explain health behavior across various groups. Doing so can also help practitioners think more deeply and critically as they guide patient care in ways that account for the social influences constraining or enabling particular behavioral choices. Finally, we conclude by emphasizing the clinical significance of health behavior and lifestyles, and by discussing ways clinicians can use this information to carry out their work more effectively. After all, the shifting health landscape of late modernity not only compels us to reconsider earlier notions of health behavior, but it is also responsible for many of the most prominent challenges practitioners will face in their work, including the notoriously complex task of helping patients change unhealthy habits.

A Renewed Emphasis on Health Behavior

Health today is not merely the absence of something undesirable (like disease or injury). Instead, it is a multidimensional concept entailing a more complete sense of not just physical but also emotional, social, and psychological well-being. The concept of health now expands beyond a default category defined by the absence of sickness to include those various, more subjective dimensions of well-being. As such, it also becomes something of an achievement—an ideal type toward which one deliberately and consciously works, or conversely, if they neglect it, risk the chance of disease or early death. These developments encourage individuals to assume greater responsibility for their own health and bodies, often by *consuming* products in pursuit of various, often somewhat subjectively defined, ideals of health (e.g., buying organic food, memberships at fitness clubs, etc.). Importantly, however, not everyone is equally able to assume that responsibility. For example, insofar as achieving health increasingly requires various practices of consumption in the chronic illness era, it is more significantly affected by socioeconomic status (SES). While social factors have always shaped disease in some way, they become even more consequential after the epidemiological transition, when health behavior and lifestyles serve as one of the most important mechanisms through which macro-level social conditions such as class ultimately affect individual health outcomes (Cockerham 2013; Hinote 2015; Wasserman & Hinote 2011).

   Health behavior can refer to any number of particular actions oriented toward the prevention of negative health conditions, the promotion of positive health and appearance, or the maintenance or management of a health or disease state. This broadly includes dietary practices, exercise, and other behavioral choices intended to prevent disease or maintain a particular state of functioning. This might also refer to specialized dietary regimens, workout routines, or herbal, vitamin, or nutrition supplements adopted to promote a healthy appearance or body image. Or it can also highlight the ways that we maintain some level of social and physical functioning amidst disease itself, like managing diabetes, high cholesterol, heart disease, hypertension, and so forth. *Health lifestyles* refer to collective patterns of these particular behaviors. For example, choosing a salad over fast food for dinner represents a health behavior. But the tendency to make a dietary decision, in conjunction with other health-related choices, over time constitutes a health lifestyle. As a result, it is no coincidence that interest in health behavior and lifestyles has surged in recent decades, precisely because the most significant health risks (including heart disease, diabetes, etc.) are so strongly tied to health behaviors and lifestyles, with broad and costly implications for patients, professionals, health care delivery, and social policy.

From an epidemiological perspective, lifestyles are the strongest predictors of disease and premature mortality for most chronic conditions. Recall from Chapter 4 that the leading modifiable risk factors for cardiovascular disease and stroke (i.e., two of the leading causes of mortality in developed societies) include hypertension, high cholesterol, cigarette smoking, diabetes, poor diet, physical inactivity, overweight, and obesity (Lloyd-Jones et al. 2010). All of these are directly tied to specific behavioral actions that coalesce into lifestyle patterns. Not only are these connected to specific behavioral profiles (e.g., diet, exercise, smoking, etc.), but the risk factors themselves (e.g., overweight/obesity, hypertension, diabetes, etc.) often arise from the repetitive enactment of negative health behaviors. As Yach and colleagues (2004:2616) note, "The current burden of chronic diseases reflects past exposures to these risk factors, and the future burden will be largely determined by current exposures." Health professionals therefore should develop a better understanding of these important sources of morbidity and mortality, as this represents an important step toward addressing disease, disability, and premature death.

Increased attention to health behavior and lifestyles also emerges from the fact that they are directly related to preventing the above-mentioned conditions, and to managing them if they develop. Consuming a balanced diet rich in vitamins and minerals, coupled with regular leisure-time physical activity, healthy social relationships, effective stress management, and other health-promoting factors, reduces the chances of developing high blood pressure, diabetes, obesity, and other conditions. However, if these conditions do indeed emerge, changing our behavior can help manage them effectively. Recent data illustrate the rising prevalence of many of these conditions in the United States. For example, overweight and obesity among men and women increased by about 3%–5% between 2002 and 2012, while nearly one-half of adults with hypertension had uncontrolled high blood pressure by 2012 (NCHS 2015). This dramatically increases their risk of heart attack and stroke. These are only two examples, among many, of significant clinical and public health priorities that are directly related to the preventative and management functions of health behavior.

Understanding why and how people make the decisions that they do is an important part of communicating with patients about their need to reconsider and reorient their behaviors toward more healthy options, and working alongside them to do so. Put another way, in many cases changing behavior is key to avoiding disease or disability or managing a condition if it is present. This seems pretty straightforward: if I continue to engage in X, then I will develop or exacerbate condition Y. Therefore, I should discontinue X to avoid Y. Unfortunately, behavior change is not so simple. We know from earlier chapters that the burden of chronic disease in the United States is not distributed equitably across populations (Bauer et al. 2014). We also know that when distinct disease patterns exist, as good scientists we are compelled to look for causes and explanations. As we will see, behavior change comes down to more than just the choices involved; it also directly relates to the chances that a person can adopt the behavior as part of their larger repertoire of available behavioral options. Moreover, the notion of *choice* itself is not simple or straightforward. Where behaviors are patterned and habituated, we should reconsider what choices really are, particularly where they are often narrowly conceptualized as rational decisions. In short, we must understand that health behavior emerges from a complex, often not fully rational process conditioned by available resources and opportunities (i.e., life chances).

Finally, interest in health behavior and lifestyles has increased because the morbidity and mortality associated with chronic illness are costly, both in terms of lives and healthy years lost, as well as in health care spending. Chronic diseases are now the primary challenge for global health (see Murray et al. 2012; Yach et al. 2004), with noncommunicable conditions responsible for nearly two-thirds of deaths worldwide (WHO 2011). This of course also applies to the United States, where chronic conditions are not only the primary cause of poor health, but also most health care expenditures. About half of American adults report at least one chronic condition, and more than one-quarter report two or more. In 2011, ten of the fifteen leading causes of death in the United States (and seven of the top ten) were chronic conditions, and about 13% of the population had a disability, including nearly half of those age 75 years or older (Bauer et al. 2014). Caring for people with chronic conditions is very costly in the American health care system, which already costs a total of about $3 trillion in 2014 (see Martin et al. 2016; Pear 2015). Additionally, there are also enormous societal costs associated with lost productivity, family instability, stagnant or downward social mobility, and other consequences of disease and disability. An overwhelming proportion of these costs are associated with chronic diseases like heart disease, diabetes, and cancer—diseases directly linked to specific behavioral choices involving smoking, diet, and exercise. Smoking alone is estimated to cost about $190 billion, and obesity is associated with annual health-related economic losses of approximately $150 billion in the United States, with estimates expected to increase in coming decades (Schroder 2014). In summary, researchers, clinicians, and policymakers increasingly focus on health behavior and lifestyles because these phenomena are so closely related to the origins of chronic disease as primary causes of morbidity and mortality; the long-term management of many common conditions; behavior modification as an element of patient care; and steadily increasing costs in an already expensive health care system.

Explaining Health Behavior

As noted above, health today is a multidimensional concept that describes many, often subjective, elements of well-being. Health behavior, in turn, constitutes a broad range of things that we do in order to influence our physical, mental, emotional, psychological, and spiritual selves. Because it constitutes such a wide-ranging and multidimensional set of actions, there are many factors that shape the contours of health behavior. These can be positive or negative and include knowledge, skills, SES, culture, beliefs, attitudes, values, religion, gender, and many more (Cockerham 2005; Hayden 2014). Gochman (1982:169) notes that health behaviors therefore include:

> those personal attributes such as beliefs, expectations, motives, values, perceptions, and other cognitive elements; personality characteristics, including affective and emotional states and traits; and overt behavior patterns, actions and habits that relate to health maintenance, to health restoration and to health improvement.

Gochman (1982:169) adds that this definition also recognizes "that these personal attributes are influenced by, and otherwise reflect family structure and processes, peer group and social factors, and societal, institutional, and cultural determinants." It is clear that health behavior encompasses a wide range of actions (as diverse as tobacco/alcohol use, brushing our teeth, unprotected sex, yoga, dieting, exercise, physician checkups, seatbelt use, etc.), with a wide range of factors that potentially affect these behaviors. Given the complexity of health behavior, therefore, various disciplines tend to study its different aspects more heavily than others. Depending on the disciplinary perspective, we may approach health behavior analytically in at least three ways (Gochman 1988). The first attempts to describe health behaviors as direct causes of disease, illness, or health status. The second approach focuses on how changing these behaviors or some combination of them produces behavioral change and improved health outcomes. And the third analyzes health behaviors as consequences of a variety of personal and social processes, and therefore as phenomena interesting in their own right, worthy of investigation and important to understand.

The interdisciplinary approach of this chapter brings these strands of thinking together, gleaning insights from multiple fields of study and practice, to understand these important health phenomena. In fact, health behavior occupies a prominent position in health education, public health, psychology, sociology, social work, and various health and medical specialties. Fields like psychology traditionally focus on changing individuals (i.e., *micro*-approaches), while disciplines like sociology tend to give closer consideration of broader social, economic, and environmental contexts (i.e., *macro*-approaches). Most however, blend elements of micro- and macro-perspectives of individuals and of social groups, and the emphasis on each (or both) changes over time. For example, health education during the 1970s and 1980s often emphasized individual behaviors as primary determinants of health, thereby neglecting broader social determinants. In a swing back toward the realm of the social, advocates of system-level changes to improve health then pushed for broader conceptualizations of health education and promotion. These calls subsequently moved health education back toward the kind of activism characteristic of early public health movements and their concern with the influences of social, economic, and political forces on health (see Chapter 1). Today, however, there is general consensus that focusing solely on *downstream* (i.e., individual) causes of health and disease to the exclusion of *upstream* (i.e., social, environmental, etc.) factors neglects important elements of health behavior, and therefore misses important opportunities to understand and improve health at both the individual and population levels (Cockerham 2013; Glanz et al. 2015; Link 2008).

Health behavior, therefore, involves phenomena much larger than just individuals and their isolated choices. Of course, there are individual-level predictors of health and disease. But those downstream predictors rarely, if ever, provide a complete picture of the various factors that influence us to behave in certain ways. As a result, they *alone* do not provide a reliable target for health professionals working with patients on healthy changes in behavior. Lifestyles, as collective patterns of health-related behavior (Cockerham 2005, 2013), illustrate this clearly where they tend to coalesce within groups of individuals that share similar characteristics. Applying the logic learned in Chapter 3, this suggests that there may be something about membership in certain groups that affects our tendencies to engage in certain behaviors and to make certain choices among similar sets of available options. Thus, while each person in a group may possess individual characteristics that distinguish them in particular ways from the group itself, their behavioral dispositions still *tend* to emanate from, and reflect, patterns and characteristics of the groups to which they belong. Despite our individuality, then, we are more likely to reflect the behavioral tendencies of the groups to which we belong than we are to deviate significantly from them. Put another way, our groups, and the characteristics and circumstances that define them, strongly influence our behaviors. For health professionals, this means that providing effective, comprehensive patient care today requires considering the larger social contexts and influences that surround the individual and the manners in which she or he makes choices about health behavior, then developing an effective treatment or guidance plan accordingly. We will conclude by elaborating on this insight, but to do so we must first explore several models of health behavior originating in sociology, psychology, public health, health promotion, and related fields.

As noted above, various explanations focus upon multiple levels of analysis along the micro–macro continuum, but all seek to better understand the dynamics of health behavior and contribute to the development of interventions that improve health at the individual and community levels. These explanations tend to differ in their relative emphasis on *cognitive* (i.e., pertaining to thoughts and beliefs) versus *affective* (i.e., pertaining to attitudes and values) determinants and on *individual* versus *environmental* determinants of behavior. Cognitive approaches tend to conceptualize behavior as a result of relatively explicit, rational thought processes, while affective approaches tend to focus more on internalized attitudes and feelings of which even the individuals carrying out particular behaviors themselves might not be fully aware. Additionally, health behavior theories in many disciplines tend to focus on individual behavior (Noar & Zimmerman 2005), while health lifestyle models tend to focus more heavily on social and contextual factors that influence health behavior. We will begin by discussing several prominent micro-approaches to health behavior, before working toward more macro-oriented explanations that consider the broader social contexts of those individual behaviors. Together, all of these models will help you think more deeply and critically about the nature and origins of health behavior and their role in clinical care, and provide tools with which to engage patients.

The Health Belief Model

One of the primary contributions of health psychology involves the development and assessment of models that explain and predict health behavior. Psychological approaches tend to employ a *motivational* component, which refers to the processes underlying an individual's willingness to change their behavior for health benefits. Health behaviors often lack an immediate reward and thereby require considerable effort and self-control. At the same time, health *benefits* are usually not noticeable until some uncertain time in the future, or may not be directly observable at all if there is no compelling proof that the change in behavior is actually responsible for the outcome (De Vries 2014). However, the *costs* of changing to healthier behaviors often are immediate and hard to resist, including cravings, habitual inertia, and giving up on previously entrenched behaviors. Take, for example, a person with a family history of heart disease, which predicts some elevated likelihood that he too will develop heart disease. Imagine then that this person adopts a range of difficult but healthy behaviors and does *not* develop heart disease. Whether or not these behaviors were responsible for avoiding the disease will inevitably remain uncertain. In short, the direct benefits associated with behavior change are difficult to assess. If not already a part of an individual's habituated set of behaviors, change can be characterized as a *cost-benefit analysis*, an approach to health decision-making expressed in the *health belief model* (Hochbaum 1958; Rosenstock 1974; Schroder 2014; Skinner et al. 2015).

At least four major considerations rest at the center of the health belief model: perceived threat, perceived severity, perceived benefits, and perceived barriers (see Fig. 6.1). *Perceived threat* (or perceived susceptibility or vulnerability) refers to the degree to which an individual considers themselves at risk for a specific condition or disorder (e.g., according to symptoms and/or risk factors—chest pain, high cholesterol, hypertension), while *perceived severity* denotes to what degree the condition or disorder is serious and/or life-threatening (e.g., a heart attack or cardiovascular disease). On the other hand, *perceived benefits* refer to the value or usefulness of the potential action for reducing the threat of disease (e.g., of a heart-healthy diet, or exercise), while *perceived barriers* include any negative dimensions of a particular behavior (e.g., financial costs, convenience, changing one's routine). In short, if a person believes (1) that they are susceptible to a negative health outcome, (2) that this outcome will have potentially serious consequences, (3) that some option available to them could help reduce the severity of and/or susceptibility to the condition, and (4) that the expected benefits of enacting that behavioral option outweigh the barriers to doing so, then the health belief model suggests that they are likely to take action to reduce the risk of poor health (Champion & Skinner 2008). As a more recent addition to this model, *self-efficacy* refers to the belief in one's ability to successfully implement and adopt the behavior needed to produce desired outcomes (Bandura 1997). Put simply, behavior is likely to change if the above-mentioned four criteria (1–4) are met, *and* the individual believes they have the ability (i.e., self-efficacy) to overcome barriers to action.

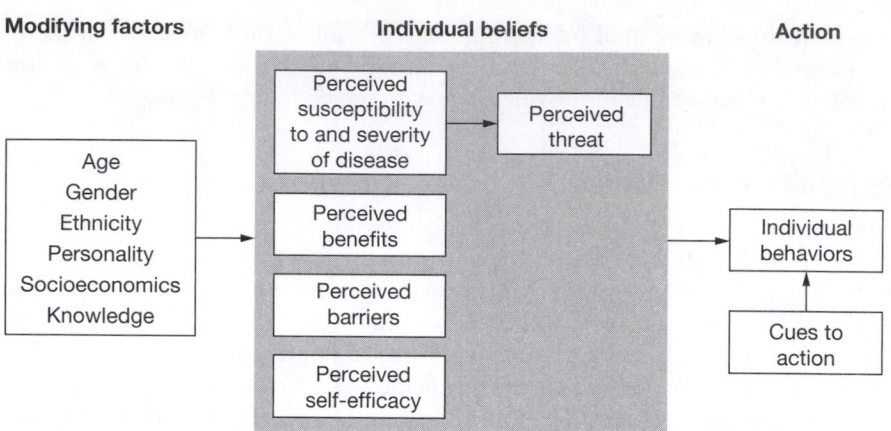

FIG. 6.1 The health belief model.

Source: Champion, Victoria L. & Celette S. Skinner. (2008). "The Health Belief Model." Pp. 45–65 in *Health Behavior: Theory, Research and Practice,* 4th edition. Karen Glanz, Barbara K. Rimer, & K. Viswanath, eds. San Francisco, CA: John Wiley & Sons.

Decisions in the health belief model involve a cost-benefit analysis, where health benefits must outweigh costs, including time, money, effort, loss of pleasure, delayed gratification, and other negative consequences. A great deal of research utilizes the health belief model as a conceptual framework. In particular, the health belief model appears useful for explaining reductions in sexual risk behavior, participation in breast and colorectal cancer screening, adopting a weight-loss diet, smoking behavior, and the like. This approach has been widely employed by researchers, both alone and in combination with other explanations, some of which we explore below (Champion & Skinner 2008; Hochbaum 1958; Rosenstock 1974; Schroder 2014).

Alternative Models

As more research accumulated since the health belief model's introduction in the 1950s, a number of other alternatives emerged with which to analyze and explain health behavior. Perhaps the most influential among them include the *theory of planned behavior* (Ajzen 1991; Ajzen & Driver 1991) and its precursor, the *theory of reasoned action* (Ajzen & Fishbein 1980). Both of these focus on individual *motivation* to engage in specific behaviors based on *expected outcomes,* weighted according to *subjective importance.* Both assume that the best predictor of action is *intention,* which expresses the overall degree of motivation to adopt a behavior (see Fig. 6.2). According to the theory of reasoned action, intention is the result of two components: one's own *attitude toward the behavior* and *subjective norm* (one's perception of others' evaluations of the behavior). For instance, the intent to diet, understood using the theory of reasoned action, is the end of a process of deliberation whereby the individual considers whether it is worthwhile to change their eating habits (the attitude) and whether and to what extent significant others (e.g., family members, peers, and partner) approve or disapprove, which influences how likely they are to support such a change (the subjective norm) (Schroder 2014).

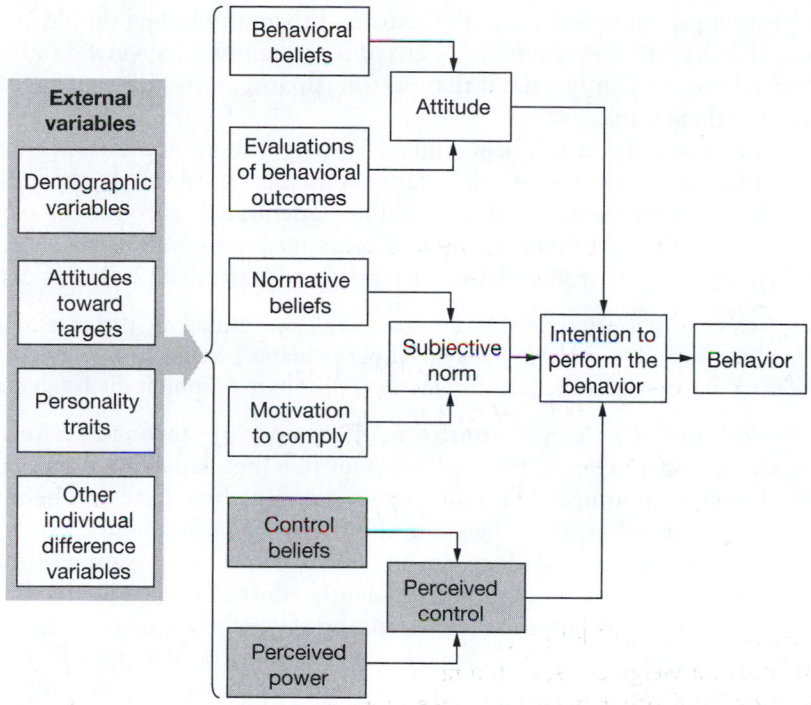

FIG. 6.2 The theory of reasoned action and theory of planned behavior.

Note: Upper light area depicts the theory of reasoned action; the entire figure depicts the theory of planned behavior.

Source: Montaño, Daniel E. & Danuta Kasprzyk. (2008). "Theory of Reasoned Action, Theory of Planned Behavior, and the Integrated Behavioral Model." Pp. 67–96 in *Health Behavior: Theory, Research and Practice*, 4th edition. Karen Glanz, Barbara K. Rimer, & K. Viswanath, eds. San Francisco, CA: John Wiley & Sons.

As we continue to work backward in Figure 6.2, we find that *attitude* is shaped by the individual's beliefs about outcomes or the attributes of performing the behavior (*behavioral beliefs*), weighted by *evaluations* of those outcomes or attributes. Someone who believes that positive outcomes will result from a behavior will tend to have a good attitude toward it and vice versa (Montaño & Kasprzyk 2008). On the other hand, an individual's *subjective norm* is shaped by *normative beliefs* (i.e., whether significant others approve or disapprove), weighted by her or his *motivation to comply* with those others. As Montaño and Kasprzyk (2008:71) point out:

A person who believes that certain referents think she should perform a behavior and is motivated to meet expectations of those referents will hold a positive subjective norm. Conversely, a person who believes that these referents think she should *not* perform the behavior will have a negative subjective norm, and a person who is less motivated to comply with those referents will have a relatively neutral subjective norm.

Put simply, if a person believes that those around them think they should engage in a particular behavior, they are more likely to do so, and the perceived opinions of others are all the more influential if that person is particularly concerned with what those around them think.

As noted above, the health belief model initially did not account for important elements of human motivation (most notably, self-efficacy). Similarly, the initial iteration of the theory of reasoned action did not adequately account for *perceived control*, a concept that includes notions of one's power to implement a particular change (*self-efficacy*) (Schroder 2014). Montaño and Kasprzyk (2008:71) continue:

> Perceived control is determined by *control beliefs* concerning the presence or absence of facilitators and barriers to behavioral performance, weighted by their perceived power or the impact of each control factor to facilitate or inhibit the behavior.

With the addition of perceived control to the theory of reasoned action, a new model was born: the *theory of planned behavior* (see the shaded boxes in Fig. 6.2).

The theory of planned behavior draws a causal link between behavioral, normative, and control beliefs to behavioral intentions and behaviors. It is assumed that other influences, depicted along the left side of Figure 6.2, operate *through* the existing model constructs, without independently contributing to the likelihood of carrying out a behavior. These ways of thinking about behavior culminated in an *integrated behavioral model* (see Kasprzyk & Montaño, 2007; Kasprzyk et al. 1998 for applications), which, as its name suggests, includes ideas and causal pathways from the theory of reasoned action, theory of planned behavior, and various other influential theoretical frameworks. As you can see in Figure 6.3, which depicts the integrated model, predicting health behavior can become quite a complicated endeavor. Just as its predecessors, the most proximal predictor of a behavior in the integrated model is *intention*, but this model adds four other direct determinants. First, even if intention is present, an individual needs *knowledge and skill* to carry out a behavior. Second, there should be few (or no) *environmental constraints* to impede adoption of the behavior. Third, behavior should be *salient*, or deemed important, and finally, repetitive enactment of the behavior can create *habit*, which can lessen the importance of intention as a behavioral determinant.

The takeaway message from various behavioral models is that a behavior becomes likely when (1) one has a strong intention to perform it, along with the knowledge and skill to do so; (2) there are no significant environmental constraints to impede performance; (3) the behavior is salient; and (4) one has performed the behavior previously. Just as in previous models, intention is shaped by one's *attitude toward the behavior* (e.g., favorable or unfavorable), *perceived norm* (i.e., social pressure), and *personal agency* (i.e., self-efficacy and perceived control). All are important, both alone and in combination, when developing potential behavioral interventions, but they may vary in significance for different behaviors within different populations (Montaño & Kasprzyk 2008). In particular, behavioral interventions must account for the ways in which upstream social determinants like SES, age, gender, and culture powerfully shape behavior, both directly and indirectly, by influencing intentions, attitudes, norms, self-efficacy, and control. All of these reflect group memberships, thereby further emphasizing the need for integrated approaches to health behavior that connect individuals to the broader collectivities and contexts of which they are a part.

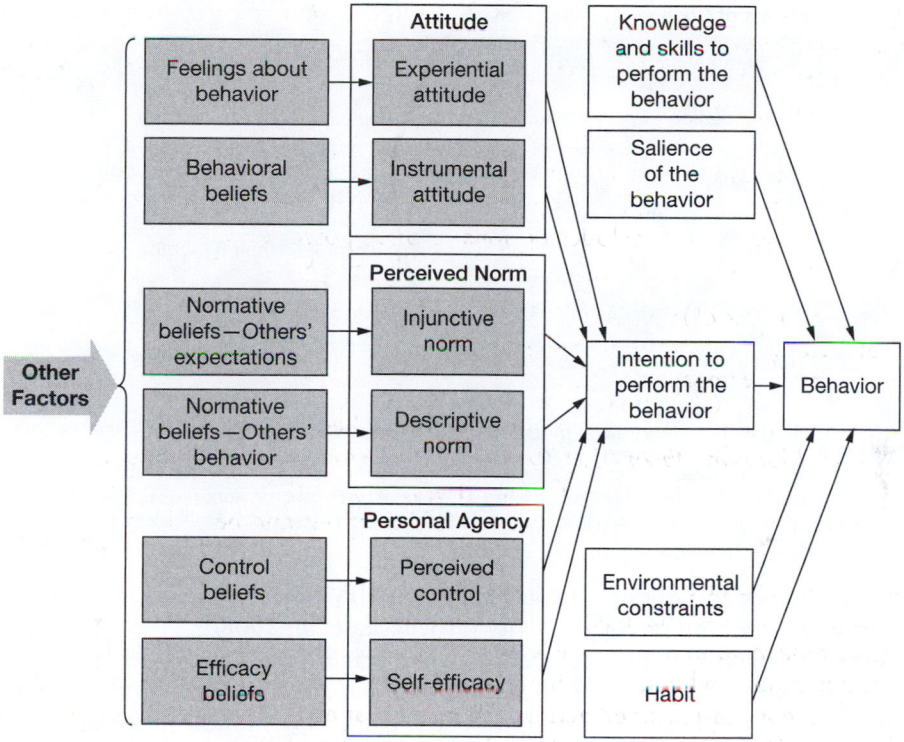

FIG. 6.3 Integrated behavior model.

Source: Montaño, Daniel E. & Danuta Kasprzyk. (2008). "Theory of Reasoned Action, Theory of Planned Behavior, and the Integrated Behavioral Model." Pp. 67–96 in *Health Behavior: Theory, Research and Practice*, 4th edition. Karen Glanz, Barbara K. Rimer, & K. Viswanath, eds. San Francisco, CA: John Wiley & Sons.

Process Models

The models of health behavior described above tend to reflect relatively static conceptualizations of health behavior. In response, *process* models have emerged to describe behavioral change as a series of stages or phases, including the *precaution adoption process model* (Weinstein 1988), the *health action process approach* (Schwarzer 2008), and the *transtheoretical model of behavior change* (Prochaska et al. 1992). The latter is arguably the most dominant of the process models and has inspired a large body of research. The transtheoretical model assumes that individuals differ in their readiness to adopt various behaviors, which may be assessed by determining in which stage of change a person is located at a given time (Schroder 2014). Accordingly, it identifies *stages of change* that integrate processes and principles from a variety of different approaches in psychotherapy and behavior modification (which is why it is called *trans*theoretical). These include *consciousness-raising* from the Freudian tradition (Freud 1926 [1959]), *contingency management* from the Skinnerian tradition (Skinner 1971), and *helping relationships* from the Rogerian tradition (Rogers 1951). Since its first application in studies of smoking, the stage approach has subsequently been adapted to other phenomena, including alcohol and substance abuse, anxiety and panic disorders, bullying, depression,

Stages of Change

Precontemplation	No intention to take action within the next 6 months
Contemplation	Intends to take action within the next 6 months
Preparation	Intends to take action within the next 30 days and has taken some behavioral steps in this direction
Action	Changed overt behavior for less than 6 months
Maintenance	Changed overt behavior for more than 6 months
Termination	No temptation to relapse and 100% confidence

FIG. 6.4 Transtheoretical model constructs: stages of change.

Source: Prochaska, James O., Colleen A. Redding, & Kerry E. Evers. (2008). "The Transtheoretical Model and Stages of Change." Pp. 97–121 in *Health Behavior: Theory, Research and Practice*, 4th edition. Karen Glanz, Barbara K. Rimer, & K. Viswanath, eds. San Francisco, CA: John Wiley & Sons.

eating disorders and obesity, dietary behavior, HIV/AIDS, cancer screening, medication adherence, and physical activity (Prochaska et al. 2008b).

The transtheoretical model identifies five stages of change (see Fig. 6.4): *precontemplation, contemplation, preparation, action,* and *maintenance*. Some iterations of this model also include a sixth phase called *termination* (discussed below). Each stage differs in its motivational parameters, and progression through these stages is not always linear, as people often move back and forth between them. These stages of change can inform any number of other behavior change models. For example, we could map these stages of change onto the theory of planned behavior to articulate how, as persons move forward through each of these stages, self-efficacy and perceived benefits increase, while perceived negative consequences decrease (Schroder 2014). In this way, the transtheoretical model's stages of change add a new process-oriented dimension to the theory of planned behavior and other frameworks. Moreover, accounting for stages of change is important because they add a temporal or time-order dimension to explanations of health behavior.

In *precontemplation*, people do not plan to take action in the near term, perhaps because they lack information on the consequences of current behaviors, or they may be demoralized due to past failed attempts to modify their behavior. They are therefore unmotivated or resistant to change, and tend to avoid reading, talking, or even thinking about their high-risk behaviors. In *contemplation*, people plan to alter their behavior in the near future (typically six months), and are aware of the advantages of changing, as well as the costs. The balance between costs and benefits often produces ambivalence and keeps many within the contemplation stage for long time periods—something referred to as *chronic contemplation* or *behavioral procrastination* (Prochaska et al. 2008). Here individuals are not quite ready for action-oriented interventions that require them to make immediate changes to behavior.

Individuals in the *action* stage have adopted specific lifestyle changes within the past six months. Still, not all change qualifies as action, because in most applications of this model, individuals must exhibit behaviors that scientists and professionals agree are sufficient to meaningfully reduce disease risk (Prochaska et al. 2008). In smoking cessation, for instance, reducing the number of cigarettes or switching to "light" or low-tar brands does not constitute action because the new behaviors still carry substantial risks of disease. Rather, only total cessation or abstinence meets the criterion of action for smoking. We might also consider dietary changes. Simply changing from one food with higher than recommended fat content to another does not constitute action, because the new behaviors carry similar risks of disease as the old. Rather, change means limiting or eliminating high-fat foods to the degree to which experts agree reduces disease risk.

In the *maintenance* stage, people maintain lifestyle changes and work to prevent relapse. Greater time leads to less temptation to return to previous behaviors, along with increasing confidence that they can continue in their new lifestyles. The maintenance stage is a period that can last from six months to around five years or more. Persons in the *termination* stage report no temptation and complete self-efficacy, despite possible present or future experiences of depression, anxiety, boredom, loneliness, anger, stress, and so on that might trigger earlier high-risk behaviors. Their behaviors have become entrenched and habituated, like buckling a seat belt almost unconsciously as you enter a motor vehicle, choosing healthy food options without considering others, turning to exercise for stress reduction instead of other harmful smoking or drinking behaviors, taking your blood pressure medication at the same time and place each day, and so on. The termination phase implies that the change process has come to a close, but some research suggests that for many people (e.g., former smokers, alcoholics, drug abusers), this stage may only represent an idealized goal because relapse temptations are so strong and sometimes never entirely disappear. As a result, a lifetime of maintenance (in the preceding stage) may be a more accurate characterization of some behavioral changes.

In addition to the stages included in Figure 6.4, the transtheoretical model also includes ten *processes of change*. While these can occur in any of the five stages, different processes of change are more salient for some of the stages than others (see Fig. 6.5). For example, as Kerstin Schroder (2014:1070) explains:

> Consciousness-raising is most likely to move a person forward in the pre-contemplation stage, prompting a process of deliberation about the benefits of behavior change, while reinforcement management refers to a self-control technique that will only impact behavior once a commitment has been made and a person has entered the action or maintenance phase.

She goes on to note that because relapse is common, this model essentially represents a spiral in which multiple attempts might be necessary before a person achieves long-term maintenance. Generally, process approaches like the transtheoretical model emphasize the need to integrate the element of time by considering where a person is with regard to changing and where they need to go in order to implement lasting, meaningful change. This is particularly important for practical settings like the clinic because it highlights the need for customized interventions according to the stage in which a person currently finds themselves, so that they can successfully move forward from one stage to the next (Schroder 2014). As Prochaska and colleagues (2008) note, systematically applying the core constructs of this model at the individual level may be key to developing high-impact programs for enhancing population-level health.

Processes of Change

Consciousness raising	Finding and learning new facts, ideas, and tips that support the healthy behavior change
Dramatic relief	Experiencing the negative emotions (fear, anxiety, worry) that go along with unhealthy behavioral risks
Self-reevaluation	Realizing that the behavior change is an important part of one's identity as a person
Environmental reevaluation	Realizing the negative impact of the unhealthy behavior or the positive impact of the healthy behavior on one's proximal social and/or physical environment
Self-liberation	Making a firm commitment to change
Helping relationships	Seeking and using social support for the healthy behavior change
Counter conditioning	Substitution of healthier alternative behaviors and cognitions for the unhealthy behavior
Reinforcement management	Increasing the rewards for the positive behavior change and decreasing the rewards of the unhealthy behavior
Stimulus control	Removing reminders or cues to engage in the unhealthy behavior and adding cues or reminders to engage in the healthy behavior
Social liberation	Realizing that the social norms are changing in the direction of supporting the healthy behavior change

FIG. 6.5 Transtheoretical model constructs: processes of change.

Source: Prochaska, James O., Colleen A. Redding, & Kerry E. Evers. (2008). "The Transtheoretical Model and Stages of Change." Pp. 97–121 in *Health Behavior: Theory, Research and Practice*, 4th edition. Karen Glanz, Barbara K. Rimer, & K. Viswanath, eds. San Francisco, CA: John Wiley & Sons.

Health behaviors obviously involve very complex sets of challenges, and it should by now be very clear that traditional methods of information, persuasion, and modes of health education (e.g., handing out pamphlets) have long been considered ineffective methods to alter high-risk behaviors. From a clinical perspective, behavior change may seem very simple and straightforward: explain the risks, then explain how changing behaviors can ameliorate those risks, and patients will alter their behaviors. But the various approaches above clarify how behavior change is not so simple. Improving and maximizing your abilities to provide effective patient care and guidance involves melding your expertise as a skilled practitioner with the patient's unique sets of motivations, attributes, and perspectives, with a keen understanding of the contexts within which that person lives, works, and plays, along with the abundance or dearth of resources available to them once they leave the quarantine of the clinic.

While they represent more robust and rightly complicated understandings of health behavior, the above-mentioned behavioral and process models have some weaknesses, particularly in underemphasizing the social contexts in which people live, and in continuing to overemphasize rational decision-making. While they all implicitly or explicitly mention environmental, personal, and behavioral components, they most strongly focus on the individual, her or his perceptions, and conscious decision-making. In fact, these models often reduce the complex processes of health behavior to a balancing act of cost-benefit analysis (though the integrated model does a better job on this account by including environment). Not only does this risk overlooking the ways that individual behavior emerges from nonrational features of one's personal and social life (e.g., habits, feelings, and attitudes), but a more comprehensive approach to health behavior should include more careful integration of various behavioral factors with social and environmental contexts (De Vries 2014). Because this requires emphasizing social, economic, and environmental contexts, we might consider these elements of health behavior fertile ground for social scientists, but sociological models of health behavior came about much later than psychological models, despite many early discussions of a more generic concept of *lifestyle* (Bourdieu [1972] 1977, 1984, 1990; Giddens 1987, 1991; Weber [1922] 1978). Still, the health lifestyles model, originating in medical sociology, provides an important complement to individualist explanations from health psychology, and accounts for various behavioral determinants at multiple levels of analysis from individual motivations and intentions to broader social and environmental influences (Cockerham 2005).

A Health Lifestyles Paradigm

Just as researchers in psychology, health promotion, public health, and other fields worked for many years to develop ways to explain health behavior, there was a distinct need for a sociological approach to health lifestyles by the end of the twentieth century. This is not to say that researchers and practitioners minimized or overlooked the significance of health behavior and lifestyles as phenomena worthy of investigation, but the more individualist focus of behavioral analysis in psychology, public health, epidemiology, and other fields diverged from the early sociological analyses of lifestyles, which explain social action amidst the enabling and/or constraining nature of life chances and other social influences. In fact, a great deal of medical discourse today overemphasizes the individualist nature of health lifestyles, thereby neglecting the inherently collective nature of these phenomena and reinforcing the traditional focus on *individual* risk factors and *individual* health education, promotion, and intervention (De Vries 2014; Frohlich et al. 2001; Hinote 2015; Link 2008). To be clear, no explanation completely denies the influence of either individual or structural influences. Rather, various models differ in the extent to which they devote greater attention to one or the other (Cockerham 2005). The task, then, is to account for both fully and simultaneously. Thus, in this section, we present a sociological complement to the health behavior and process models above.

Building on classic and contemporary sociological thinking, Cockerham (2005:55) shifts focus from individual health behaviors to aggregate patterns. He notes that "health lifestyles are not the uncoordinated behaviors of disconnected individuals, but are personal routines that merge into an aggregate form representative of specific groups." He goes on to define health lifestyles as "collective patterns of health-related behavior based on choices available to people according to their life chances." While the above models focus upon the motivations and intent

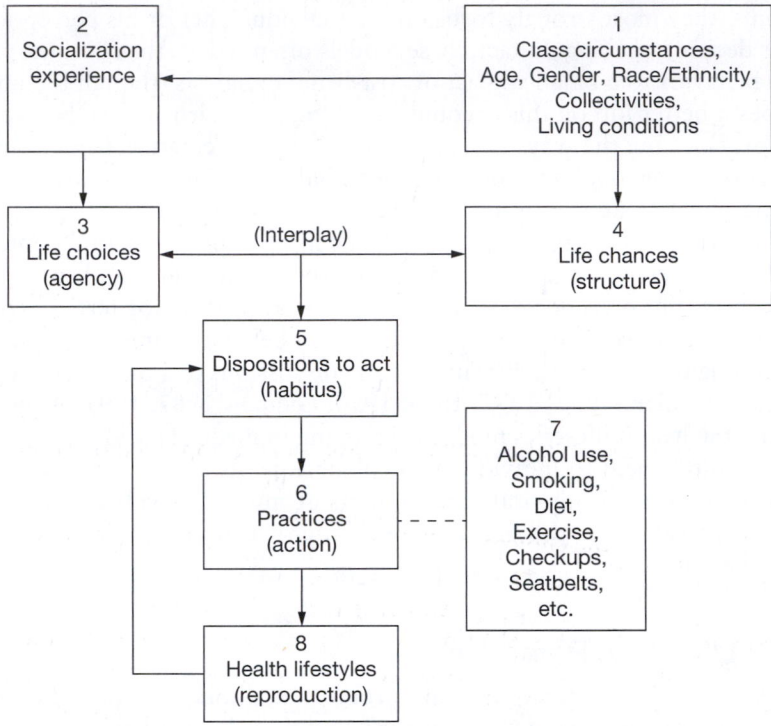

FIG. 6.6 The health lifestyles paradigm.

Source: Cockerham, William C. (2005). "Health Lifestyle Theory and the Convergence of Agency and Structure." *Journal of Health and Social Behavior* 46, 51–67.

of the individual in adopting this or that behavior, the health lifestyles paradigm[1] (see Fig. 6.6) works deeper into the social features that underlie motivation and intent. At the core of this model is the concept of *habitus* (Bourdieu 1984, 1990). Habitus is essentially a cognitive map, or set of dispositions, that simultaneously reflects, and routinely guides, an individual's health choices. These dispositions generate behavior that is not only normative (i.e., consistent with peer group expectations) but also habitual (i.e., repetitive and entrenched) and intuitive (i.e., almost subconscious). Habitus characterizes the deep-seated, attitudinal roots of health behavior for individuals, but importantly, it is also characteristic of the groups to which they belong. The habitus thereby connects individuals to others like them through various group memberships or *collectivities* (Fig. 6.6, Box 1), based upon age, gender, SES, religion, race/ethnicity, culture, and so on. We internalize the norms, perspectives, aspirations, and opportunity structures (i.e., life chances) associated with these collectivities during socialization and through our subsequent life experience (Box 2). The health lifestyles paradigm thereby sets up two general pathways through which we develop attitudes toward the world (through habitus). The first results from socialization, which affects how we cognize the world around us and

---

[1] We use the term *paradigm* to denote a more general analytical model that lacks the precise empirical specification and operationalization of several *theories* described above.

identify the choices we perceive that we have within it (Box 3). The second is a direct product of our social position, whereby our class, neighborhood, gender, and the like affect what sorts of access we have to resources and opportunities—life chances (Box 4). Because life chances and our perceived range of available choices emerge from the same structural conditions, we are significantly more likely to adopt a habitus (Box 5) that is consistent with our social background, family of origin, and/ or peer group. In turn, the habitus as a general set of dispositions to act in particular ways strongly influences the behavioral practices (Boxes 6 and 7) that constitute our health lifestyle. While the behaviors associated with habitus are somewhat open to change (through life experience and conscious decision-making), they are also remarkably durable, because they are both habitual (Box 8) and emerge from intuitive, rather than rational and fully conscious, understandings of our world.

Habitus therefore represents a cognitive resource for individuals, providing them with an *agenda of plausible choices* (i.e., a perceived set of available options) as well as a *code of choosing* (i.e., guidelines for what is approved or appropriate in a given situation), both of which originate in our life chances and are internalized during socialization and social interaction (Bauman 1999; Hinote 2015). In other words, habitus shapes the choices available and recognizable to us, as well as what, in turn, should be chosen. As such, the practices emerging from habitus (Fig. 6.6, Boxes 6 and 7) might be based on deliberate rational calculation (i.e., cost-benefit analysis, described above)—selecting lower-fat dietary options, despite possible time, cost, or information barriers associated with preparation, because such a diet might lessen the risk of developing disease at some unknown time in the future. But more likely, our lifestyle practices might emerge from habit and/or intuition— selecting dietary options from the repertoire of choices that we are accustomed to making with relatively little conscious deliberation. Many of our choices, whether healthy or unhealthy, may be so deeply ingrained into our routines that we enact them with little or no conscious thought. For example, under conditions of stress, one person might reach for alcohol or tobacco (or even a specific type or brand of either), while another might go to the gym, or for a jog through their neighborhood. In any event, these are perhaps best described less as choices than as semiconscious habits emerging from an internalized way of living. A cost-benefit calculation clearly points us toward the more healthy option (i.e., exercise), but we do not always (if ever) make decisions in such a fully rational way. Moreover, because things like repetition and access to valued resources also play an important role in the decisions we make in the real world, we can observe large behavioral variations when it comes to health lifestyles. And these variations are very often patterned along demographic lines, particularly SES. In fact, many of our preferences typically align quite closely with SES, which is why we observe so many class-based lifestyle profiles (and morbidity and mortality gradients) in the United States and other developed nations.

Take the following hypothetical example: Ray Carpro grew up relatively poor and with a high degree of food insecurity. The types of foods he eats consist of high-fat processed meats, cheap grains and breads, and so on. His mother frequently prepared casseroles and the like because they are cost-effective and could feed all of the members of the family with leftovers. Chili dogs at the diner down the street were considered a special treat. Over time, habitus predicts that he will develop a taste for these kinds of foods. These options emerge from his class background, but he is also socialized into these dietary practices. That is, his food consumption may originate in considerations of affordability, but, over time, as he internalizes this particular style of eating it will likely become his own preference. As an adult, Ray becomes solidly middle class and can afford any kind of food he wants, but while his material wealth and his corresponding ability to access resources such as healthy food has changed, his underlying dispositions toward food (i.e., the tastes and preferences that developed much earlier) are relatively durable. Even when he might rationally know that a kale salad is healthier, chili dogs are still the thing that makes his mouth water because of his deep-seated dispositions toward food. The key here is that what might originate as simply a matter of affordability over time can become an internalized matter of taste and preference. As a result, the habitus is incredibly durable because it is not simply a matter of what is affordable, but the ingrained dispositions that have become part of a person's subconscious cognitive frameworks.

As a result of these processes, individuals with quite different social backgrounds (like the factors discussed in Chapters 4 and 5) will predictably tend to make different choices when confronted with a similar range of options. The behavioral tendencies underlying those choices emerge from habitus, which is conditioned by the resources and environments to which we have access. As in the example above, for those without the resources to pay dues for a gym or health club, or without an exercise-friendly neighborhood for jogging, other less healthy options might appear more feasible or desirable in a particular time and place, and with a specific peer group. This is particularly true when those less healthy options often offer immediate psychological and physiological gratification, like high-fat sugary foods, alcohol, or tobacco, in the absence of other realistically attainable options. And when these behavioral choices, conditioned by so many of the factors we have discussed thus far, are repetitively enacted over time, they feed back into habitus and are more likely to become part of the behavioral repertoire from which future behaviors emerge (see Fig. 6.6). Habitus and the health lifestyles paradigm therefore explain why many lifestyles are remarkably durable over time and thereby difficult to modify—because they emerge from deeply ingrained dispositions of which we are not fully conscious. Moreover, because habitus is transmitted through socialization and other group interaction, this approach also helps us explain behavioral patterns that stretch across generations and socioeconomic groups over time. For example, obesity is "inherited" not just through genetics, but also as lifestyle patterns are passed on through socialization and experience.

Finally, the factors that converge around habitus illustrate how seemingly unrelated health behaviors tend to cluster together within similar groups and even in the same individuals. For example, individuals who do not regularly brush their teeth are also less likely to wear a seat belt. On the surface, these may appear unrelated. However, both correspond to the same underlying disposition, what we might call *health fatalism*—feelings of powerlessness or the meaninglessness of one's own efforts, often accompanied by notions of fate or destiny—which predicts both behaviors (Keeley et al. 2009). Habitus is therefore important because it explains how sets of health behaviors coalesce into a lifestyle consistent with a person's personal and social life and characteristics. We will return to the clinical significance of these insights at the end of this chapter.

Although it is a somewhat recent development, the health lifestyles paradigm quickly garnered a great deal of interest (e.g., Cockerham et al. 2006b; Fitzpatrick & LaGory 2011; Hinote 2015; Hinote & Webber 2012; Korp 2008; Phelan et al. 2010). Like the fundamental cause explanation, this framework formalizes many of the general premises of fields like social epidemiology and medical sociology, particularly by illustrating how social factors have great potential to affect individual- and population-level health. Health lifestyles are one of the principal mechanisms through which these social factors work. This approach therefore provides an important set of ideas to help explain exactly how individuals make behavioral choices amidst a host of socioeconomic and environmental influences, and even how those influences affect the very psychology of choice itself (i.e., motivations, values, and intent). It is clear that these ideas push our thinking away from a singular focus on the individual and the notion of health choices as entirely rational and internal, but it is important to note that the individual is not lost in these processes. To be sure, we all have choices, but some of us have more choices (i.e., options from which to choose) than others. Moreover, the range of choices we have over time can become an internalized way of looking at the world, which significantly affects the health behaviors in which one engages. All of these features have important implications for clinical practice.

Implications for Health Care Practice

It has always been relatively clear that social conditions influence health. Even in premodern times, based on patterns that were plainly observable, there was talk about how diseases clustered among certain social groups. But the advent of modern medicine encouraged an increasingly individualistic focus for medicine and health care in part because infectious diseases and acute injuries could be effectively treated on an individual basis with pharmaceutical and surgical interventions. So the success of modern medicine forestalled, to some extent, the development of broader social–psychological accounts of health and illness. After the epidemiological transition, however, the individualist paradigm became increasingly insufficient as chronic diseases became more prevalent sources of morbidity and mortality. This shifting epidemiological landscape necessitated accounts of health behavior because chronic illnesses often result from hundreds of thousands of small decisions that individuals make across their life course (i.e., what types of foods they eat each day, whether they exercise or watch TV, etc.). As models from health psychology emerged to explain these behaviors, they grew more robust and complex, coming to include various aspects of internal motivation and behavioral intention, along with the various forces that act on an individual's psychological orientation toward those factors.

Medical sociologists further contributed to understanding health behavior by emphasizing how these psychological processes, while partially internal to the individual, are nonetheless socially structured. Among a variety of concepts in this literature, the notion of habitus articulates how socialization processes, which originate in the family and proceed within defined group settings (i.e., by SES, culture, race/ethnicity, etc.), lead to the internalization of opportunity structures such that individuals develop cognitive expectations and evaluations of the world (and the choices it offers them) that are consistent with their groups of origin. The habitus, as a general cognitive orientation, is linked to a range of practices that can be more or less healthy. Structural influences affect not only material access to health resources, but also internal cognitive orientations that manifest in psychological processes such as sense of self-efficacy. These influence not only health behaviors but also the likelihood and success of behavioral change. While this is a necessarily complex picture, its multidimensional nature ultimately provides a number of insights that are relevant for clinical practice.

Perhaps the most fundamental insight for practitioners emerges from the sociological nature of chronic illness and conditions closely related to health lifestyles. While modern medicine was built around treating individuals in the quarantined clinical environment, contemporary health care practice must consider the social contexts in which patients become ill, and in which they carry out long-term illness management. This instantly raises a number of questions with which practitioners should be concerned. For example, a pediatrician seeing an obese child might naturally and reasonably recommend that the child get more exercise. But without considering the social environment in which the child lives, this recommendation may not be fully effective. If the child lives in a poor, inner city neighborhood, they may have limited opportunities for physical activity such as safe parks or similar environments.[2] We already addressed some of these considerations in Chapter 4 with respect to the physical and material barriers that low-SES presents for achieving health, but we can now add that exposure to limited opportunities creates internal dispositions toward less healthy behaviors (precisely because today many healthy behavioral choices depend upon those same opportunities). That is, the pediatrician treating the obese child may need, in their treatment plan, to account for the fact that limited access to safe physical activity opportunities may have resulted in an *internal disposition* toward sedentary practices, and likely throughout an entire family. Perhaps this practitioner meets the first challenge by demonstrating some calisthenic exercises that the child can do in the home, thereby mitigating limited outdoor activity opportunities or unaffordable exercise equipment. But the models of health behavior described above also tell us that other psychological and sociological aspects of health behavior should also be addressed.

The transtheoretical model informs a practitioner, for example, that the physical activity messages they deliver during clinical visits should be matched with the cognitive stage of the patient. If the obese child and her parents are not even contemplating exercise, then providing them with a detailed exercise program is not likely to be effective. At that point, it is probably better to spend time on consciousness-raising. Moreover, the notion of habitus tells us that individuals' dispositions are highly durable. They are unlikely, particularly in the short term, to adopt lifestyle practices that are dramatically different than those to which they are accustomed. This too is informative for working with, rather than against, patients' deep-seated cognitive

---

[2] Recall from Chapter 4, for example, that while urban neighborhoods often have more parks, they tend to be less safe both in terms of crime and in terms of the equipment and infrastructure of the parks themselves (Suminski et al. 2012).

orientations. For example, rather than providing a dietary plan for the obese child that radically subverts the family's food practices, working with them to cook healthier versions of those same foods is likely to be more effective. As highlighted above, tastes tend to change slowly. Health behavior changes will likely be more effective to the extent that they align with individual tastes in the short term.

Alongside patients, individual practitioners clearly confront powerful social forces in their work today—forces that undeniably shape health more strongly than ever before. Ultimately, there are limits to what an individual practitioner can do to modify habitus, poverty, living conditions, group norms, and the like. Still, it is possible to target various social and psychological influences that modify choice, intention, self-efficacy, perceived control, salience, contemplation, and other important factors discussed above. In doing so, one can positively affect individual health behavior by helping patients refocus cognitive dispositions and psychological tendencies toward healthy behaviors. The various health behavior and process models, along with the health lifestyles paradigm, highlight many factors and insights that can sensitize[3] practitioners to the influence of social and psychological factors on a patient's health and health behavior, and thereby inform more effective treatment plans.

CHAPTER 6 ACTIVITY

Habitus and Health Behavior: How Can You Get Janek Polakow to Diet and Exercise?

Janek Polakow is a 67-year-old patient whom you are seeing for a yearly physical. As a longtime patient of your practice, you know him quite well.

Janek is the son of Polish immigrants and grew up in a Pennsylvania coal-mining town. At the age of 15 he ran away from home and joined a lumber camp. At 17 years old he joined the army and served in Vietnam. He has substantial hearing loss from this time, and while he has hearing aids, his wife complains that he never wears them. He also has limited motion in his left thumb as a result of getting it caught trying to clear a jam in his M60 machine gun. "There was no doctor with our platoon, just an 18-year-old medic who picked out

the pieces of bone and stitched me up," he once laughingly told you, with a slight air of pride for the battle scar. He spent the remainder of his career as a police officer and after retiring from the police department, he earned extra money as a handyman around his neighborhood. He and his wife moved to Florida in 1995, but divorced several years later and he remarried shortly after. His current wife comes to every appointment with him.

Mr. Polakow (as he prefers to be called by "young people such as yourself") had two heart attacks in the mid-1990s, but his blood pressure and cholesterol have been well managed with dietary changes since then. He recently had both

[3] We return to *sensitizing concepts* in the book's conclusion. Briefly, as noted in Chapter 3, practitioners face a paradox where they know that social conditions affect the health of their patients, but at the same time they must avoid reductionism in applying that knowledge. The notion of sensitizing concepts (Blumer 1954) provides one suggestion for steering between reductionist approaches to the social determinants of health and equally unappealing individualistic models that ignore those broader contextual influences. For now, understanding the ways that social structural factors influence health should not dictate treatment for any individual patient, even if they live with or in those social conditions. Rather, that knowledge can open up appropriate lines of inquiry for practitioners to ascertain how those factors might be affecting a particular individual patient. They then can specify a treatment plan that accounts for them.

knees replaced and complains of severe back pain, but refuses to take pain medication for it, citing that he does not want to be "all doped up." Otherwise he is in good physical health for his age.

At the visit today, however, you notice that he has gained a significant amount of weight. When you ask him about it he doesn't seem to hear you clearly, but before you can ask him in a louder voice, his wife chimes in. "He's not walking like he used to. He used to go around the block twice a day, but now he just sits in that Lazy-boy chair with that TV blaring full blast, always on the History channel. I can't hear myself think!" she chuckles. In a louder voice, you say to Mr. Polakow, "Tell me about what you're eating these days." He hears you this time, and responds, "Same as always, I guess. She makes good casseroles, these great stuffed cabbage rolls, meatloaf ... regular food, I guess. My back has been hurting more lately, that's for sure. I don't sleep so well anymore either. But hey, I'm almost 70. That's just what happens."

Discussion Questions

1. Articulate what the concept of habitus adds to your understanding of Mr. Polakow's dietary practices and attitudes toward health and physical decline.

2. Using the theory of planned behavior, what domains might be most important to target when working with Mr. Polakow (i.e., attitude, subjective norms, perceived control, etc., and the facets of each of these)?

3. Using the framework of the transtheoretical model, at what stage of change would you say Mr. Polakow is most likely situated? How does this inform how you might begin to work with him on lifestyle changes?

4. Suppose at his next appointment, Mr. Polakow says to you, "I've been thinking lately, there's not a damn thing wrong with me other than my knees and back ... I'll probably live to 90. So I probably better get my weight back down." At what stage of change would you say he is most likely situated now? How would this inform your consultation with him about diet and exercise?

5. Suppose at a third appointment, Mr. Polakow says, "I've been going to that Silver Sneakers group you mentioned. The workouts are good and I can usually keep up with everybody, even the ones that are still in their fifties. But some days my back just hurts too bad to go." At what stage of change would you say he is most likely situated now? How might what he says inform your treatment recommendations for him at this appointment? What might you need to recommend so he will be less tempted to relapse into a sedentary lifestyle?

6. What additional information would you want to know about Mr. Polakow and how might the answers to those questions about his lifestyle, social history, and the like inform your treatment plan?

PART III

Social Science in Clinical Practice

Power, Medicalization, and Clinical Practice

Introduction

Among the overarching themes of this book is that medicine and health care are at least as much social enterprises as scientific ones. In this chapter we discuss how arrangements of power affect the definitions and experiences of illness in various facets of clinical practice. Recall from Chapter 2 that risk estimation, as opposed to calculation, amplifies the influence of personal and social values on understandings of health and illness. As one example, the ambiguity of chronic illness presses fractured health beliefs into enclaves organized around various lifestyles. One result of these processes is that a variety of social forces have more impact on dispositions toward health and the body. Similarly, social forces affect how we define illnesses, especially when they are much more ambiguous. While there is consensus that a broken leg is in need of treatment, defining heart disease or type 2 diabetes is more complicated, and the classification of obesity or alcoholism as disease even more contested. Yet over time we have reshaped these and other disease phenomena to fit changing expectations of health, social functioning, and individual behavior. In short, the contours of illness have a significantly social character. Particularly in the chronic illness era, when many major disease profiles are less discrete and more multifaceted, the social forces underlying how we approach and define them become more influential, and arguably more problematic, for clinical practice.

Examining the influences that shape definitions of disease is critical to understanding not only the dynamics of health care, but also how patient experiences of illness might differ dramatically from the professional gaze of clinical practitioners. In what follows, we will discuss various ways that power is threaded through health care provision, including the process of medicalization and how diagnoses can represent forms of social control. We will conclude by discussing the dilemmas that these present for clinical practitioners.

Medicalization

Medicalization generally refers to a social process by which previously nonmedical conditions come under the purview of medicine and health care. Multiple social phenomena drive this process, including scientific advances, economic interests, consumerism, managed care, and an expanding professional terrain of clinical practice. While medicalization is discussed extensively in the literature as exemplary of the social nature of health and medicine, its clinical relevance has been underappreciated. Recognizing that defining disease is not merely an objectively scientific exercise raises a number of important social and ethical issues for clinical practitioners. This is true not only where clinical professionals benefit by recognizing the impact of various social forces on patient care, but also where they have an obligation to participate in the shape and direction of their respective professions. Medicalization provides a lens through which we can understand how power shapes the landscape of health and disease, both clinically and professionally, and therefore provides practitioners with important tools for both.

Childbirth and alcoholism are particularly illustrative examples of medicalization. Childbirth historically occurred in the home under the supervision of midwives, or women in the family or community experienced in assisting with the process. Over time, however, childbirth increasingly came under the supervision of physicians and moved from the home into hospitals where technological interventions were more prevalent. Of course, part of this has to do with the availability of the technology itself. Nonetheless, the terrain of medicine and its capacities to monitor and treat conditions exerted influences that reshaped the meaning of childbirth from something that was a normal, communal phenomenon integrated within home life, into a highly technological event that was perceived as especially risky and therefore quarantined in the clinic and overseen by physicians.

Of course, there are real risks associated with childbirth. But recall from Chapter 2 that a paradigmatic characteristic of modernity is that risks can and should be managed by human ingenuity. That is, before medical science could manage risks, they were in some sense taken for granted. The concept of medicalization adds to this picture the idea that as modernizing societies develop an orientation toward risk management, they do not do so in only a reactive way. As the capacity of science for managing risk grows, so do our expectations of the risks we expect it to confront. That is, as socioscientific advances subdue high-risk phenomena, other phenomena that previously were less concerning become the new frontiers of risk management. Put simply, health and medical professions, like all professions, are subject to a sort of mission-creep where, in the process of dealing with threats to human health, there naturally is an underlying drive to continue to identify new threats that must then be confronted.

Where childbirth has been pathologized—that is, turned into an object of medical intervention, even where there is low risk of complications—clinical practitioners and patients experience it differently.[1] Certainly there are benefits to medical management, particularly for high-risk pregnancies and for unforeseen complications that, while relatively infrequent, do occasionally arise. At the same time, there are downsides, including rising costs without significant gains in safety and at the expense of a variety of experiential factors that are valued by many patients (e.g., compliance with their birth plans, control of the environment, the presence of family, etc.). Data from the Centers for Disease Control and Prevention (CDC) show that rates of Cesarean section (C-section), even for low-risk pregnancies, not only mirror the rates of all pregnancies (including high-risk), but also vary by a number of factors that are ostensibly unrelated to medical risk (Fig. 7.1; Osterman & Martin 2014). For example, rates of Cesarean vary significantly by state. In 2007,

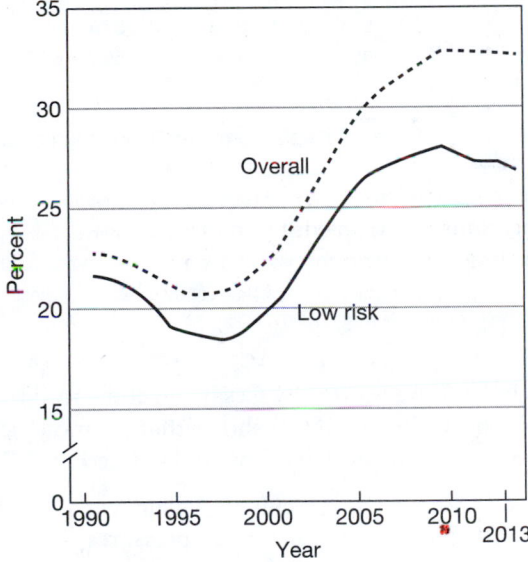

FIG. 7.1 Overall Cesarean delivery and low-risk Cesarean delivery: United States final 1990–2012 and preliminary 2013.

Note: Low risk is defined as nulliparous, term, singleton births in a vertex (head first) presentation.

Sources: CDC/NCHS, National Vital Statistics System; Osterman, Michelle J. K. & Joyce A. Martin. (2014). "Trends in Low-Risk Cesarean Delivery in the United States, 1990-2013." *National Vital Statistics Reports* 63, November 5, Centers for Disease Control and Prevention.

---

[1] There also is a gendered history to the medicalization of childbirth, in particular, where midwifery, as a profession historically dominated by women, was at odds with the *historically* patriarchal character of modern medicine.

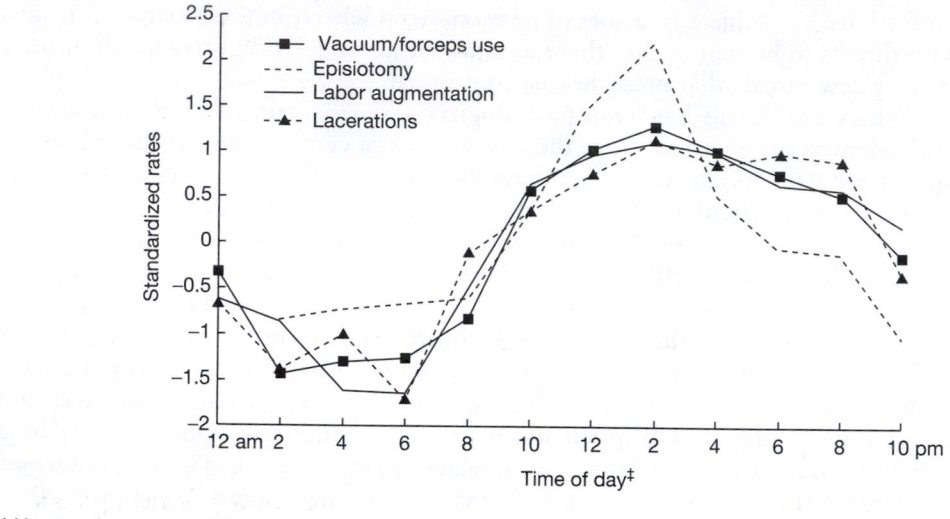

% Vacuum foreceps -   9.3   7.1   7.4   7.5   8.4   11.1   12.1   12.6   12.0   11.5   11.1   9.7
% Episiotomy* - 24.7   24.3   24.5   24.5   24.7   26.3   28.3   29.4   26.5   25.6   25.6   24.0
% Augmented† - 25.7   24.4   21.0   20.8   26.3   34.4   37.7   39.3   37.9   34.3   34.0   30.7
Lacerations‡ - 43.7   37.3   40.8   34.4   48.9   53.3   56.7   60.3   57.8   58.8   57.9   46.8
(per 1000 births)

FIG. 7.2 Rates of vacuum/forceps use, episiotomy use, labor augmentation, and severe lacerations by time of delivery.

Note: * Labor augmentation and episiotomy rates pertain only to spontaneous vaginal deliveries.

†Refers to the occurrence of third and fourth degree tears per 1,000 deliveries.

‡Values on *x*-axis refer to the two-hour time period beginning with hour shown.

Source: Webb, David A. & Jennifer F. Culhane. (2002). "Time of Day Variation in Rates of Obstetric Intervention to Assist in Vaginal Delivery." *Journal of Epidemiology and Community Health* 56, 577–78.

22.2% of births in Utah were done by Cesarean, compared to 38.3% in New Jersey. A study by Webb and Culhane (2002) shows that technological interventions in the birthing process vary significantly by time of day (see Fig. 7.2). They note:

> the results would seem to be difficult to explain, without reference to the influence of "time" itself—that is, to the increased pressures on doctors and hospital staff to "clear" patients at times when they have other patients to see and/or when the hospital census is high. Busy doctors in busy hospitals may simply have less tolerance for the otherwise time consuming natural progression of labour and delivery during "high demand" hours, and thus are more willing during these times to perform procedures that hasten the labour and delivery process. (Webb & Culhane 2002:577–78)

We would add that these various social factors are particularly influential against a backdrop of the medicalization of childbirth, that is, where childbirth is seen *typically* as something in need of medical intervention. Childbirth is now classified as a condition over which medicine exercises considerable authority, which in turn catalyzes a propensity for the types of interventions observed by Webb and Culhane (2002).

Medicalization therefore affects health care practice in a number of ways. Much of the literature focuses on how medicalization benefits the health professions and industry, but the issue is not so one sided. The medicalization of childbirth, for example, certainly has benefited the health professions and even created new ones. While obstetrics is one of the oldest branches of medicine, insofar as men were often barred from attending childbirth, doctors were not summoned until midwives believed there were otherwise insurmountable problems (Drife 2002). With the development of new techniques for dealing with breeched babies, obstetrics textbooks exposed physicians to midwifery practices, and later antiseptic procedures and antibiotics, which were especially important to the survival of the mother following C-section. As a result, physicians gained greater control over childbirth and certainly benefited financially and professionally. These advances ultimately led to the organization of obstetrics and gynecology as its own specialty in the early 1900s, where it continued to expand its domains of practice. Although in recent decades we have witnessed something of a resurgence in midwifery in the United States, a biomedical paradigm is now well established in this field (Johanson et al. 2002). But clinicians are not the only engines driving the medicalization of childbirth. Where technological intervention in virtually all circumstances is now normalized, it has also become the expectation of many patients. For example, many women request scheduled C-sections even when there is no medical indication to justify it. But as MacDorman and colleagues (2008) point out, few, if any, of these decisions are made outside of the context of an interaction with providers and a larger framework of medical norms. Additionally, legal pressures encourage intervention. Johanson et al. (2002) note:

> Given that the NHS in the United Kingdom is facing a bill for medical negligence of £2.6bn ($5.9bn; €4.2bn)—double the amount for 1997—it is reasonable to ask whether professionals are encouraged to act "defensively" (particularly as 70% of litigation relates to obstetrics). Most obstetric cases relate to labour ward practice, and 99% of these relate to "failure to intervene" or "delay in intervention."

In the end, patients-as-consumers and serious professional and financial threat from legal actions also drive high levels of biomedical, technological intervention, placing pressure even on practitioners who would be otherwise disposed. Conrad and Leiter (2004) point out that direct-to-consumer marketing of drugs such as Viagra and Paxil created a groundswell in demand that was then facilitated by physicians, insurance companies, and regulatory bodies who evolved to meet consumer demand. This is a cyclical phenomenon that we discuss further below. Still, it is particularly important for practitioners to recognize not only their own dispositions and patterns of practice, but other contextual forces as well. As only one example, the medicalization of childbirth shows us how clinical practices are not only affected by scientific evidence, but also shaped by powerful social forces. Professionals should be able to critically reflect on where their own practices stand in relation to these norms and patterns.

While defining pregnancy as a medical condition in need of medical intervention raises many social and moral questions, the intersection of medicalization and moral judgment is perhaps made clearer in the case of alcoholism. Schneider (1978:361) notes that the evolution of alcoholism follows a common pattern, "wherein a form of non-normative behavior is labeled first a 'sin,' then a 'crime,' and finally a 'sickness'." This is especially true where evidence of a genetic component of addiction has fostered the construction of alcoholism as a disease. As with childbirth, there are significant benefits to this construction, particularly where moral judgments are mitigated within a disease framework, at least compared to notions of "sin." Additionally, the definition of alcoholism as a disease helps marshal professional resources that can help individuals who want to stop drinking. Insurance coverage for treatment and increasing numbers of professionals specializing in addiction treatment certainly represent catalysts to "recovery." While it is now common to hear things like alcoholism is "just like cancer" (Erchak 1992:158), and indeed there is utility in the metaphor, there remain significant differences between addiction and other diseases.

Whether or not alcoholism is, by some objective standard, a disease is less important here than the fact that its character (from a sociological perspective) empowers some approaches, groups, and professions over others. For example, within a disease framework medical professionals have authority over diagnosing and treating alcoholism. As a result, treatments that employ a disease framework are given preference over others, even when other treatments or lifestyle changes might be more efficacious or less risky. There also are important moral, social, and financial consequences to these definitions, as they shape not only the experience of patients, but also the practices of those in health care. Stigma associated with drinking may be lessened in lieu of a disease framework, but that sort of biological determinism might also eclipse any sense of moral responsibility and autonomous control over behavior. As with childbirth, it is important to be reflexive and critical not only about how social forces shape one's own clinical perspective and practices, but also the way in which utilizing a disease perspective and enacting corresponding treatments affect a patient's sense of self and experience of illness (see Chapter 8).

There are many other examples of medicalization, and we will return to another (ADHD) later in this chapter, but each of them illustrates the ways that powerful social forces clearly shape our constructions of disease and illness, in terms of both patient experience and professional practice. In the next section we explore notions of power, particularly how subtle and insidious forms can often problematically operate in a clinical encounter. At the heart of medicalization lie subtle forces of social power that we often fail to recognize, forces that shape the health landscape in which we work in significant ways.

Power in the Clinic

Two Forms of Power

We typically think of power as something overt, something obvious, and even something physically present in a situation. A person who pulls out a gun in a bank and tells everyone to get on the floor has decidedly clear power in that moment. And later, when they are locked behind bars for the crime, the criminal justice system demonstrates a compelling amount of power. Someone with a significant amount of money often also wields significant power. After all, they can use their resources to influence other individuals and events. Sociologists sometimes refer to the kind of power that is wielded by guns or money as *material power*. Material power is physical and tangible, and its influence is very direct: "that guy has a gun; I'm going to do what he says" or, "my boss can fire me; I'm going to do what she says." The force of power in these situations often goes from the source to the consequence very directly and with relative immediacy.

While he certainly did not deny that material power was an important social force, Michel Foucault (1963 [2003], 1975 [1995]) argued that power in industrialized societies had become far more subtle and insidious. For him, the *physical* consequences of acting outside of social norms was only a starting place for how power functions in society. That people internalize those norms, and the negative sanctions associated with failing to follow them, was a far more complicated social phenomenon, called *disciplinary power*.

Take this example: You are walking through the mall with two 5-year-old children, when one pushes the other to the ground. You stop and scold the offending child, and tell him that because of his actions, he will not get an ice cream that you had promised. You have exercised material power. That is, you have used your physical attributes in both scolding him and depriving him of a treat (i.e., an object they value) in order to get him to conform to behavioral norms. Assuming that you are interested in more than just the satisfaction of dominating a small child, however, you likely have a larger goal in mind. That is, you are trying to teach the child how to behave (i.e., conforming to the accepted norms of social behavior). Your goal in reprimanding the child is not just to make him behave in that moment, but for him to internalize those norms so that he behaves accordingly even in the absence of the physical punishment. This is of course what we mean by *discipline*. While discipline is a relatively commonplace term, if we unpack its deeper power dimensions, we uncover a more robust concept. Discipline is when we act in accordance with certain norms even in the absence of positive and negative sanctions; it is when we exercise power over ourselves.

Foucault went further with this analysis to say that in the modern era, much authority is derived from expert knowledge. Experts are individuals who have knowledge that is not possessed by, and perhaps not even available to, the average person. In a very literal sense, experts can see things that nonexperts cannot. This is where the concept of disciplinary power becomes critically related to medicine. Examine the x-ray below (Photo 7.1). A person with limited knowledge of physical medicine cannot discern what, if anything, is problematic in this image. However, a trained diagnostician will immediately see any number of

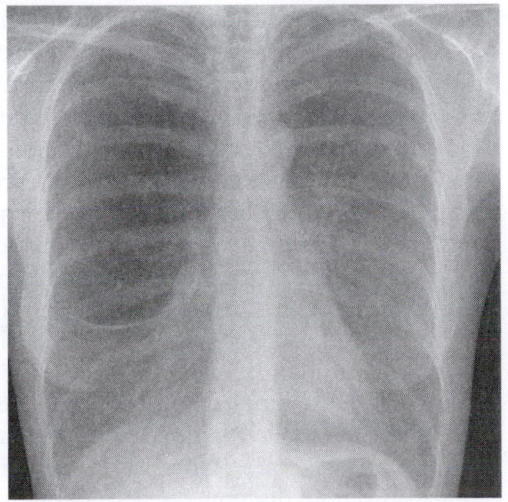

PHOTO 7.1 Photo X-ray of lungs of a person with early COPD (emphysema).

problems and, perhaps along with other pieces of information, diagnose this person with early chronic obstructive pulmonary disease (COPD). That is, because of their expert knowledge, they can see something in this image that others cannot. Accordingly, when a clinical practitioner gives a diagnosis, the average patient really is in no position to dispute it (at least not rationally, though they may exhibit denial-like behavior). Patients cannot contest an expert's observations, at least not on any logical diagnostic grounds, because they cannot see what experts can. At best, they can solicit another practitioner with expert knowledge for another opinion. But ultimately, because clinicians have the ability to see things that patients cannot, the latter are, to a great degree, at the mercy of their knowledge. To reduce this back to a cliché, but which readers now hopefully understand at a much deeper level: Knowledge is power. In fact, Foucault often combines the two words into a single concept, *knowledge-power*, because they are inextricably linked in modern society.

In Chapter 1 we briefly discussed instances in which symbols operated as powerful social forces. Recall that in the Milgram experiments, the researchers specifically and intentionally neutralized the effect of the payment to the subjects—that is, material power—by telling them it was theirs to keep no matter what. Yet the symbolic assertions of authority—the white lab coat worn by the researcher, his authoritative tone, the expectations of their role as teacher, and so on—continued to influence a significant number of participants. None of these symbols exerted physical force, but they were extremely powerful nonetheless. The concept of disciplinary power adds to this picture the notion that symbols operate as forces of power because we have *internalized* their meaning. In effect, the symbols are powerful because of how we conceptualize them in our own minds. In clinical practice, these symbolic forces also are present, and we see patients often behaving in ways that are very deferential. While that has advantages in some instances, it also can obviate important information that practitioners might need if patients are unwilling to be assertive in a clinical encounter. We will see an example of this below.

By most accounts, clinicians have historically wielded a lot of power. In recent decades, however, physicians report feeling increasingly powerless as the demands of managed medicine and its bureaucratic requirements have caused the professional power of doctors to contract. And it is true that practitioners today do not feel imbued with a great deal of material power: they feel helpless to get their patients to comply with medical advice, they feel powerless to affect policy changes that enable them to better care for their patients, and they often feel comparatively powerless in the face of insurance companies and administrative policies and procedures that define greater and greater portions of their daily practice. But power in the practitioner–patient relationship is a far more complicated social phenomenon that largely involves disciplinary, not material power. The kind of power that can complicate the practitioner–patient relationship is an inherent feature of the asymmetrical knowledge between the expert-practitioner and the nonexpert-patient. At the same time, practitioners are subject to disciplinary forces as well, and while these shape the expert lenses they use to examine problems, they can also promote disconnects with patients who are experiencing their illnesses in very different ways.

The Clinical Functions of Power

Material power is comparatively rare in clinical practice. Of course, there may be times that practitioners use physical force to compel patients. For example, patients who threaten to kill themselves may be forcibly committed to a hospital for observation and treatment. But disciplinary power is common to every clinical interaction and while it is far subtler, it is critically important to understand its potential to complicate, confound, or even corrupt the practitioner–patient interaction.

Examine carefully the following transcript that we have adapted from an actual patient encounter (reported in Clair 1990), including notations about body language and other nonverbal behavior:

001 Doctor: Hello.

002 Patient: Hey Doc.

003 Nurse: Mr. Levario was just telling me that he can't believe he was scuba diving only a year ago.

004 Doctor: Oh yeah? <Looks down at chart for 5 full seconds> How is the fluid in his lung?

005 Nurse: Not any better.

006 Patient: I'm not struggling to breathe but I just can't breathe real deep, ya know?

007 Doctor: I was planning to use Bleomycin for the cancer, but I can't because of the severe obstructive path you have.

008 Patient: (softly, confessing tone) Yeah, I know.

009 Doctor: (softly, almost to himself, stuttering at first) I-it's a real severe obstruction.
<Ten uncomfortable seconds of silence pass while the doctor reads the chart.>

010 Patient: Yeah, the human body is a funny thing. Just a little over a year ago, I was still scuba diving.

011 Nurse: Wow, I've always wanted to do that. Is it hard to learn?

012 Patient: You just start slow, you know a little at a time. Pretty soon, you're going pretty deep. I got pretty good at it over the years. Can't do that anymore, I guess.

013 Nurse: Well...

014 Doctor: <Looks up from the chart and interrupts the nurse> We need you to eat more okay? When you were home last time you weren't eating much. We've got to build you up some.

015 Patient: (sighing) Alright.

016 Doctor: <Turning to the nurse> Will you schedule Pulmonology to come drain his lung?

017 Patient: <Looks at the nurse with a "shrugged face"> See ya.

018 Nurse: (To the doctor) Sure. (To the patient) I'll see you later today, okay? <Leaves the room>

019 Doctor: Alright, we're going to get that lung taken care of and get some good food in you and then we'll see about the medicine after that okay?

020 Patient: Okay.

021 Doctor: <Looking back at the chart> Do you have any questions for me?

022 Patient: Nope.

023 Doctor: Okay, I'll see you tomorrow. Bye now.

024 Patient: Later, Doc.

While an ordinary reading of this dialogue does not immediately signal power issues, a deeper exploration emphasizes important features of disciplinary power and its relation to patient care.

In Jeffrey Michael Clair's (1990) discourse analysis of physician encounters with terminal patients, from which this dialogue was adapted, he notes that the discomfort felt by the physicians led them to manage the discourse in particularly interesting ways. In the first place, health care providers go into their fields to cure people, not to watch them die. While they will inevitably experience the latter, there remains a sense of failure when it occurs. They often feel helpless and inadequate, and often unconsciously attempt to regain a sense of control by managing the discourse with patients in particular ways. In the dialogue above, the physician is struggling with his role in the context of a patient who is terminal, while the patient is feeling disconnected from and ignored by his physician. The patient attempts to engage his care providers in a discussion about his past experiences in scuba diving. While the nurse is receptive to the discussion, the physician almost completely ignores it, returning focus to the physiological features of the patient's condition (e.g., lines 004 and 014). Toward the end of the discussion, the patient "gives up" his attempts to talk about scuba diving and becomes passive.

We can see disciplinary power operating first in the way the physician manages the discourse. By redirecting the conversation back toward biomedical issues and away from the personal issues that the patient appears to want to talk about, the physician, though likely without conscious intent, signals that those sorts of personal aspects of the patient's life are not relevant, and, by implication, unimportant. The patient gets the message and desists his attempts to talk about his personal life, but not without feeling somewhat rejected in the process and disengaging from the physician. The physician also signals that the patient's engagement in the encounter is largely unnecessary when he asks if the patient has any questions, but does so while looking back at the chart (line 021). That is, he signals that he is not genuinely interested in the patient's questions. Additionally, the physician, again without consciously knowing he is doing so, exerts his authority throughout the conversation by interrupting the conversation between the patient and nurse (line 014), and by holding out long silences followed by nonsequiturs (lines 004, 009, and 014). In the business world, when one is having a difficult time in a negotiation, a good strategy is to call for a break, leave the room, and make sure to be the last one to come back in at the end of the break (Parker & Lambert 2008). Psychologically, this signals to everyone else, "I've returned and we can get started again," placing that person symbolically in a position of power. Without knowing it, the physician in this encounter was engaging in a very similar micro-level discursive strategy. He takes a break from the discourse with long silences, and reenters the conversation after a break with a statement that does not fit in with what the nurse and patient are discussing. This signals, "I've returned to the conversation and what I'm saying is more important than what you were saying," symbolizing his power and authority in the interaction.

In the above scenario, we can see the patient being disciplined to avoid discussion of things that are personal into a very passive, disengaged role in the encounter. However, thinking more broadly, we can understand that the way the physician is acting also results from disciplinary forces. Until recently, medical training gave scant attention to the social and psychological elements of patient care, focusing nearly exclusively on the biomedical aspects of health and illness. That is, this physician was likely trained to hone a biomedical focus, so it is not surprising that this forms the dominant lens through which he sees this patient. In cases like this where the physician is feeling uncomfortable in the face of an inability to cure the patient, he may especially resort to that dominant biomedical framework that gives some semblance of control and certainty, rather than wading into the murky waters of the social and psychological elements of the patient's life. Moreover, just as the technological and medicolegal environment disciplines childbirth practices for obstetricians, this physician may encounter professional constraints that mitigate his ability to do the social and humanistic work needed in this encounter. Time constraints, the financial demands to provide billable services, and the like may create a professional habit of ignoring the more ambiguous terrain of the social and psychological elements of the individual patient. Here, it is important to recognize that material power (i.e., the demand to produce revenue by seeing patients and providing billable services) represents disciplinary power when clinicians internalize material constraints as habits of professional practice, and then enact those constraints themselves. In other words, the structural constraints in which we practice can become part of how we conceptualize our own practices (this echoes heavily the notion of *habitus* discussed in Chapter 6).

While we typically think of clinical encounters as places where practitioners have greater power compared to patients, examining this scenario illustrates that the functions of power are much more complex. Certainly the patient is subject to the subtle disciplinary forces in this encounter, but it is important to recognize that practitioners are as well. The professional roles of practitioners come with particular role expectations, and in the modern period, the clinician's role has been widely recognized as curing disease. The inability to do this destabilizes that role in the encounter, and it potentially creates a great deal of existential discomfort, where the clinician has internalized the role of "curer," as opposed to another, potentially broader role that would enable him or her to more easily conceive of a way to engage the patient who cannot be cured. In short, he is disciplined by the expectations of his or her role as one who cures diseases.

The implications of this scenario are critically important for patient care. We can understand the divergence between patient and physician fundamentally as a mismatch of the identities each was offering in the encounter (Wasserman 2014).

Talcott Parsons 1951 [1991] used the notion of the *sick role* to capture essential aspects of being a patient. When people get sick, according to Parsons (1951 [1991]), their behavior deviates from societal norms but in a patterned way that tends to reflect institutionalized expectations.[2] Specifically, Parsons (1951 [1991]) suggested that when one enters the sick role they have two rights and two responsibilities:

Rights:

1. The sick person is excused from normal social roles.
2. The sick person is not blamed for their condition.

Responsibilities:

1. The sick person should try to get well again.
2. The sick person should seek professional help.

Importantly, Parsons explored the meaning of being sick in the context of functional social relationships. That is, his concept of the sick role accounts for the relationship of the sick person to their social system and inherently assumes that they will return to serving their social functions (or at least attempt to do so). However, as noted by Varul (2010:72), "Parsons' sick role concept has become problematic in the face of the increased significance of chronic illness and the growing emphasis on lifestyle-centered health promotion." This is both because medicine proper increasingly has to share terrain with other players in the health landscape (see Chapter 2) and because the incurability of chronic illness renders the requirement of healing and returning to social functions difficult and sometimes impossible. Similarly, in the scenario above, the patient is terminal. That is, the sick role no longer has any functional utility for him. We can therefore read his assertions about scuba diving, not as irrelevant chatter, but rather as his attempt to exit the sick role and return to a sense of himself as a whole person (Wasserman 2014). As later critics have pointed out, Parsons' concept hinges on the acceptance of the role by the person who is sick. In this case, the patient is beginning to reject the sick role because it no longer offers any benefit; he cannot fulfill his responsibility to get well again and that likely will no longer be his goal. This is disruptive to the physician who appears to be continuing to exercise the functions of a "curer."

For his part, the physician appears unable to recognize the significance of the patient's behavior and the deeper implications of his talk about scuba diving. Put another way, while the physician's curative identity is well matched to a patient fully engaged in the sick role, the relationship falls apart when the curer cannot understand the whole person who is giving up the "responsibilities" of the sick role. If the physician recognized this feature of the discourse, a number of very positive things could have unfolded. For one, he may have been able to more easily initiate a discussion about transitioning the goals of care toward providing the patient with comfort and dignity at the end of his life. Moreover, while the goal of curing this patient's cancer may no longer be possible, there are other goals that are evident. For example, the physician wants the patient to eat more, but he misses the opportunity to connect with the patient personally in a way that may facilitate that goal. For

---

[2] Parsons considered this a form of sanctioned deviance, an *accepted* deviation from normal behavior.

example, the physician might have been able to capitalize on the patient's identity by saying, "I want you to eat like you used to when you got back from scuba diving all day," rather than ignoring it as irrelevant.

To be clear, power differentials are inevitable in clinical practice. The entire basis of each health profession stands on the fact that each has its own body of knowledge, skills, and specialized training. Where knowledge differentials double as power differentials, power will always be asymmetrical, but it is important to recognize the complexity of these dynamics. While practitioners exercise power in both direct and subtle ways, they also are subject to many kinds of power that condition how they practice and even what they see in their patients. Thus, even though power differences may be inevitable, it is important to be conscious in clinical practice, not only of how one might unknowingly exercising power in ways that might be problematic, but also how one's habits of practice are conditioned by a variety of powerful influences. In the next section we examine how medicalization emerges from these kinds of disciplinary social forces.

Medicalization, Social Control, and Overdiagnosis

At its heart, medicalization works through the powerful social influences that create norms and pathologize deviation from those norms. Within the context of medical care, we tend to act as though sickness is defined in objectively scientific terms, and certainly there are conditions that are so devastating and disruptive that it would seem impossible to define them any other way. However, we can also discern many illnesses that are more clearly social in character. This is perhaps most clear for conditions that have a behavioral component (like alcoholism, discussed above). Where particular forms of behavior are pathologized, we gain a glimpse into how defining and diagnosing diseases can operate as a form of social control. While unintentional and often unseen among practitioners, it is important to recognize that the diagnostic process can reflect social norms just as much as biomedical markers, and therefore can function as a disciplining force. Being reflective about this element of clinical practice raises important social and ethical questions for practitioners concerning the relationship between their care of individual patients and the functions they serve in broader social contexts. Understanding the influence that social norms bear on the practitioner–patient relationship is important for protecting its integrity and also promoting the ability of each to be reflective about the meanings and experiences of illness.

Childhood attention deficit/hyperactivity disorder (ADHD) provides an excellent example of the potential for diagnosis to serve as a social control. There is intense debate about the factors that influence the prevalence of ADHD in society. Rates of ADHD vary significantly between cultures and classes, and have risen significantly over time. Since the late 1800s there have been numerous diagnostic classifications for sets of behavioral symptoms in children that now belong to the ADHD diagnosis. In 1902, Dr. Richard Still observed the behavior of twenty children whom he described as having a "defect of moral control," whereby they knew right from wrong but lacked the willpower to control their behavior (Reeve & Wright 1996:I-1). From the 1920s through the 1960s, practitioners and researchers focused on brain pathology resulting from disease (especially encephalitis) or injury, including diagnosing children displaying symptoms of hyperactivity with "minimal brain damage" (MBD). In the 1970s the focus shifted to more behavioral concerns, and variants of the term *hyperkinesia* were used to describe children who had difficulty sitting still, would fidget, lacked impulse control, and the like. In the 1980s, the focus shifted again toward the ability to pay attention, with or without hyperactivity. In 1994, the American Psychiatric Association (2013) defined ADHD as, "a neurobiological, developmental disorder" essentially characterized by, "a persistent pattern of inattention and/or hyperactivity-impulsivity that is more frequent than is typically observed in individuals at a comparable level of development." The *Diagnostic and Statistical Manual of Mental Disorders* (DSM-V) updated criteria to include the diagnosis of ADHD in adults as well as children.

The current diagnostic criteria for ADHD require that symptoms interfere with functioning and development; are present in at least two settings (e.g., school and home); have direct negative consequences for social, academic, and/or occupational functioning; and that several symptoms are present before age 12, and that six or more symptoms have persisted for at least six months. In order to be diagnosed with ADHD, a child should exhibit six or more symptoms from either of the following two categories taken from the *DSM*-V (American Psychiatric Association 2013):

Inattention

- Fails to give close attention to details or makes careless mistakes
- Has difficulty sustaining attention in tasks or play activities
- Often does not seem to listen when spoken to directly
- Often does not follow through on instructions
- Often has difficulty with organization
- Often avoids, dislikes, or is reluctant tasks requiring a lot of thinking
- Often loses things necessary for tasks or activities
- Is often easily distracted by extraneous stimuli
- Is forgetful in daily activities

Hyperactive-impulsive

- Often fidgets with or taps hands or feet or squirms in chair
- Often leaves seat in situations when remaining seated is expected
- Often runs about or climbs in situations where it is inappropriate
- Often unable to play or engage in leisure activities quietly
- Often acts as if driven by a motor
- Often talks excessively
- Often blurts out an answer before a question has been completed
- Often has difficulty waiting his or her turn
- Often interrupts or intrudes on others

The diagnostic process centers on interviews not only with the child, but also their parents, and ideally their teachers, counselors, and the like, along with direct observation and reports about behaviors from teachers or classroom observation by an educational psychologist. This process also is intended to incorporate a clinical exam to rule out vision and hearing difficulties, which might otherwise explain many of the above symptoms.

While there are some neurological conditions associated with ADHD, the substantial increases in the rate over time have given rise to concerns that the disease is overdiagnosed. One large meta-analysis found a pooled ADHD prevalence estimate of 7.2%, making it one of the most commonly diagnosed childhood conditions (Thomas et al. 2015). Rates of diagnosis vary by a number of factors such as sex and race/ethnicity, with boys diagnosed significantly more than girls and white children diagnosed at a significantly higher rate than African American and Hispanic children (Morgan et al. 2013). Taylor (2004:9) points out that, "Individual differences in hyperactivity have known physical counterparts" including genetic variations that, "work in interaction with the environment ... to set the course into adjustment or disorder." Timimi (2004:8), however, counters by noting, "The immaturity of children is a biological fact, but the ways in which this immaturity is understood and made meaningful is a fact of culture." In particular, the definitions of ADHD, where the diagnostic process is grounded, depend on social expectations of behavior in an academic environment that require even very young children to have a certain level of focus and stillness. It is against such a backdrop that child behavior is defined as problematic and those sorts of social contexts determine where we draw the line between normal and pathological behavior. The social process of defining disease in general, and ADHD in particular, is a complex process influenced by a number of macro- and micro-level social forces.

Because ADHD is fundamentally a matter of child behavior deviating significantly from our expectations of what is normal or functional, the environmental backdrop against which we are evaluating behavior is critical. For example, increased academic evaluation at earlier grades, particularly in the form of standardized state testing, causes a shift in our expectations of school children. Children whose behavior would be relatively unremarkable in a less structured educational environment, for example, have functional difficulties in a highly structured one. Additionally, as the educational goals and evaluation metrics shift expectations of classroom behavior, parental expectations of behavior may also shift accordingly.

Complicating the environmental backdrop against which ADHD is given meaning are professional and industrial shifts in health care, including where "the profit-dependent pharmaceutical industry and a high-status profession looking for new roles [contribute to] the ideal cultural preconditions for the birth and propagation of the ADHD construct" (Timimi 2004:8). Anyone even casually familiar with American television will be familiar with direct-to-consumer marketing by pharmaceutical companies, which highlights various "symptoms" that a given drug can treat. Indeed, patient requests for particular drugs significantly increase the likelihood that a clinician will prescribe them (see, e.g., Kravitz et al. 2005). Moreover, prescribers get much of their information about particular drugs from pharmaceutical company representatives themselves (known as *detailers*). Detailing and the distribution of free samples also influence prescribing practices (Gönül et al. 2001). Add to this a shift in American psychiatry, "away from a focus on context to an approach that essentialized and biologized mental illness" (Vallée 2011:93) and we can see that there are powerful social forces that influence the boundaries between normal and pathological behavior.

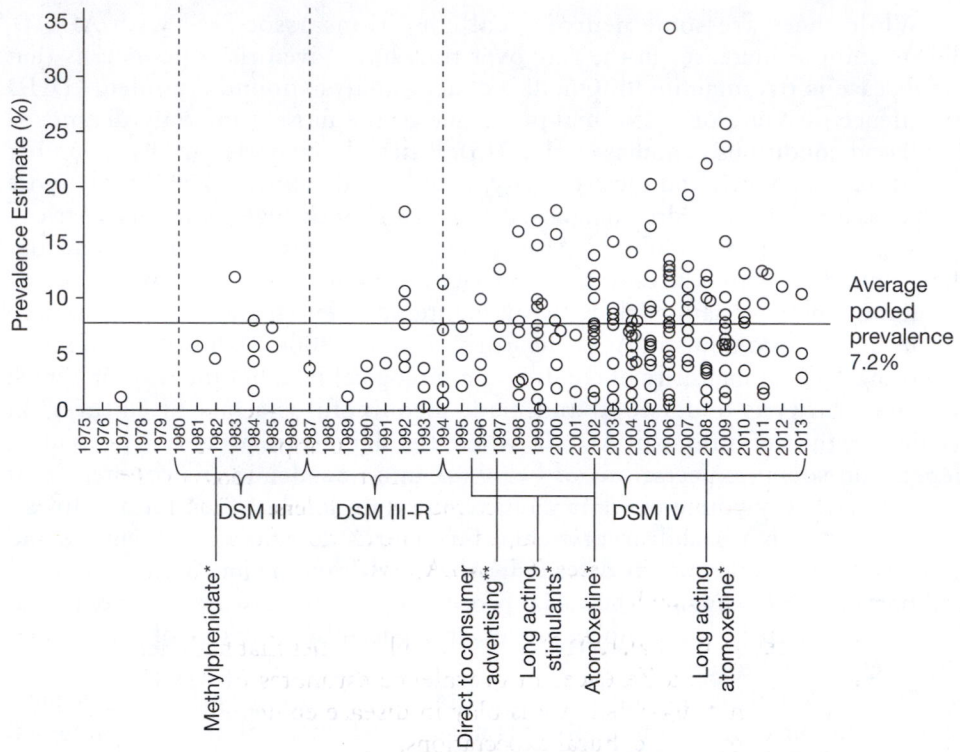

FIG. 7.3 Prevalence of ADHD over time (with benchmarks for approval of key drugs, direct-to-consumer advertising, and *DSM* version).

Note: * U.S. Food and Drug Administration approval year.

** Direct-to-consumer advertising to the United States.

Source: Thomas, Rae, Sharon Sanders, Jenny Doust, Elaine Beller, & Paul Glasziou. (2015). "Prevalence of Attention-Deficit/Hyperactivity Disorder: A Systematic Review and Meta-analysis." *Pediatrics* 135, e994–1001.

The diagnostic process for ADHD involves relatively subjective criteria and is influenced by the subjective perspectives of a variety of observers (Kirk 2004). As described above, the *DSM* provides various criteria and thresholds for diagnosis (e.g., meeting at least six criteria in at least two settings), but these criteria have been revised across different editions of the *DSM*. Thomas et al. (2015) found that studies using the *DSM*-III-R manifested significantly lower prevalence rates of ADHD than those using the *DSM*-IV (see Fig. 7.3). Of course, this does not necessarily signify that changes to the diagnostic criteria *cause* increases in prevalence; they might simply covary (see Chapter 3). Moreover, one might argue that if criteria are improved over time, as is implied by any such revision, and in turn more accurately identify conditions, then it is not surprising to see prevalence rates rise. Still, it is important to recognize the role that diagnostic criteria have in shaping the definitions, meanings, and, ultimately, the rates of an illness. Bastra and Frances (2012:486) argue that the recently revised *DSM*-V will further inflate these rates "by adding new impulsivity criteria, lowering the percentage of criteria needed for the diagnosis, lowering the number of criteria needed for individuals older than

17 years, applying criteria with untested wording to adults, increasing the latest age of onset from 7 to 12 years, and switching the focus from impairment to displayed behaviors before that age."

The role of measurement was highlighted in an article on the popular *Psychology Today* website claiming, "French kids don't have ADHD" in which the rate of ADHD among children in France was reported to be only 0.5% (Wedge 2012). This prompted a flurry of responses to the contrary, many citing a study by Lecendreux et al. (2010) that placed the prevalence between 3.5% and 5.6%, a range similar to other countries. What was really at issue, however, were the differences in measurement. Vallée (2011:95) suggests that psychoanalysis exerted a consulting, rather than diagnostic, influence on the culture of French psychiatry. He continues:

> While some French child psychiatrists realized the DSM-III's classificatory approach offered potential benefits for epidemiological research, leaders within the profession believed the DSM-III was wholly inappropriate for the French setting, as the classification was overly reductionistic and at odds with French child psychiatry's developmental approach to mental disorders.... The [French Federation of Psychiatry] task force developed the French classification system for child and adolescent mental illnesses (CFTMEA), which they released in 1983, and updated in 1988 and 2000.

The study by Lecendreux et al. (2010) reviewed only studies that had used the *DSM*.[3] The resulting dramatic differences in prevalence estimates of ADHD in France highlight the role that diagnostic tools play in disease epidemiology, particularly because they operationalize cultural expectations.

Assessing whether a child, for example, "struggles to follow through on instructions," in a way that is normal or abnormal is inevitably a matter of judgment. The incorporation of assessments from teachers, counselors, and parents may give a more holistic perspective; however, these assessments nonetheless hinge on subjective judgments. For example, Havey et al. (2005) found that teachers identified ADHD in their students at much higher rates than the expected based on national estimates of prevalence. More striking is that class size was significantly associated with the likelihood of identifying ADHD at a high rate (Havey et al. 2005). This likely suggests that teachers with larger class sizes have less tolerance for nonconforming behaviors, which lowers their threshold for perceiving a child's behavior as problematic. Ultimately, however, this demonstrates how various social factors can affect the diagnostic process.

There is little doubt that some children suffer from the symptoms that comprise the diagnostic label of attention deficit and hyperactivity in ways that are debilitating and in need of medical intervention. It is also clear, however, that there are social forces that shape the boundaries and meanings of ADHD. We could examine any number of illnesses in the same way, sketching the social factors that surround how these diseases emerge and how their meanings change over time. Ultimately, the picture of medicalization is complex, involving systemic forces (e.g., economics, marketing, or educational policy), cultural forces (e.g., our expectations of normal

---

[3] Perhaps not incidentally, this study also was funded by Shire Development Inc., which raises questions about conflicts of interest, particularly where there may be financial benefit associated with greater rates of diagnosis.

child behavior), and interpersonal dynamics (e.g., subjective observations in the diagnostic process; see Conrad 1975; Vallée 2010). However, the complexities of the medicalization of behavior have a core underlying disciplinary function. That is, with the help of marketing and policy forces, we internalize expectations, which condition how we view behavior. These conditioned perceptions, in turn, cause us to look for ways to "correct" behaviors in children that deviate from the norms we hold. Put simply, medicalization reflects a form of social control (Conrad 1992), both where systemic forces condition our expectations and where we ourselves enact those expectations on our social world.

Some diagnoses might also significantly affect a person's understanding of their own identity. We more fully address issues of illness experience in Chapter 8, but insofar as diagnoses give meaning to an embodied experience that often is existentially significant to the patient, a diagnosis has the power to affect how patients see themselves. With respect to ADHD, the diagnosis can affect how children conceptualize their behavior vis-à-vis their identity. This is not to say, as some might assume, that the children internalize the diagnosis itself as a core flaw in their moral identity. Singh (2007:176) reports, "A majority of children felt that at their core, there was persistent 'badness'. Medication could help to overcome badness, but not entirely." It is unclear how much of this developing sense of self is internalized from feedback these children receive about their behavior from parents and teachers versus how much of it, if any, is their own self-assessment. At the same time, this shows that diagnosis and treatment are powerful social vectors intersecting a complex system. That is, diagnosis and treatment enter a complicated landscape where children are developing a sense of self, being conditioned by their environments and the reactions of others to their behavior. While diagnosis and treatment could undermine an "authentic sense of self" among these children, Singh (2007) illustrates that this could be a positive thing, if children are developing a sense that they are morally flawed. In that case, diagnosis and treatment might help the children develop a sense that their impulses are not indicative of their character. Additionally, this shows that the foundations of medicalization are not exclusive to practitioners and the health care industry, but function in tandem with broader environmental factors and social expectations. While there are any number of alternative possibilities, the critical point here is that the ADHD diagnosis is a powerful social force that not only conditions behavior of children with the goal of making them more functional within a social system, it also affects their developing understandings of themselves, specifically their perception of their own moral character (Singh 2007). Again, this highlights the immense power, and corresponding responsibility, that clinicians should appreciate as they engage with these patients.

The cyclical nature of medicalization as a form of social control (where our cognitive frameworks are conditioned and where we then condition social life accordingly, which reinforces the norms we hold, etc.) represents an important moment of reflection for health practitioners. Often, clinicians are postured as one of many agents of medicalization, part of the problem. But this dramatically oversimplifies the complexity of the process. In fact, in a study by Rushton et al. (2004), 55.3% of physicians surveyed felt that teachers pressured them to make an ADHD diagnosis and 71.3% agreed that teachers expected them to prescribe medication. With respect to diagnosing and treating illness, particularly those with diffuse and subjective criteria, practitioners find themselves in a complex and contested landscape with social pressures emerging from multiple directions. The influence of those social forces and the subjective qualities of the diagnostic process likely are inevitable. But it is important for practitioners to recognize the social nature of diagnosis and to be conscious of the ways these social forces might affect them. Critically reflecting on these features of health care practice can empower clinicians to work creatively and reflexively with individual patients.

As shown above, illnesses with criteria that are measured subjectively (such as ADHD) provide good examples of how social forces shape the boundaries of illness. Yet it is not only psychological or contested illnesses that are subject to the various forces of medicalization. These processes also apply to those conditions that we see every day. In their book *Overdiagnosed*, Welch et al. (2011) explore a variety of conditions for which the diagnostic boundaries have expanded, corresponding to rising prevalence rates and greater numbers of people treated, thereby turning people into patients overnight, even in the absence of symptoms. They point out that until relatively recently, practitioners did not diagnose diseases in the absence of outward symptoms and therefore did not treat them. However, as we have discussed, in the era of chronic illness, disease has shifted from being a matter of the presence or absence of some infectious agent, toward a matter of having too much or too little of something that is normal (e.g., cholesterol, blood sugar, etc.). These diseases of degree, such as hypertension, can be misleading. We use epidemiological data to set standards for normal and abnormal blood pressure and then classify everyone above the standard (e.g., diastolic BP > 90 mm Hg) as hypertensive. But where we reify the categorical diagnosis, we can forget that there remains a significant difference in degree of severity. That is, we can easily decide simply to treat everyone who is hypertensive with a dose of medication to lower blood pressure. While we will calibrate the dosage and kind of medication to their condition, the decision to treat often can follow unreflexively from the fact that they fall on the side of the line that has been deemed abnormal.

Welch and colleagues (2011) point out that in the case of hypertension, degree matters a great deal not just in terms of how much medicine one gives, but whether it makes sense at all to treat the same condition in all clinical cases. They point out that there are diminishing returns to treating less severe cases of hypertension (and other conditions) that become at least questionable at some point, particularly since medications also have well-known risks. For example, in data from early studies of hypertension (also discussed in Chapter 3), those with severe diastolic hypertension (115–129 mm Hg) exhibited a 72% chance of benefiting from the treatment over five years (i.e., avoiding a significant cardiac event), while those with mild diastolic hypertension (90–104 mm Hg) exhibited only a 9% chance of benefit. Those with very mild cases (90–100 mm Hg) only showed a 6% chance of benefit.[4] Put another way, for those with very mild hypertension, eighteen people have to be medicated for only one person to benefit, while seventeen additional people bear the risks of treatment with no benefit (i.e., they were overdiagnosed). In short, patients with milder degrees of abnormality typically have a lower chance of treatment benefit,

---

[4] Categories for mild and very mild hypertension overlap in this example, due to different measurement definitions for these categories in the multiple studies from which the Welch et al. (2011) data are drawn.

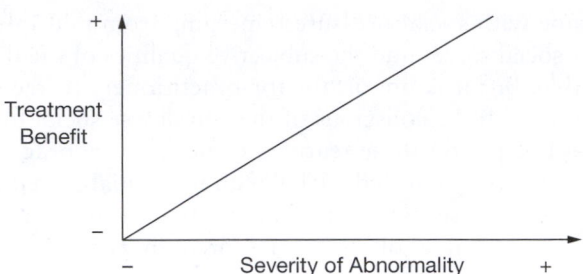

FIG. 7.4 Relationship between degree of abnormality and potential treatment benefit.

Source: Welch, H. Gilbert, Lisa M. Schwartz, & Steven Woloshin. (2011). *Over-Diagnosed: Making People Sick in the Pursuit of Health.* Boston, MA: Beacon Press.

and vice versa (see Fig. 7.4). Of course, part of the issue is that we cannot tell who will and who will not benefit. But at the same time, what becomes clear is that creating categories of disease out of conditions of degree engenders a slippery slope of more treatment in a population, despite often-questionable effectiveness. This too is a form (and outcome) of medicalization. More importantly, it reminds us that epidemiological evidence is not a substitute for reflexive clinical judgment. In particular, practitioners need to be thoughtful not only about what kind of treatment a person needs, but also about the question of whether they need treatment at all, that is, whether the treatment is indeed sufficiently beneficial (refer to Chapter 3 for further discussion of the VA hypertension studies, evidence-based decision-making, and incorporating the notion of reflexivity vis-à-vis research findings).

Conclusion: Dilemmas of Difference

At its heart, navigating diagnosis and treatment and the social forces that influence those clinical practices is a matter of delineating normality and abnormality. As noted in Chapter 2, with chronic illnesses this becomes especially difficult where it involves matters of degree (i.e., how much LDL cholesterol is too much?), rather than the presence or absence of a discrete condition or infectious agent. In this chapter, we showed that this also is the case where other conditions, and often, social behaviors, are pathologized. Ultimately, in all of these instances we make a decision about what constitutes a normal lab value or behavior, and what constitutes an unacceptable deviation from those norms, with the latter naturally engendering treatment. But despite increasing utilization of evidence in making these judgments (which, as noted in Chapter 3, typically is derived from studies of groups and therefore still has to be adapted and applied to individual patients), they have an unavoidably social component. Because defining illness is a matter of making judgments about what is normal and abnormal, health care practitioners wield significant power, and they in turn have an ethical responsibility to exercise it judiciously.

Medicating behavioral deviations, for example, risks a move toward the intolerance of difference that practitioners should bear in mind. Historically, the eugenics movement (particularly in the first half of the twentieth century) sought to improve the health and fitness of the population, either by promoting procreation among "desirable people" or by eliminating "undesirable people," through sterilization or outright genocide (Kevles 1995). While eugenics is widely considered an historical shame and associated largely with Nazi Germany, we ought to bear in mind that eugenics was pioneered in the United States and that practices of opposing and eliminating differences continue even today. At the same time, some differences and deviations clearly are unfavorable. Certainly it would be unreasonable to say that a cancerous growth is just a "difference," without making any normative judgment about it. However, while that sort of nihilistic view of health and the body is problematic, drawing the lines between "abnormal" and simply "different" is not easy and requires sensitivity to the way social forces might influence such determinations. This poses a significant dilemma for practitioners.

For example, deafness is widely defined as a disability, at least by hearing society. However, members of the Deaf[5] community often see it simply as a difference and view themselves as a subculture; their deafness simply is a part of who they are. After all, the Deaf community has strong in-ties, its own language (e.g., American Sign Language, or ASL) with a unique syntax, along with its own social institutions, arts community, and so on. With the advent and increasing success of cochlear implants, many in the hearing world are shocked to discover that Deaf parents often have strong opposition to getting the procedure for their children.[6] Dolnick (1993:38) writes, "So strong is the feeling of cultural solidarity that many deaf parents cheer on discovering that their baby is deaf. Pondering such a scene, a hearing person can experience a kind of vertigo." However, just as these parents feel a strong attachment to Deaf culture, they want to share that culture with their children, to have an identity connected to them in that way.

The idea that deafness ought not be treated, or at least that treatment is not a foregone conclusion, is challenging for the institution of health care whose very ethos drives toward fixing problems. Deafness certainly represents a disadvantage in contemporary society, including reading and literacy deficits in children and later employment and earnings disadvantages in adults (Harris & Terlektsi 2011; PepNet2 2014). The argument that naturally follows suggests that if we can mitigate these disadvantages using medical technology, then we ought to do so. This reasoning has prima facie appeal, but as Levy (2002) points out, many (though not all) of these disadvantages are the results of discrimination and social stigma, not deafness itself. If society were more accommodating, these disadvantages would be significantly mitigated. Moreover, when this logic is extrapolated to other groups who also face disadvantage, it is less palpable. African Americans, for example, also face educational attainment and income disadvantages in the United States. These disadvantages also result from past and present discrimination and the structural accumulation of disadvantage (Chapter 5). Few would be comfortable with medically intervening to make African American children white, if such a treatment existed.[7]

---

[5] The capital "D" is used to distinguish a culture from the physiological fact of deafness.

[6] The procedure is still very common owing significantly to the fact that the vast majority of deaf children are born to hearing parents, without the kind of cultural attachments to deafness as Deaf parents.

[7] In fact, in the late 1800s, there were attempts to deal with the "Negro problem" by whitening the skin of African Americans (Kevles 1997). Today, such an idea is repugnant to most.

At the same time, the entirety of race/ethnic disadvantage can be accounted for by discrimination and stigma, whereas deafness arguably represents a real, physical disadvantage (Levy 2002). Here we see how health care practice is caught between avoiding the oppressive enforcement of social norms on the one hand, and a sort of health nihilism on the other. That is, if we consider all physical conditions simply to be differences and reject the idea that we ought to use medical science to correct them, we face a reduction to the absurd, where health care ought never to intervene. Of course, there are reasonable middle options to these polar extremes. Practitioners might consider counseling patients about the features of their conditions, including the social disadvantages, while at the same time respecting the idea that patients' perspectives and values might differ significantly from their own, even where there is widespread social consensus. Moreover, the "dilemma of difference" ought to give practitioners pause with regard to the momentum of interventionist medicine. As we grow in our ability to treat various diseases, we also need to remember that we partially are acting out a particular set of conceptions of normality. This is a form of social power entrusted to clinicians who have the responsibility to be judicious and reflexive about the social forces involved in their practice.

CHAPTER 7 ACTIVITY

Risks, Benefits, and Perspective: Navigating the Autism Spectrum

It's 2026 and you are a clinician working at the Eleanor Olivia Center for Behavioral Pediatrics and you specialize in autism spectrum disorder.

Today, you are meeting with Ethan and Eliot Tyne, the parents of a 5-year-old child, Madeline, who has been undergoing a number of tests at the Center. You reveal to them your diagnosis that Madeline has a mild form of autism spectrum disorder.

The parents are distraught. Eliot immediately begins to cry, while Ethan appears angry with you for being the bearer of bad news. You emphasize that the condition seems mild and that therapeutic interventions have advanced greatly over the last several decades, noting that you think the prospects for Madeline to live a healthy and productive life are good. Little you say to them seems to put them at ease, but eventually they gather themselves and head home.

A week later, you notice that the Tynes are on your patient schedule for the day. When you meet with them, Ethan hands you a stack of papers printed from various websites about new therapies for treating autism.

"What do you know about intrathecal infusion of hematopoietic stem cells as a therapy?" Ethan asks.

You reply, "Well, it was approved about five years ago. It helps in the pathophysiology of the disease, but the benefits appear to decrease over time. Additionally, we see the biggest benefits in the most severe cases, so it's typically not recommended for milder forms of autism because the risks don't outweigh the benefits."

"We'd like to try it," Ethan says firmly, "The stories we've read have been incredible. So many people have reported that their children improved tremendously."

"Before we head down that road, let's talk about what the condition really is and what it really means," you respond, trying to defuse some of the tension in the situation. You think back to an article you read early in your career by autism researcher and neuro-scientist Laurent Mottron (2011:33–35) who wrote:

> As a clinician, I also know all too well that autism is a disability that can make daily activities difficult. One out of ten autistics

cannot speak, nine out of ten have no regular job and four out of five autistic adults are still dependent on their parents. Most face the harsh consequences of living in a world that has not been constructed around their priorities and interests.

But in my experience, autism can also be an advantage. In certain settings, autistic individuals can fare extremely well. One such setting is scientific research. For the past seven years, I have been a close collaborator of an autistic woman, Michelle Dawson. She has shown me that autism, when combined with extreme intelligence and an interest in science, can be an incredible boon to a research lab

As a result, my research group and others believe that autism should be described and investigated as a variant within the human species. These variations in gene sequence or expression may have adaptive or maladaptive consequences, but they cannot be reduced to an error of nature that should be corrected.

You think that perhaps getting these parents to consider the diagnosis from this other perspective may be helpful, particularly since you believe that less invasive and risky treatments will be sufficient to address the social disadvantages that come with Madeline's mild version of the condition.

Finally, you say to them, "The newer cognitive behavioral approaches we are using still try to help children with autism manage sometimes dysfunctional aspects of their condition, but we focus more now on how they can grow and develop their innate talents."

Eliot, who has been very quiet throughout the meeting, looks up at you asking, "What do you mean? It sounds like you're saying autism is a good thing."

Discussion Questions

1. Discuss whether autism spectrum disorder is overly medicalized. That is, are people too quick to see all forms of it as in need of medical intervention (i.e., as something to be normalized)?

   Helpful Hint: Your perspective on this, like autism itself, does not have to be "all or nothing" with regard to understanding it as a medical condition in need of intervention. There are degrees of severity in the condition and therefore potential degrees of intervention.

2. How would you respond to Eliot's question? How would you approach these parents, who are clearly struggling to deal with this condition and how it is affecting their family? If the parents insisted on proceeding with the more aggressive therapy, how would you make the decision about whether to agree and refer them for the procedure?

   Helpful Hint: Some of the material on illness experience and grief in Chapter 8 and on patient–provider communication in Chapter 9 might be helpful as you think about your approach.

3. Do you agree with Mottron (2011)? Should we abandon the notion that autism is an "error" (or a disease) and see it instead as a "variant" with good and bad attributes?

4. To what other diseases might we apply these same questions? Should we abandon the notion of those conditions as "error" as well? What are the benefits and consequences of doing so?

   Helpful Hint: Think about how seeing various conditions through a medical lens can cause us to miss the potential positive aspects in various conditions, but at the same time, how the opposite extreme might obscure real disadvantages faced by people with those conditions for which they may need and want treatment.

The Illness Experiences of Patients and Families

LEARNING OBJECTIVES

After reading this chapter, students should be able to

- Articulate the differences between a disease and an illness and elaborate on how professional approaches to a disease can become disconnected from patients' experiences of illness.

- Discuss common social–psychological experiences of illness including the experience of grief and the impact of a significant illness on one's identity.

- Explain the social factors that influence caregiver burden and the outcomes associated with it.

- Describe various ways in which clinical practitioners can intervene in caregiver burden and demonstrate an appreciation for the need to do so.

In Chapter 2, we discussed how the underlying perspective of modernism narrowed the scope of clinical practice, how it receded from a sense of the whole person nested in a larger cosmic context to a compartmentalized physical body. As Foucault captured it: "'What is the matter with you?'... was replaced by that other question: 'Where does it hurt?'" In this chapter we explore a number of important implications of this transition. For patients, sickness has remained a holistic, embodied, and lived experience that is often inseparable from how it affects their social functions and identity. Moreover, illness is not experienced exclusively by the patient but also, in very real terms, by their families. Yet modern medicine has largely ignored such features of the patient experience in its narrow focus on biomedical features of the disease and the sick body. This has created a significant divergence in how patients and families experience illness and how providers approach disease.

Fundamentally, what is required for providers to bridge the gap between their own professional gaze and the paradigmatically different experiences that patients and families have of illness is a recurring theme of this book: a sociological imagination.[1] More specifically, a provider has to be able to *exit*, so to speak, the

---

[1] Keep in mind that even though it was termed the "sociological" imagination by Mills (1959), he argued (and we agree) that it represents a core way of thinking for the social and behavioral sciences in general, particularly in the ways in which these are utilized by medical and allied health practitioners.

framework through which he or she views the disease in professional terms, and *enter* the world in which the patient and their family will experience illness, how it affects their identities and transforms their social relationships, etc. Some decades before C. Wright Mills (1959) captured the essence of the social sciences in the concept of the sociological imagination, Max Weber (1904 [1949]) articulated the notion of *verstehen*. Its literal translation is *interpretive understanding*, but Weber's concept is better described as *taking on the role of the other*. For Weber, this was an essential aspect of studying culture, particularly for coming to understand how those who are not like us experience the world from within their own perspective. *Verstehen* is, therefore, an important element of the sociological imagination that is useful for beginning to conceptualize how we can cross the gaps between our own perspectives and those of others, to understand the frames of reference with which people who see the world differently make sense of their experiences. Of course, providers and patients are usually not entirely alien to each other. After all, they often (although not always) share a great deal with regard to cultural background and community affiliation. But in health care contexts the distance between them can nonetheless become quite large, particularly because they are very differently positioned around the ailment that has brought them together. In health care, substantial differences between the provider's professional experience of the disease and the patient's lived experience of the illness represent such a disconnect.

In what follows, we explore illness experience, in which social and psychological experiences of illness, for both patients and families, are seamlessly interwoven with the biophysical. As a basis for the ability of providers to take on the role of patients (i.e., to begin to employ the methodology of *verstehen*), we examine several key frameworks of illness experience, including grief and the intersection of illness and identity, with respect to both physical and mental illnesses. We then examine the illness experiences of families, in particular the burdens they face as caregivers, and potential places for providers to intervene in the stress process that comes along with caregiving.

The Illness Experience of Patients

Social scientists have for a long time distinguished *disease* from *illness* (Kleinman 1973, 2013). Building upon Parsons' work on illness as acceptable deviance (see Chapter 7), Freidson (1970:223) notes that, although we often confuse the two, disease is physiological, while illness reflects a wide range of meanings and signals dysfunctions that must be understood in terms of social relationships:

> the etiology of *illness is not biological but social*, stemming from the current social conceptions of what disease is, limited perhaps by whatever few biological facts are universally recognized, and ordered by organizations and occupations devoted to defining, uncovering, and managing illness. As social deviance, illness may be expected to vary in its content and organization fairly independently of biophysical reality. (emphasis added)

While biophysical markers largely, if not entirely, constitute disease, the boundaries of illnesses billow out into larger, more ambiguous, social spaces. Moreover, the contours of illness are defined by social forces in ways that may or may not align with the physiology of disease. Put crudely, while disease is relatively objective, illness is significantly subjective. The former is defined by physical states: a broken bone, contusion, abnormally high lab value, systemic functioning, and the like.[2] The latter, however, is defined by the experience and impact of a physiological condition on expectations of our own functionality. In Chapter 7 we discussed how the meanings of illnesses such as attention deficit hyperactivity disorder (ADHD) must be understood against a backdrop of social expectations (e.g., "normal" child behavior). But every disease doubles as an illness in this way. That is, it has meaning for someone only in the context of how they expect to live and function. Put another way, they experience disease as an intricate part of their social life; the disease expands or diminishes the boundaries and meanings of their social world. As Scambler (2014:1215) puts it: "one can be ill without having a disease, and have a disease without being ill."

The conceptual gap between disease and illness has become more significant after the epidemiological transition, largely because so many chronic diseases are asymptomatic for long periods of time. For example, one can have high cholesterol and high blood pressure without experiencing any significant impact on normal daily functioning for years. Particularly if that person does not, from their own perspective, view themselves as sick, we might say they have a disease, but not an illness. Conversely, many individuals live with "contested illnesses," which affect their social functioning but are not "officially" recognized as disease (Brown et al. 2012). Illnesses such as irritable bowel syndrome and chronic fatigue syndrome, particularly insofar as they have unspecified causes and somatic profiles, might not be recognized as disease from a physiological standpoint if associated physical markers cannot be detected. But from the standpoint of individuals who live these somatic experiences, especially where they experience significant dysfunction or pain and suffering, the illnesses are very real.

There is a great deal of work on the social construction of illness that shows how patients and practitioners both navigate the meanings of illness, and indeed the definitions of disease amidst a complex sociopolitical landscape. While providers often engage patients through a lens of disease with which they are trained to diagnose and treat, patients approach those same encounters through a lens of illness. Where these fail to align, there rests the potential for problems in the provider–patient encounter. Perhaps the clearest expression of the gap between disease and illness concerns the specific gap between pain and suffering. In the clinical setting the former often may be reduced to physical pain, while patients often experience pain in a holistic way such that its physical, social, and psychological aspects may, for them, be indistinguishable. We use the term "suffering" here to set such experiences apart from the narrow concept of pain that literally is measured in the clinic on a scale of 1 to 10 cartoon faces (see Fig. 8.1).

---

[2] It's important to remember that in the era of chronic illness, where disease sometimes can be defined as having too much or too little of something (e.g., cholesterol, Hemoglobin A1c), what *ought* to fall within a *normal* range is what we might call a matter of diagnostic judgment, hopefully buoyed by a solid statistical imagination (see Chapter 3). After all, such ranges are decided based on epidemiological data on human populations, which suggests that particular thresholds correspond with particular health outcomes.

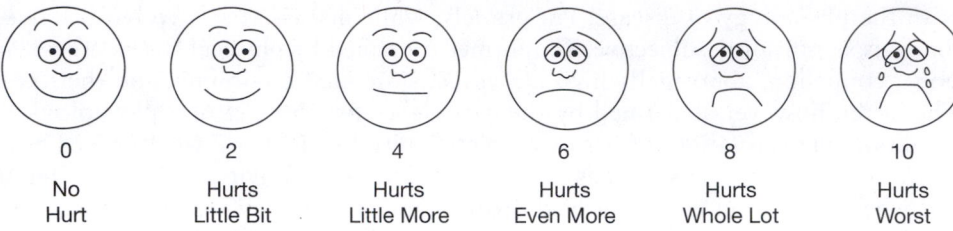

FIG. 8.1 Wong-Baker FACES® Pain Rating Scale.

Source: Wong-Baker FACES Foundation (2015). Wong-Baker FACES® Pain Rating Scale. Retrieved July 7, 2015 with permission from http://www.WongBakerFACES.org.

We do not debate the utility of measuring the transitory experience of physical pain in the clinical context, which can vary between patients even with the same conditions, insofar as they have different levels of pain tolerance. And, of course, this is the properly limited intention of the Wong-Baker scale.[3] At the same time, such scales symbolize the reductionist approach to suffering in the clinical context. They highlight how the complex experience of suffering can be lost in an attempt to quantify the experience within the narrowly constructed notion of physical pain in clinical settings.

Eric Cassell (1991) writes of one patient's experience with a recurring and physically devastating breast cancer that had metastasized to a number of locations in her body. Her physical pain was caused by widespread damage from the cancer (a pathologic fracture of her thigh, nerve damage in her shoulder, etc.). It was also caused by her medical treatment itself, in particular, the devastating effects of radiation, as well as the nausea and vomiting from chemotherapy. But her suffering extended still further beyond these boundaries. As a sculptor, she became depressed when a tumor caused nerve damage to her shoulder that affected her work. Cassell (1991:30) notes, "At one time, she had watery diarrhea that would occur unexpectedly ... sometimes when visitors were present." And finally, she faced not only a fear about future declines, but also an existential suffering that almost always accompanies serious illness. While her physical pain arguably was undertreated, her larger experience of suffering was nearly totally ignored. Cassell (1991:31) summarizes:

> This young woman had severe pain and other physical symptoms that caused her suffering. But she also suffered from threats that were social and others that were personal and private. She suffered from the effects of the disease and its treatment on her appearance and her abilities. She also suffered unremittingly from her perception of the future.

The breadth and complexity of this patient's suffering certainly is not well captured on a scale of 1 to 10. That is, suffering constitutes the more expansive, diffuse, and embodied experience of pain and includes a variety of social and psychological features in addition to physiological stimuli. Suffering breaks free of the more limited boundaries that circumscribe the notion of pain in the same way that illness generally breaks free of the more limited boundaries that circumscribe disease.

[3] Use of such scales to assess pain is also a Joint Commission requirement.

To connect with patients, providers must understand that while their training in the physiology of disease empowers them in all sorts of critically important ways, it can also blind them to the larger illness experiences of the patients. Recall from Chapter 7 that disciplinary forces construct lenses for providers that can make it easier for them to stay focused on the physiological features of disease and treatments. It is what they know best and where they may feel like they have the most control. But while the larger terrain of illness and suffering is ambiguous, subjective, and even perceptibly chaotic, it is important to remember that the patient's embodied experience of illness naturally and inevitably includes the social, psychological, and existential. Later we will highlight that understanding and attending to these wider experiences of illness helps one care for the patient. In the next section, however, we explore several of these aspects of illness experience in more detail.

Grief in Health Care

Early work in the grieving process focused squarely on dying. Elizabeth Kübler-Ross' (1969) seminal work delineated stages of grief experienced by those coping with a terminal illness or the death of a loved one. The five stages are

Denial: A shock-like state where one refuses to acknowledge the reality of the death or the inevitability of the diagnosis.

Anger: Where one expresses extreme frustration, which often manifests in blaming others (including God).

Bargaining: Where an individual attempts to make a sort of cosmic exchange, such as promising to become a better person if God will cure them of their ailment.

Depression: During this stage a person often retreats into a deep sadness over their loss or the inevitability of their death. They may say things like, "what's the point?"

Acceptance: In this stage, terminal patients or those surviving the loss of a loved one come to terms with the event. They often become reflective about their own lives and demonstrate feelings of peace concerning the loss.

This framework matriculated widely into the public consciousness. It has clear utility for understanding the experience of dying patients and their families and it seems to capture very common reactions. In terms of clinical communication the stages of grief can shape patient–provider encounters in important ways and help avoid pitfalls. For example, a discussion about transitioning the goals of care for a terminally ill patient from more aggressive treatment toward providing comfort as they die likely would be misplaced with a patient who is experiencing denial or anger. Patients might not be in the right frame of mind to make those sorts of judgments. While these stages were identified by Kübler-Ross (1969) based on interviews with dying patients and their families, she later argued that they applied to any significant loss (e.g., divorce, job loss, other significant medical events). Indeed, we would argue that since it fundamentally revolves around matters of life and death—after all, that is the whole point of it—*that grief is ubiquitous in health care.*[4]

---

[4] We are borrowing this phrase, with permission, from our colleague Dr. Ami Harbin, at Oakland University.

Some years ago, a physician–administrator at a hospital told a story about the day he learned of his child's autism diagnosis. He obviously was highly educated and prepared to understand everything about the diagnosis, recommended therapies, promising research, and the like. Yet when the treating physician launched into a description of a potential clinical trial just after breaking the news to the parents, he said, "I didn't understand a word he said. All I could think was, 'where can I get a drink?'" On the provider's part, recall from Chapter 7 how this likely reflects a conditioned (i.e., disciplined) response, a retreat into the technical and functional aspects of his training as opposed to engaging the social–psychological aspects of care. On the part of the child's family, one can imagine how various experiences of grief might have followed. While it is not a terminal diagnosis, parents of children with developmental deficits such as autism often experience grief. They grieve the loss of the future they anticipated for their child, for the impacts it might have on their other children, and for the struggles that they know await the child they love as he or she grows up in a world that is not always accommodating. Here again, understanding the five stages of grief can be clinically useful. If one understands that parents of a newly diagnosed autistic child might experience denial, anger, or bargaining, one can better gauge how to tailor communication. The clinician above failed to recognize that the father was not cognitively ready to consider enrolling his child in a clinical trial. Even though this father also was a highly educated physician, in his role as the child's parent, the diagnosis did not connote a disease, but an illness experience inseparable from the social context of his family and the future that he had envisioned for his son.

Even when they seem relatively innocuous, a medical diagnosis can trigger grief-like reactions. Take, for example, a 63-year-old man diagnosed with atrial fibrillation. It is a relatively common diagnosis, occurring in about 2% of men this age, and while it is associated with other conditions, it is not usually life threatening and can be successfully treated. This might not, on its own, seem a likely trigger for grief. But consider the larger context in which this patient might experience the illness. It may be his first clear sign of aging and associated bodily declines. The diagnosis may therefore trigger a psychological confrontation with his own mortality, in ways that seem disproportionate to the features of the disease itself. He may demonstrate signs of grief that, while not as obvious as in someone diagnosed with a terminal illness, nonetheless display similar key features. Wrestling with our own existence can be traumatic because we spend a great deal of time and energy denying or ignoring the inevitability of death.[5] These thoughts can be triggered by any number of health events, not only those that seem objectively significant, because a patient's diagnosis is inextricably connected to a larger social context, psychological experience, and reflection upon his or her own life course.

While the work of Kübler-Ross (1969) and others on grief and illness experiences surrounding death (see, e.g., Glaser & Strauss 1965) is now almost half a century old, the examples above show that it retains utility for clinical practice. At the same time, it is important to recognize the limitations and dangers of drawing

---

[5] Studies in *terror management*, in fact, build upon Ernst Becker's work to suggest that a great deal of human behavior is motivated by the urge to suppress a constantly lurking sense of our own mortality and our anxiety about it (see, e.g., Solomon et al. 1991; see also Becker 1973).

on that framework in an unreflexive way. It is easy, for example, to allow normative judgments to color our perceptions of the stages of grief, as though acceptance is a morally superior stage than anger or denial. This is particularly problematic when those sorts of normative judgments are imposed on patients where we want or even expect them to demonstrate a dignified and stoic, if not cheerful, resignation. These expectations are captured in the clinical context when providers compliment the brave or cheerful patient, but never the depressed or angry one. Friends and family can unintentionally pile on in this way when they say things like, "Be brave! You can beat this!" The implicit expectation to have a particular attitude and orientation toward one's illness becomes an additional burden that an ill person has to face. Arthur Frank (1991 [2000]:65–66) expresses this clearly, writing, "Too few people, whether medical staff, family, or friends, seem willing to accept the possibility that depression may be the ill person's most appropriate response to the situation ... What makes me saddest is seeing the work ill persons must do to sustain [the] 'cheerful patient' image." It is more helpful to the patient to acknowledge that each reaction to grief is valid. While we may be required to work differently with the patient at different stages of the experience (such that we can do things with a patient who is experiencing acceptance that we cannot do with one who is experiencing anger or denial), it is important not to label such reactions as deficient, but rather to recognize and address them. Frank (1991 [2000]:67) continues describing the "costs of appearances" during his own illness experience:

> When I tried to sustain a cheerful and tidy image, it cost me energy, which was scarce. It also cost me opportunities to express what *was* happening in my life with cancer and to understand that life. Finally, my attempts at a positive image diminished my relationships with others by preventing them from sharing my experience. But this image is all that many of those around an ill person are willing to see. (italics are original)

While seemingly supportive, statements celebrating an ill person's efforts to fight the illness or their cheerful nature in the face of illness signify social expectations. These normative expectations reflect a lot about the needs of those surrounding the ill person to not have to confront the darker sides of illness and suffering. But for their part, a patient can easily feel alienated from their own experiences of anger or denial, which are normal and reasonable forms of reaction to serious illness.

Other updates to the stages of grief model also are important to recognize. For example, more recent work has suggested that some people do not grieve, or not deeply, at tragedy. If we take the stages of grief model rigidly, we may mistake such behavior as a sort of permanent denial. However, research suggests that some individuals display health resilience such that they do not experience grief associated with loss (Bonanno 2004). Additionally, later work has suggested that the term "stages" is misleading, not only in that it inherently suggests a moral hierarchy (e.g., that acceptance is better than bargaining), but also because it implies an orderly progression that is not consistent with how people often experience grief (Neimeyer 2001). Rather, individuals experience different stages at different times, in different orders, moving from one to another and back again. Those caveats aside, maintaining a flexible and reflexive understanding of the many different reactions that patients have to illness, particularly when it connotes significant loss, remains clinically useful because such reactions can sensitize practitioners to the potential socioemotional experiences of patients.

Patients do not experience illness purely, or even primarily, as disease. A diagnosis therefore is not circumscribed by its physiology but inextricably linked to its social consequences and the patients' social relationships. Take as a final example, a married woman who has not had any sexual encounters outside of her marriage, who is diagnosed with gonorrhea.[6] She might naturally react, "I don't understand how this could have happened!" Of course, this is not literally true. In all likelihood she knows precisely how one acquires a sexually transmitted infection. Rather, she is grieving the infidelity of her partner. Understanding this experience, how the diagnosis is linked to her social relationships, to the image she possessed of her family life, is critical to creating a good clinical encounter. Launching into the pathogenesis of gonorrhea would, of course, be ill advised. In Chapter 9 we will explore some good communication practices, but for now, it is important to recognize that those good communication practices have to be built on a foundation of understanding the patient's experience of illness. We continue the development of this foundation in the next two sections, the first of which explores the intersection of illness and identity, and the second which explores the impact of illness on families, particularly those involved with caregiving.

Illness and Identity

While we have discussed how illness is nested in social relationships and social functions, the examples above also suggest that the illness experience intersects our sense of who we are. That is, illness challenges and shapes our identities.[7] Our concepts of self are shaped throughout our lives, particularly by our social activities. Musician, athlete, intellectual, boating enthusiast—any number of interests and endeavors can become significant parts of not only what we do with our lives, but also how we perceive and define ourselves. Other core social identities are also defined in terms of our relationships with others: mother, father, wife, husband, daughter, son, and so on. In acting out these roles, each of us puts our own personal twist on them; our role performances have meanings that are consistent with the identities that we assert (Burke & Reitzes 1981). A father, for example, might take his daughter hiking to spend time with her. However, this is not only a matter of hiking itself, or even just of spending time with his daughter, but an assertion of the kind of father he wishes to be, the particular *father-identity* he wants to express. Those types of activities therefore become special markers of our identity. But because illness can so significantly disrupt the role performances

---

[6] Credit for this example belongs to Dr. Elysa Koppelman-White of Oakland University, who, in turn, credits it to her husband, an OB/GYN.

[7] The way illness intersects with identity certainly depends on the type of illness we are speaking about. Congenital ailments may be inextricable parts of one's identity from the beginning. Also, the distinction between acute and chronic illnesses is important here. The latter intersects with identity over longer periods of time and often has an evolutionary character with respect to identity. Acute illnesses, on the other hand, depending on their severity, may be either unremarkable in our lives or might engender existential reflection that affects the way we see things.

we use to signify and confirm who we are (to both ourselves and others), illness often disrupts our identity.

Kathy Charmaz's (1991) seminal research on the experience of physical chronic illnesses highlights that patients travel through a three-stage *odyssey of self*, as they navigate the relationships between their body, their illness, and their identity (Charmaz 1995:675).[8] These stages include (1) *experiencing an altered body*, (2) *making bodily assessments and subsequent identity trade-offs*, and (3) *surrendering to the sick self ... and flowing with the experience of it* (Charmaz 1995:657).

In the first stage, an ill person begins to take notice of their functional impairments. Fundamentally, they notice that something about their current body is diminished. They also often feel estranged from their bodies, as though their bodies have betrayed them. The encroachment of these functional limitations reaches a threshold where one seeks professional help, which is a complex process of assessing these insurgent discomforts. Zola (1973) notes, "Virtually every day of our lives we are subject to a vast array of bodily discomforts. Only an infinitesimal amount of these get to a physician." Impairment alone does not cause an ill person to seek professional care, but rather a variety of social and psychological "triggers," including

> (1) the occurrence of an interpersonal crisis; (2) the *perceived* interference with social or personal relations; (3) sanctioning [where one is motivated by some sort of external reward for seeking help or punishment for not doing so]; (4) the *perceived* interference with vocational or physical activity; and (5) a kind of temporalizing of symptomatology [an assessment that the length of the impairment or discomfort is too long to endure, or will only get worse over time]. (Zola 1973:683; italics in the original)

As chronic illness impairment begins to limit the functions that are attached to identity expressions, and also to reshape the physical body, they spark a confrontation between the illness and identity that takes place on the terrain of the body.

Diagnosis also plays a significant transitional role during the first stage, giving definite shape to an inchoate set of sensations and impairments, which are codified into symptoms and a named *disease* (see Karp 1996). Diagnosis can be a double-edged sword for persons experiencing illness—who at this point become patients—because it confirms the unfortunate reality of disease, but at the same time offers relief as it makes sense of the variety of sensations they have been experiencing that previously were, to them, characterized by a high degree of mystery (e.g., "maybe these are related," "maybe this signifies something serious," "maybe this will go away on its own"). After diagnosis, the ill person can feel some relief in finally knowing what "it" is. When Venus Williams, a professional tennis player, was diagnosed in 2011 with Sjogren's syndrome, she noted, "I think I've had issues with Sjogren's for a while. It just wasn't diagnosed" (Moisse & Childs 2011). She added, "The good news for me is now I know what's happening."

In the second stage, ill persons undergo a process of "making bodily assessments and, subsequently, identity trade-offs, as ill people weigh their losses and gains and revise their identity goals" (Charmaz 1995:657). In this stage there is an explicit

---

[8] Remember here that one can have a disease without an illness (e.g., heart disease that is currently asymptomatic). Thus, when we refer to "chronic illness" in this section, we are assuming that it entails some level of functional impairment (even though chronic *disease* might not).

focus on social functions and relationships. That is, while in the first stage the ill person is experiencing new limitations and trying to make sense of their symptoms, in the second stage, they explore redefinitions of their identity in light of what they *can* do given the functional limitations of their illness. Insofar as our identities are tied to our role performances, however, this is a very important part of the illness experience. We might say that these functional self-assessments set the limitations for one's new roles and identities. Take, for example, a person who is a passionate runner for whom "athlete" has always been a significant part of his or her identity, but who develops severe lupus with chronic joint swelling and fatigue. The functional limitations of the disease naturally will cause that person to trade what he or she can no longer do for that which he or she can. In the process, the person will often significantly modify his or her "athlete" identity, or trade it out altogether, for an identity that one can successfully perform in light of one's functional impairments. For Williams, even though Sjogren's syndrome did not immediately end her athletic career, it has significantly affected her performance, and she has altered her training and playing style in light of it (Masters & Cash 2014). In fact, on her website, she refers to the later stage of her career as "Venus A.D.," meaning "Venus After Diagnosis," signifying the extent to which a significant illness can reshape our identity.

The third stage that emerged from Charmaz's (1991, 1995) research on chronic illness and identity finds ill persons "surrendering to the sick self by relinquishing control over illness and by flowing with the experience of it" (1995:657). While in the first stage, individuals maintain, "firm separations between their impaired bodies and their self concepts," and in the second, they make identity trade-offs predominantly centered around functional activities (Charmaz 1995:663), the third stage finds ill persons, "(1) relinquishing the quest for control over one's body, (2) giving up notions of victory over illness, [and] (3) affirming, however implicitly, that one's self is tied to the sick body" (Charmaz 1995:672). One woman in Charmaz's (1995:674) study remarked about the meaning of "surrendering to the sick self":

> It means that I don't have—I can't control it [ill body] and [it means] to look at what it has to teach me. Just … let it tell me what it needs to tell me. You know, that willingness and that acceptance …. So it didn't come instantly, but I was willing to surrender and to look at what was going on. But it did come; it did happen. And I'm always much more at peace after I'm able to do that anyway.

There are parallels here to the acceptance stage in Kübler-Ross' (1969) stages of grief, particularly where this stage is punctuated by a kind of existential reflection and peaceful settling into reality, an accepted embodiment of the illness by the patient. As with our discussion of the stages of grief above, Charmaz (1995) is careful to point out that the three stages that emerged from her research should not be routinely expected from, or forced onto, patients, who could move through them quickly, oscillate between them, or skip stages altogether. As explained above, illness experiences are inextricably linked to social functions and social identities. Thus, where ill persons do experience these stages, they may do so with a high degree of variation. Each person's experience is unique to their personal history, perspective, and the conditions of their social life.

At the same time, these stages provide a valuable conceptual framework for understanding the illness experience, particularly for chronic illnesses. As with the stages of grief, clinical providers should find them useful in understanding patients' behaviors as they react to their diagnoses, carry out their treatment plans, and experience continued declines over time. With respect to patients who first appear with symptoms, practitioners should understand the dual experience of diagnosis—the simultaneous experience of grief and relief. Patients in the second stage may desire more functional interventions, assistance with maintaining altered versions of the functions they are used to performing, or support as they transition to new roles. Practitioners should bear in mind the efforts at identity trade-offs as they develop treatment plans with patients, such that treatment supports rather than interferes with the patient's recalibration of identity-related goals. Referrals to support groups may be especially helpful in these earlier stages when patients are engaged in struggles against the illness. Finally, patients in the third stage may be ready for longer-term planning and establishing goals of care and contingency plans for various situations. In earlier stages, when the focus is more immediately on making sense of one's functional declines (stage one) or adapting to those changes (stage two), discussions about long-term goals may be more difficult (though still perhaps necessary if one's prognosis suggests the potential for rapid decline). As a general theme, Charmaz's three stages of negotiating illness, body, and identity suggest a transition that begins with externalized experiences where there are physical sensations happening *to* the person or where the body is postured against, or at least separated from, the self. As the negotiation between illness and identity proceeds into the terrain of the body, the illness moves toward identity, passing first through the social functions and relationships to which a person is connected and finally being internalized and woven into their concept of self.

Interestingly, David Karp's (1996) study of depression elucidates a very similar process occurring for mental illnesses. Karp (1996:57) writes:

> Every person I interviewed moved through these identity turning points in their view of themselves and their problem with depression:
>
> 1. A period of *inchoate feelings* during which they lacked the vocabulary to label their experience as depression.
> 2. A phase during which they conclude that *something is really wrong with me.*
> 3. A *crisis stage* that thrusts them into a world of therapeutic experts.
> 4. A stage of *coming to grips with an illness identity* during which they theorize about the cause(s) for their difficulty and evaluate the prospects for getting beyond depression. (Italics are original)

He concludes, "Each of these career moments assumes and requires redefinitions of self." The term "career" is interesting and useful because, as with a person's work career, it articulates that persons grow and develop in their experiences with illness both internally, with respect to their identity, and externally, with respect to their social relationships and interactions with health care professionals (see Goffman 1959).

Just as with physical illness, persons struggling with mental illness begin by noticing things that are happening to them (though within them). As before, a particular level of severity or a particularly poignant event is needed to trigger care-seeking from professional providers (Zola 1973). From there, they negotiate how the illness fits into their social life and how it intersects with their concept of self. Karp (1996:75) concludes, "People's experience with clinical depression is an exercise in negotiating ambiguity and involves the evolution of an illness consciousness often extending over many years." The clinical utility of understanding this career also is similar to that of physical illness as illustrated by Charmaz (1995). In short, a provider must adapt their language and discourse, as well as their goals of care, to where a person is with respect to their illness career.

Families and Caregiving

It is difficult to underappreciate the roles that families play in providing care for those who are sick. This is especially true in the chronic illness era, where people are living with illnesses for longer periods of time, particularly at the end of their lives. In fact, families often assume the bulk of the responsibility for filling in where illness creates limitations for the patient. They not only bathe, feed, and transport loved ones, but also often assume primary responsibility for monitoring their condition and providing treatments that are frequently administered in the home. However, the relationship between families and providers is less straightforward. In the world of child health it is perhaps clearer, since parents have responsibility for the health and health care decisions of their minor children. But the relationship between practitioners and the family members of adult patients is rather complicated. On the one hand, the ill person is their patient, while family members are informal supports. On the other hand, the significance of that support to the health and well-being of that patient is immeasurable, and family caregivers therefore often become explicit and utterly necessary parts of the care plan. Because of this vital role, the illness experience cannot be fully understood without addressing the experiences of family caregivers. For their part, practitioners need to be mindful of caregivers' experiences of their loved one's illness in order to foster relationships that promote the best outcomes in their care. In short, understanding the experiences of family caregivers is a critical part of patient care.

Caregiving Burden

Providing care for ill family members is a widespread phenomenon, particularly as the population ages; that is, as greater numbers of individuals are living longer. Recent estimates suggest that family caregivers provide over 90% of in-home care to ill adults (Adelman et al. 2014). In fact, of adults receiving long-term care in their homes, 78% are *exclusively* cared for by family members, while another 14% receive care from family members in addition to some professional in-home care (Thompson 2004). Nearly a third (32%) of family caregivers spend more than 20 hours a week providing care to their loved one. And while the overwhelming majority report feeling appreciated by the family member they are caring for, 30% felt torn between their "patient" and other members of their family, while 21% reported declines in their own physical health (Donelan et al. 2002; Thompson 2004). Of course, stress, anxiety, depression, and related illnesses are particularly salient (Hodges et al. 2005; Bruhn & Rebach 2014). Perhaps most striking, Adelman et al. (2014:1054) note, "Caregiving burden [has been] identified as an independent predictor of caregiver mortality with a 63% increased risk of death."

While increases in male caregiving are arguably attributable to the increased demands of an older population with more prolonged caregiving needs combined with slowly changing gender roles (Bruhn & Rebach 2014; Drentea 2014), women still disproportionately bear the burdens of caregiving (Johnson & Lo Sasso 2000). Interestingly, as women entered the workforce in greater numbers in the mid-twentieth century, their caregiver burden remained relatively stable. In the United States there was a shift from the "male breadwinner/female caregiver" model to the "dual breadwinner/female caregiver" model (Bruhn & Rebach 2014). In turn, there are significant financial costs associated with caregiving, not only in terms of expenditures for the caregiving itself, but also in terms of time lost in the workforce. Johnson and Lo Sasso (2000:27) write, "for those who do provide informal care the costs are high. The loss of 459 annual work hours for women translates on average into about $7,800 in lost wages per year in 1994 dollars."

Caregiving often represents a sociocultural obligation. Moreover, it is an obligation that is socially structured so that some have a greater propensity to bear those burdens directly (e.g., women and individuals in lower socioeconomic status brackets). As a result, Drentea (2014:204) suggests that, "*carework* is a more accurate way of describing a relationship that is not always voluntary and freely given" and moreover disproportionately affects some groups more than others (italics added).

Just as gender shapes the contours of caregiving itself, the experience of caregiving is affected by other social structural conditions that surround it. Socioeconomic status, for example, obviously can mitigate some caregiver burden, particularly those related to financial strain. However, culture also shapes the structure of family life and our expectations of our social responsibilities within the family structure (Knight et al. 2002). Latino caregivers, for example, report lower levels of social support and high levels of caregiving-related distress (Adams et al. 2002). African Americans, on the other hand, tend to report less stress and more positive emotional experiences of providing in-home care for a relative despite facing disproportionate socioeconomic disadvantages (Cox & Monk 1996).

The illness experiences of family caregivers are also shaped by cultural norms and must be understood against a backdrop of cultural expectations. In particular, when cultural norms promote closer intergenerational family relationships and intergenerational cohabitation, caring for an ill family member may be experienced more as an anticipated feature of one's life and less of a jarring disruption. For example, second-generation immigrants from cultures with strong filial ties (e.g., Latino, Asian, etc.) often experience a sort of role conflict, where traditional expectations of taking in and caring for elder relatives may conflict with more contemporary Western norms with which second-generation immigrants more strongly identify in contrast to their first-generation relatives (Sharma et al. 2011). As Knight et al. (2002:75) write, "it appears that culture... does not directly affect appraisal of caregiving as burdensome, [but affects] precursor variables such as familism, and familism (a cultural value) was associated with lesser burden." That is, culture sets a stage upon which we develop our values and social expectations and, in turn, our values and social expectations constitute a lens through which we understand and experience caregiving. When one values family relationships more and expects to care for relatives during their life course, caregiving stress likely is reduced. When one values relative independence and does not have such expectations, caregiving stress likely is greater.

Conflicts within families can often attend caregiving for an ill or severely impaired family member. For example, adult siblings who are caring for aging parents often experience conflict over caregiving roles and the distribution of burdens. This is particularly true when some siblings, by virtue of geography, for example, bear a greater proportion of the caregiving burden than others. Younger siblings of ill or impaired children often experience not only deficits in attention and resources from their parents, but also the burdens associated with assisting in the caregiving itself (Cohen 1999). Lamorey (1999) notes that the "parentification" of siblings of children with severe disability or chronic illness puts them more at risk for internalizing illnesses such as depression and social isolation, as well as externalizing illnesses such as aggressiveness and oppositional behavior.

Finally, just as the onset of significant illness generates identity struggles for the afflicted person, caregiving places enormous strain on the identities of caregivers. This is true not only when caregiving functions begin to consume the time previously dedicated to other activities, such as paid work outside the home, but also where family roles must be renegotiated. A common manifestation of this occurs when adult caregivers and their ill parents both experience a sort of role reversal. Parents are used to caring for their children, giving them advice about decisions, and being the stalwart of wisdom and experience for their children. However, as they become more dependent on their children while experiencing physical and mental declines, they often struggle with a sort of *role conflict*. The identity shifts that come with family caregiving can therefore be difficult to navigate.

The Stress Process Model

From the above, it should be clear that the burdens of caregiving are complex and affected by a host of sociological and psychological factors (Folkman 1984; Lazarus 1993; Pearlin 1989; Pearlin et al. 1981). Social positions affect the propensity of becoming a caregiver, while financial resources, as well as the values internalized from cultural systems and a psychological ability to cope with stress, all affect the amount and quality of caregiving burden that someone will experience. The various factors involved in this complex process have been summarized in the *Stress Process Model* (Pearlin et al. 1981; see Fig. 8.2, from Turner 2010).

The stress process model elaborates factors that ultimately result in tangible mental or physical health outcomes. This is particularly important because social conditions increase or decrease the likelihood of experiencing a stressful life event, but even more critically it highlights that the same stressful event can affect individuals differently when they occupy different social positions (e.g., high or low socioeconomic status), have differing levels of social support, or are simply more or less psychologically resilient. Put another way, social conditions affect how likely we are to encounter stressful situations while social circumstances and psychological resources influence how well we deal with them, thereby mediating how much they ultimately affect our health.

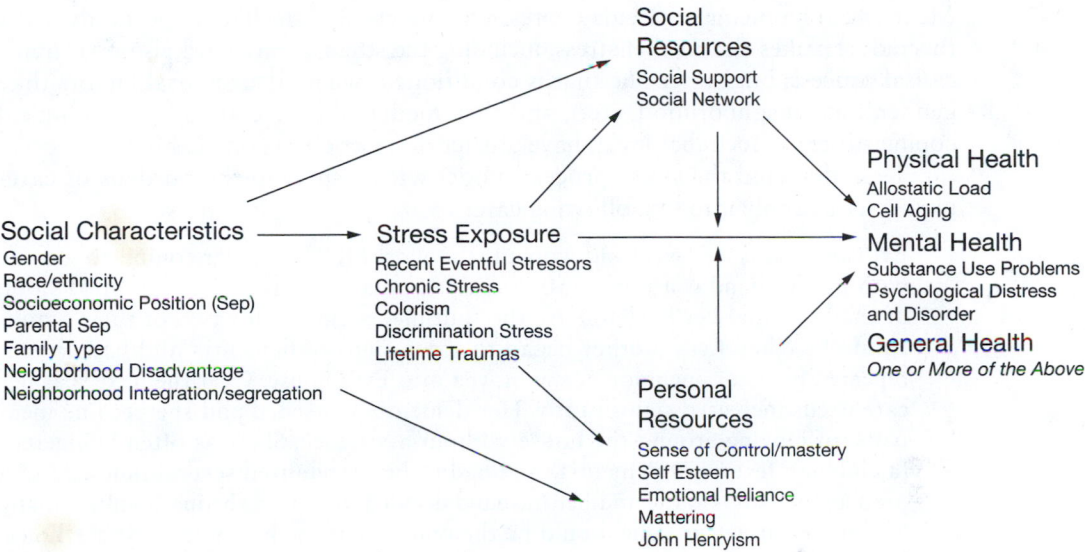

FIG. 8.2 Stress process model.

Source: Turner, R. Jay. (2010). "Understanding Health Disparities: The Promise of the Stress Process Model." Pp. 3–21 in *Advances in the Conceptualization of the Stress Process: Essays in Honor of Leonard I. Pearlin.* William, R. Avison, Carol S. Aneshensel, Scott Schieman, & Blair Wheaton, eds. New York: Springer.

Moving from left to right, the social characteristics set the conditions in which we are more or less likely to encounter stressful situations. Because we are socialized within our own particular sets of social characteristics, they also condition the expectations that we hold, which, as discussed above, can attenuate or amplify how stressful we judge a situation to be. Stress exposure can either be acute or chronic. An acute stressor, like the sudden death of a loved one, usually occurs as a spike in stress followed by its gradual reduction as one copes with it. Chronic stress, however, is persistent. Of course, these two can interact, particularly where chronic stress can amplify the effects of acute stress.

Figure 8.2 then moves to the right in two directions reflecting different ways of coping (Turner 2010). Social resources represent relatively tangible, external capital that a person can dedicate to coping with stress. A person whose car breaks down may be stressed by that event, but a person who has the money to hail a cab or a friend who can pick him up is better positioned to cope with that stressor by virtue of his social resources. On the other hand, personal resources reflect internal, cognitive coping abilities. How well one copes psychologically with stress can amplify or attenuate its ultimate effects on health.

To the far right of this figure we see physical and mental health outcomes. Physical health outcomes related to stress include obesity and heart disease, secondary to high levels of cortisol and even aging at a cellular level, where telomeres at the ends of chromosomes are shorter in persons experiencing chronic stress.[9]

[9] This includes, for example, individuals who live in environments with high levels of neighborhood disorder such as crime or those who experience chronic racial bias (Chae et al. 2014; Needham et al. 2014).

Mental health outcomes include depression, anxiety, and the like. Importantly, what this model makes clear is that stress, including the stress of care work, is not a simple causal process, but rather one that is conditioned by social structural factors (like gender, race, neighborhood, etc.), and then mediated by social and psychological coping strategies such that it can have greater or lesser effects on health.

To understand the stress process model with respect to the burdens of caregiving, let us apply it to the following case:

> Evi Rickomo is a 54-year-old woman who works full time. Her combined income with her husband is around $50,000 a year, but she makes only about $12,000 of that. She and her husband are the fulltime caregivers for two of their grandchildren. When Evi's mother began to show signs of dementia and had several repeated bouts of pneumonia, she moved into Evi's house. Over the next year her care needs increased significantly. Her dementia worsened and she became incapable of moving around the house without assistance. She was often belligerent (a common feature of dementia) and had to be hospitalized several times. After a particularly bad fall, Evi and her husband decided that since she made substantially less money at her job, she would be the one to quit so she could be at the house full-time. Over the next couple of years, Evi herself was diagnosed with high blood pressure and diabetes.

Evi is in a position in which many adult children find themselves. She is "sandwiched" between caring for young children and aging parents in a dual-income household. Evi appears to assume the majority of the care work in her house, reflecting a gendered construction of caregiving. Moreover, her socioeconomic position means that she likely cannot afford in-home care. Given the costs of that care, it made more financial sense for Evi to leave the workforce to provide that care instead, but of course this also may reflect the social force of gender insofar as women earn less than men on average, and are typically expected to take responsibility for carework across the entire family unit. The family's socioeconomic position set the stage for this scenario, as opposed to one where her mother might move into a tiered senior living community, something that can be quite costly. In short, we can say that the social construct of gender and the social condition of socioeconomic status set a stage for exposing Evi to a high level of caregiving burden.

Evi's life as the caregiver displays the daily chronic strains of care work, punctuated by the acute stress of intermittent medical events (e.g., her mother's hospitalizations, falls, etc.). While her gender and socioeconomic position condition her exposure to these various stressors, they also condition to a large degree how well she can cope with caregiving burden. This is true not only where she may have greater or lesser degrees of social support, but also with respect to her psychological resources. How thoroughly she sees herself as a caregiver and whether she expected to be providing this much care for family members at this stage in her life, along with her self-esteem and perception of how much she matters to others all mediate her experience of stress and related health outcomes. With regard to social support, Evi's extended family may also share her working-class socioeconomic position, which may affect how much assistance she can expect from them, both financially and in terms of time spent participating in caregiving. On the other hand, if she is connected to a religious community, she may receive important social support from other congregants or clergy. In terms of personal resources, Evi may have internalized a role as caregiver that normalizes her current situation, which may reduce her perception of her care work as burdensome. At the same time, even though her mother's belligerent behavior results from dementia, it may nonetheless impede Evi's ability to cope psychologically with the demands of her care. It is critical to note that at each stage of the stress process model, there are a variety of factors that can strengthen or weaken the force of stress on Evi's physical and mental health, which appear to be declining under the weight of her caregiving burden.

Understanding that the multifactorial system involved in the stress process is not only sociologically interesting, but also clinically useful. Examining the various dimensions of the stress process model is informative both for providers with patients for whom family caregivers are playing a significant role, and those providers whose patients are themselves caregivers (See also Bevans and Sternberg 2012). With respect to the case above, the providers who are caring for her mother, along with those who are caring for Evi, would be well advised to consider the ways in which she experiences her mother's illness and the social psychological burdens she faces as a caregiver. These are germane to both Evi's and her mother's health.

The stress process model applied to caregiver burden also helps clarify where practitioners can intervene. Even when health care providers are sensitive to the social determinants of health (see Chapters 4 and 5), their implications for clinical practice are not always clear. Obviously, practitioners cannot rectify the socioeconomic burdens or gender disadvantages faced by their patients. However, the stress process model emphasizes areas that are ripe for clinical intervention. For one, providers ought to be sensitive to how social characteristics can set a stage for a differential experience of stress. That is, they can understand how the experience of stress is nested in sets of social conditions, such that something that might not seem objectively stressful is indeed a salient event for particular patients. Additionally, practitioners can use this deeper understanding of caregiver burden to address potential coping strategies. In the area of social resources, this might include recommending support groups or home care services that may fit a particular budget or counseling patients about seeking support from their own communities where they might be reluctant to do so. It often includes consulting social work services that may be able to assist with developing and implementing many of these strategies.

With respect to psychological resources, providers, even when not specifically working in the area of mental health, should be sensitive to how well a patient is coping psychologically with the burdens of caregiving. This is relevant to any number of mental and physical health outcomes, placing it squarely in the domain of almost every provider. While not every provider can or should become a full-time counselor, each needs to have at least a baseline sensitivity to these features of the illness experience of family caregivers, if for no other reason than to identify problems when they occur and to refer the patient to someone who can help them.

Adelman et al. (2014) provide a number of discussion questions that practitioners can use to assess caregiver burden in a clinical encounter (see Fig. 8.3). Notice how the question domains align with those components of the stress process model on which providers can successfully intervene. Additionally, based on the results of numerous other studies on caregiving burden interventions, Adelman

Caregiver health

To provide the very best patient care. I find I need to also pay attention to my patients' caregivers. Can you tell me a bit about how you are feeling/doing?

We know that caregivers often neglect their own health. When was the last time you saw your physician?

Do you have your own physician? Is she or he aware of your caregiving situation? What has she or he advised about it?

Quality of life

I know that many family caregivers find the role to be very stressful.

How are you coping with these responsibilities?

How would you describe your quality of life these days?

How often do you get out?

What do you do for fun?

Support

Many caregivers don't want to burden others-especially their children, Are there times when you really need help but don't ask for fear of being a burden?

Who gives you support? How helpful is this support?

We work with a social worker who is an expert in assisting caregivers. May I refer you to this individual?

Caregiving is a very hard job and the best way to do it well is to take advantage of some of the resources available for help. Are you using any of these? May I help you with a referral?

In case of emergency

If anything should happen to you, have you made arrangements for someone to take care of [name patient here]?

FIG 8.3 Discussion catalysts for engaging family caregivers.

Source: Adelman, Ronald D., Lyubov L. Tmanova, Diana Delgado, Sarah Dion, & Mark S. Lachs. (2014). "Caregiver Burden: A Clinical Review." *Journal of the American Medical Association* 311, 1052–59.

et al. (2014:1056) compiled a set of practical recommendations for intervening to reduce caregiver burden:[10]

1. *Encourage the caregiver to function as a member of the team.* This includes bringing caregivers into the conversations about the illness experience of their loved one, along with treatment decisions and goal planning. Moreover, these processes should always account for the needs and capacities of the caregiver as well as the patient.
2. *Encourage caregivers to improve self-care and maintain their health.* This includes the recommendation to schedule consecutive visits for patients and family caregivers to assist in care planning that accounts for the needs of both.

[10] The items themselves are quoted, but the explanations of them are in our own words.

3. *Provide education and information.* Educating caregivers about their loved one's illness and its likely long-term trajectory is essential not only so they can perform the needed daily caregiving tasks, but so that they can observe and report important somatic information and so that they are prepared for the care decisions that will have to be made along the course of the illness.

4. *Use the support of technology.* The burdens of care can be significantly reduced by technology. Lifts can help a person navigate stairs; GPS monitors can help locate dementia patients who wander; Internet communities can help reduce isolation; and so on.

5. *Coordinate and refer for assistance with care.* This includes knowing various support services that are available to the caregiver and patient, both those to which they are formally entitled to and other private support services that they may be able to access in their area, such as home care, legal assistance, family counseling, and the like.

6. *Encourage caregivers to access respite care.* Where many individuals are reticent to ask for help, this recommendation is as much about encouraging them to do so as it is about actually connecting them with day programs, or having someone else (e.g., a family member or home care provider) stay with the ill person to give some relief to the primary caregiver.

A number of things become clear from these recommendations. First, illness experience is not exclusive to the patient, but it is a significant, stressful, and even traumatic experience for their families, particularly those who assume a substantial caregiving role. Second, providers can successfully intervene to reduce stress associated with care work by remaining sensitive to differential stress experiences conditioned by social structure, and then by addressing the social support systems and the cognitive resources that caregivers use to cope. Finally, this is an important function for practitioners because the burdens of caregiving not only affect the care provided to the ailing person, but are also intricately linked to significant health outcomes for caregivers themselves.

Conclusion: Disease and Illness, Patients and Persons

As patients and their family members experience illness, they do so through a variety of lenses. Their social experiences, their expectations for their lives, the meanings they find in suffering and their views of death—all of these shape how they receive a diagnosis, experience impairment, renegotiate their identities, execute treatment plans, and make choices as they die. Where medical and allied health professionals are largely trained to understand and treat disease, they can be cutoff from their patients' more holistic, embodied experiences of illness. There is now greater emphasis on social science and humanism in health care in the medical and allied health curricula (i.e., the impetus of this book) because practitioners need the skills to navigate the complex space between disease and illness. Resting in that space, we find a variety of material conditions like socioeconomic position and symbolic understandings of illness, which result from socialization within a specific cultural framework.

Throughout this book, we have intermittently discussed issues of culture. Above, for example, we discussed how cultural norms shape expectations of caregiving and how these affect caregiver burden and resulting health outcomes. Indeed, cultural competency is a significant feature in the content standards and learning objectives of every medical and allied health profession. But cultural competency education very often centers on learning about customs and perspectives of different cultures. This approach is useful in some ways, but problematic in others. For one, there are too many cultural groups for this to be very efficient. Practitioners cannot double as professional anthropologists, and even if they could, the variations between cultural groups would render it impossible to learn enough to prepare oneself for every possible clinical encounter. Certainly, though, one can (and should) learn about dominant cultures in one's particular practice area. For example, if there is a large Vietnamese population surrounding the clinic in which you work, it certainly is a worthwhile endeavor to learn, in general terms, their customs, norms, and ways of seeing the health, the body, and the larger universe (see Chapter 2). At the same time, a new version of the gap between practitioner and patient emerges with this approach. That is, in practice one must work with an individual patient who may or may not take up all of the proclivities of their cultural background. Assuming that a member functions in lockstep with the customs and norms of their group is a form of stereotyping called *reductionism*, a view that reduces a complex individual to the themes of a group to which they belong. Put another way, taking a reductionist view of cultural competency does not allow you to bridge the gap between a set of expectations based on group *tendencies* and the actual experiences, perspectives, habits, and idiosyncrasies of the individual patient in front of you.

So while understanding cultural norms can sensitize us to what we *might* expect from a patient affiliated with a particular group, they should not *dictate* how we understand that patient's experience or how we care for them. Balancing the understanding of social processes at an aggregate level with our need to deliver individualized care to patients is therefore a tricky problem. But we can begin to address it when we realize, for example, that culture is only one of many things that affect how individual patients experience illness or how their family reacts to the burdens of caregiving. Perhaps the most useful way to avoid reductionism is to remain reflexive about how social factors interface with individual patient experiences. Put more simply, our understanding of social factors should sensitize us to the kinds of things that might be pertinent—they should stimulate our clinical thinking—but the clinical dialogue with the individual patient is necessary to clarify how each person sees the world in general (and their health in particular), along with how they individually relate to their social conditions and cultural backgrounds. In Chapter 9 we focus directly on patient–provider communication as a way to bridge the gap between the disease perspective of biomedicine and the illness experience of patients, as well as a way to bring together one's knowledge of the social–psychological tendencies of various groups with the actual perspectives and behaviors of individual patients.

CHAPTER 8 ACTIVITY

The Illness Experience of Patients and Families

Diya Majumdar and her husband Ravi are the parents of three teenage boys living in San Diego, California. Ravi works as a systems analyst making about $75,000 a year. Diya has always stayed at home to take care of the boys, but she had planned to go back to school and get her master's degree in audiology once they were older. Both have been very active members of the Shiva Vishnu Temple, where Diya gave Kathak dance lessons for many years. However, about two years ago, Ravi's father passed away. Shortly thereafter, Ravi's mother, Abha, began to have issues with mobility and moved in with the family.

At first, Abha was a big help, particularly with household chores. She cooked delicious traditional meals for the family and did all the laundry for the three boys. But although she tried not to let it show, Diya was irritated, particularly when Abha would sometimes undermine her, for example, by cleaning the boys' rooms even though the rule was that they had to do it themselves. Abha could sense Diya's frustration and would often say things under her breath like, "In my day, a wife respected her husband's mother; she would never be made to feel like a bothersome guest in her own son's house."

Over the next few years, Abha's health continued to decline, her eyesight worsened, and she began to experience bouts of dementia. She would often forget things, repeat stories several times in the same day, and began to have difficulty finding things in the house. Sometimes she would even become lost when trying to find the bathroom or her bedroom. One afternoon she left a hot pan on the stove and laid down to take a nap, leading to a fire that destroyed a set of cabinets in the kitchen. After that, Ravi told her she could not cook anymore without someone's help. Abha resented this a great deal, saying, "I've been cooking for this family for 75 years and now you say I can't? I guess I'm no use to anyone anymore."

Shortly after the fire incident, Abha began to have problems with incontinence. This was particularly hard for Ravi to deal with and he began staying later and later at work. Abha began to need nearly constant supervision and so Diya put off her plans to go back to school and took on most of the duties of cleaning and caring for her. Diya stopped teaching dance at the temple and although she stayed in contact with friends by phone, Ravi became upset if she talked to them about their struggles with Abha. "Keep our family business in our family," he would admonish her.

Discussion Questions

1. Discuss the differences between Abha's *illness* and her *disease*.

2. Try to take on Abha's perspective. What do you think she is feeling? How is her illness affecting her sense of her own identity?

3. Try to take on Ravi's perspective. What do you think he is feeling? How is he dealing with the declines he is seeing in his mother? Characterize his response using the stress process model.

4. Try to take on Diya's perspective. What do you think she is feeling? In what way could gender or cultural norms affect her caregiving stress? How is she coping with the burdens of caregiving? Characterize her experience using the stress process model.

5. If Abha was your patient, how might you need to work with the family on the issues they are facing? What advantages and disadvantages do they face in terms of providing care to Abha? Using the stress process model, at what points might you intervene to improve the situation for the family?

CHAPTER 9

The Social Dynamics
of Clinical Communication

LEARNING OBJECTIVES

After reading this chapter, students should be able to

- Describe various social structural conditions and how they affect clinical interactions and communication.

- Elaborate five best practices of clinical communication and describe how these can mitigate problems associated with social conditions and inherent power differentials within clinical interaction.

- Demonstrate appreciation for how a well-developed sociological imagination can benefit clinical communication, foster stronger patient–provider relationships, and improve health outcomes.

In Chapter 8, we used the contrast between disease and illness to discuss how an experiential gap can emerge between providers and patients. The conceptual distance between the two is important to recognize because it mitigates the effective provision of care and support, particularly where the illness experience of patients and their families is reduced to a physiological phenomenon within a rigidly defined disease perspective. The biomedical aspects of illness certainly are important to providing good care, and it's even reasonable that they are the practitioners' primary focus. Nonetheless, recognizing that, for patients and their loved ones, illness is not limited to those physiological aspects promotes a broader and more informed perspective of what it means to provide care. Indeed, patients may be much more concerned about the social and psychological conditions that attend their illness experience. As a result, the different experiences and social positions of patients and providers create gaps that can confound communication between them. This is especially problematic where communication is the conduit through which important clinical and diagnostic information flows. Alternatively, good patient–provider communication can also bridge the gap between clinicians and the illness experience, including its social and psychological features, from the patient's point of view.

Not only is good communication essential for providing good health care experience for patients, but a great deal of diagnostic information also relies on patient self-reports. Good rapport with a patient, then, is not simply a matter of making them feel good about the encounter; rather, it is a requirement for diagnosing disease, establishing a treatment plan, and executing it successfully. While interpersonal communication is complicated in its own right, complexity pervades within clinical contexts. First, many factors shape our ability to communicate with another person (i.e., what we might call our *discursive relationship* with them). Where our social characteristics (and the perspectives shaped by those attributes) dispose us toward different experiences in life, we often have greater distances to cross in communicating with those whose experiences are significantly different from our own. The call for cultural competence in medical, nursing, and allied health education, for example, speaks precisely to this particular experiential gap between patients and providers.

Too often, communication training in these fields focuses on what to say and how to say it. Historically, communication in health care settings was reducible to "bedside manner," a term that casts the social activity of providers in relatively superficial terms. Moreover, there have long been questions about whether we can teach good interpersonal communication skills, beyond the simple dictates of professional etiquette. Many believe that the ability to connect socially with others is inborn or at least ingrained by the time one reaches postsecondary or graduate training. While personality traits like "extraversion" may be in some part hardwired or the products of early socialization (and they certainly confer benefits with respect to one's bedside manner), good communication is a far deeper process of crossing the distances between provider and patient. This is not a function of a bubbly or engaging personality as much as it is a function of robust awareness about the patient as a person.

Certainly good communication is essential to crossing the various degrees of social separation between providers and patients. This means, however, not only improving how we speak and interact with someone, but also a deeper awareness and recognition of the ways that social positions can create interpersonal distances. It also means cultivating the ability to put ourselves into the role of the other, and to see the world from those perspectives, to the greatest extent possible (recall the concept of *verstehen* from Chapter 8). Only upon these foundations can we meaningfully address how to speak and behave in a clinical encounter so that it promotes trust, connection, and rapport with a patient. Put another way, a good sociological imagination is at the core of good clinical communication because it allows us to envision the range of issues and ways of seeing that we need to explore during the clinical interview. In this sense, good communication does not reduce to speaking well to a patient and does not come to someone as an inherent personality trait, but it is a learned capacity to see things about others that are often obscured by the biomedical paradigm of disease. In short, we believe this awareness is indeed something we can teach.

In this chapter, we will begin by discussing how various social structural conditions confound communication and micro-interactions within a clinical context. These include age, gender, socioeconomic status (SES), race/ethnicity, and culture. We will then elaborate a paradigm for thinking about clinical communication, drawing from the literature on narrative practices. On these foundations, we will highlight some best practices in clinical communication, concluding with a discussion of the significance these practices have in promoting a variety of good outcomes in patient care.

The Social Structure of Clinical Encounters

Increasing complexity in clinical communication is largely a consequence of the various social influences that shape micro-level interactions between practitioners and patients. While the clinical encounter appears quite personal, a broad array of research illustrates that age, gender, SES, race, and other cultural factors enter the room with both providers and patients, and strongly influence how they speak, how they exchange information, and how they understand each other. A good sociological imagination helps us remain conscious of how we carry these larger influences with us into clinical encounters, even when those interactions appear to be wholly private and personal.

A tremendous body of research suggests that clinical communication varies based on the social characteristics of both the patients and the providers. In a call to fellow physicians to recognize the social structural determinants of clinical decision-making, Eisenberg (1979) elucidated four influential sociological factors emerging from what was, at the time, a burgeoning body of research: (1) the characteristics of the patient, (2) the characteristics of the clinician, (3) the clinician's interaction with his or her profession, and (4) the clinician's relationship with the patient (i.e., the two as a dyad constituting something more than just the combination of the individuals). Subsequent decades of research demonstrate the persistent influence of social factors in shaping clinical communication, both in terms of what each party brings to the encounter and what together they become as a micro-social system (Bloom 1965). Szasz and Hollender (1956), for example, classically identified three types of physician–patient dyads (see Table 9.1). While these are a useful starting point for thinking about how clinical relationships might unfold, we should remember that dynamic interactions between providers and patients rarely, if ever, fall neatly into one of these categories. Nonetheless, we might better understand problems of clinical communication, at least in one important sense, by examining how various social forces can press clinical communication into a

TABLE 9.1 Three Basic Models of the Physician–Patient Relationship

Model	Physician's Role	Patient's Role	Clinical Application of Model	Prototype of Model
Activity-passivity	Does something to patient	Recipient (unable to respond or inert)	Anesthesia, acute trauma, coma, delirium, etc.	Parent-infant
Guidance-cooperation	Tells patient what to do	Cooperator (obeys)	Acute infectious processes, etc.	Parent-child (adolescent)
Mutual participation	Helps patient to help himself	Participant in "partnership" (uses expert help)	Most chronic illnesses, psychoanalysis, etc.	Adult-adult

Source: Szasz, Thomas S. & Marc H. Hollender. (1956). "A Contribution to the Philosophy of Medicine: The Basic Models of the Doctor-Patient Relationship." *AMA Archives of Internal Medicine* 97, 585–92.

guidance-cooperation or activity-passivity model, even in clinical situations for which these are not suitable (e.g., chronic illness management).

At the same time, these categories remind us that, despite the more recent glorification of shared decision-making between patients and providers (along with various other attempts to equalize power within clinical practice), power differentials in these contexts are inevitable (see Chapter 7), and practitioner authority retains importance and utility in decision-making in a number of situations (emergencies, as well as situations that arguably call for "beneficent persuasion"). In the end, clinical communication is a complex process whereby players are differently positioned by virtue of their personal and social characteristics, as well as their roles in the encounter (e.g., expert or patient), and together they navigate various conditions of health and illness. Throughout this process, the character of the social system they are co-creating oscillates in response to how they act with and upon each other. In this section, we discuss how age, gender, SES, race, and culture each influences clinical communication as these relationships are established and evolve.

The Influence of Age

Age represents a particularly important social structural factor that influences clinical communication in at least two key ways. First, age is associated with a *cohort effect*, meaning that an age differential between a provider and a patient connotes a different set of experiences in the world that are distinctly age-dependent. For example, a patient who is 95 years old in 2015 would have been 9 years old at the beginning of the Great Depression. Those events undoubtedly shaped their childhood experiences in significant ways. At the same time, their 42-year-old physician would *not* share those experiences. Second, there are stereotypes associated with becoming older. Often referred to as *ageism*, these biases can affect not only the way that providers speak to older patients, but also the very treatment decisions that they make in providing care to them (Butler 1969; Clark et al. 1991). Age thus represents a potential confounding factor for clinical communication not only because of biases we hold toward aging, but also because age is a proxy for a set of social experiences that are not shared by people whose socialization occurred in a different time period.

In their seminal work on the function of ageism in clinical communication, Greene and colleagues (1986:113) write, "Specific ageist assumptions about older people are legion: they can't hear, they can't remember, they can't think for themselves, they are depressing, they are non-productive, they are infantile." In their examination of age-related clinical communication dynamics, these authors found that despite no significant differences between young and old patients in terms of assertiveness, friendliness, and expressiveness, physicians were significantly more egalitarian, patient, engaged, and respectful when interacting with younger patients when compared with older ones.

More recent research suggests that similar patterns persist. A systematic review of articles on ageism in health care between 2005 and 2015 demonstrates persistent stereotyping based on age. Though not exclusively directed at older people (e.g., there was bias directed toward particularly young mothers), themes in the literature make clear that, like other marginalized groups, older patients regularly face negative stereotypes and often receive poorer care (Kydd & Fleming 2015). Several research studies in this review also highlight that closing clinics and wards focused on geriatric care has redistributed the care of older persons to larger acute hospitals, which often lack specialized expertise in the care of older persons (see also Eymard & Douglas 2012).

Ageism also can manifest as *self-stereotyping* where older patients themselves make decisions based on social constructs of old age (Kagan 2008; see also Eymard & Douglas 2012). Makris et al. (2015:41), for example, point out that a belief in the "age-related inevitability of restrictive back pain" is a key reason that older persons do not seek care for the condition. Perhaps most clinically relevant, *beneficent ageism* refers to situations where providers or family members make decisions they believe are protecting the older patient, but which undermine the patient's actual wishes (Kagan 2008). This sort of paternalism is often grounded on questions about the capacity of older people to make decisions for themselves, but of course, age bias can confound our ability to assess fairly their capacity in the first place (see also Chapter 11).

For these reasons and others, providers can find clinical care and communication with older patients quite challenging. Not only can their biases engender bad communication, but they also report "feeling challenged" by older patients because of the often complex and multifaceted nature of their medical problems. This may be especially true if providers with particular specialties focus only on certain aspects of the patient's care, while needing at the same time to coordinate recommendations with multiple other treatment plans.[1] Additionally, remaining mindful of potential cognitive declines while often simultaneously dealing with more intricate involvement from family members can frustrate and perplex many practitioners (Ekdahl et al. 2012).

Kydd and Fleming (2015) conclude their systematic review by noting that a focus on individual, patient-centered care can undercut these problematic biases in the care of older patients. Below we discuss strategies for precisely that sort of work. Nonetheless, without recognition of these biases and how they affect care, it will be difficult for providers to move beyond the confounding effects of age differences, to get to a truly individualized perspective. The need for health care providers to remain reflexive about their own biases is a critical first step toward patient-centered communication.

The Influence of Gender

Social norms surrounding gender appear to be some of the earliest that we internalize through the process of socialization. The worlds of young children are often color coded by gender (i.e., blue or pink) before they can really even see color, and

---

[1] This challenge is exacerbated by a declining number of geriatricians even among an aging population in the United States:

Pediatrics and other specialties seem to have historically responded to market needs. The specialty of geriatrics has definitely not taken the same path, despite a demographic imperative that has seen an unprecedented growth in the number of older people in the United States, fueled by the same baby boomer population that fueled the growth of pediatrics " Not only are the present number of geriatricians far below the present and expected need, but the number has actually been declining. (Wasserman 2015:100)

even before they are born. As a consequence, gender norms structure much of the world around us and how we perceive and interpret it. For example, suppose you were presented with the following list of sports and asked to sort them by whether they were masculine or feminine: figure skating versus ice hockey, or baseball versus softball. Nearly everyone could sort those neatly across gendered categories, and there would be very little variation between individuals doing so. Despite the fact that all of these sports are independent of gender as a concept, we nonetheless internalize gendered constructs to form a lens through which we see the world. This conceptual lens colors our social life such that we often learn to act in ways that accord with our biological sex.[2] Boys, particularly after a certain age, may be sanctioned for playing with dolls or doing ballet. Alternatively, though at slightly older ages, girls often are sanctioned for being too tomboyish or "butch." Media images reinforce gendered notions of the world around us, even specifically with regard to health. "Texts such as *Men's Health* and *Shape Magazine*," for example, "contribute to the production of gendered health discourses" (Brenton 2014:648). Later in life, gender not only conditions how we behave, but also how we interpret and even influence the behavior of others.

Communication, therefore, is also a distinctly gendered phenomenon. Men tend to be more assertive, interruptive, and quick to jump into a problem-solving role in a discourse (see classic work by Tannen 1991, among others). Women, on the other hand, tend to listen without interrupting and exhibit greater empathy without jumping in too quickly to intervene. While we learn gendered norms from our social environments, we also practice and therefore perpetuate gender as we play it out in interactional situations. As West and Zimmerman (1987) write, "Doing gender involves a complex of socially guided perceptual interactional, and micropolitical activities ..." Insofar as the clinical encounter represents an interactive moment nested in particularly influential social contexts (e.g., see Chapter 2 regarding the structure of the clinic and a history of medical paternalism), gender plays a major role in clinical communication.

A large body of research consistently links the gender of practitioners to an array of clinical communication habits. A systematic literature review by Roter et al. (2002) found that female physicians engaged in *patient-centered communication* to a significantly higher degree than male physicians. This included greater engagement with psychosocial issues (both in giving information and asking questions), more actively creating partnerships by encouraging patient participation and attempting to equalize status differences, and greater utilization of *positive talk*, including encouragement and reassurance (see also Roter & Hall 2004). Visits with female physicians lasted nearly four minutes longer with male patients (compared to male physicians seeing male patients) and more than seven minutes longer with female patients (compared to male physicians seeing female patients; Hall et al. 1994). Gendered notions of appropriate communication often disempower or disadvantage women in some contexts (e.g., women are less likely to

---

[2] Sex is generally regarded as biological while gender is generally regarded as a social construct. However, the issue becomes more complicated where some social–psychological tendencies appear to be rooted in genetic and physiological features of sex biology, while at the same time the physiology of sex is hardly deterministic and its meanings and classifications are rooted heavily in sociomedical norms (West & Zimmerman 1987).

ask for raises, owing significantly to gender socialization that associates passivity with femininity; see Babcock & Laschever 2003). But in a clinical context where historical power inequities favor providers (see Chapter 7), clinicians who are women often exhibit tendencies that counterbalance the paternalism historically inherent to medical practice.

While the gender of providers is clearly influential, the characteristics of patients also are important. As a result, gender dynamics unfold differently between providers who are men and women, depending on the gender of the patients. For example, male patients rated the tone of female physicians as more anxious and less friendly, perhaps signaling discomfort or ambivalence with a situation where traditional gender hierarchies preferencing men were undercut by the power dynamics of the traditional practitioner–patient relationship (Hall et al. 1994). At the same time, contrary to what traditional gender constructs might lead us to predict, research nonetheless suggests that men and women create an equal number of empathic opportunities in clinical encounters and clearly express emotions while doing so (Bylund & Makoul 2002; Hall & Roter 2002). This highlights the important insight that gender constructs are not deterministic. Rather, they affect the contours of clinical communication in complex ways, and interact with other, sometimes countervailing social forces in the process.

Internalized social constructs are not neatly parsed across different categories but are instead interwoven with one another. Age, gender, class, and race all intersect in a complex interactive social dynamic (see Chapter 5). In fact, Bertakis and Azari (2012) found that female physicians utilized patient-centered communication significantly more frequently than male physicians overall. But when they controlled for sociodemographic factors, health risk behaviors, pain, and health status, gender differences in physician use of patient-centered communication decreased dramatically to the point that they were statistically equivalent between men and women. It is thus important to think about how some social structural conditions may amplify or attenuate the influence of others.

The Influence of Socioeconomic Status

In Chapter 4 we discuss how SES is associated with a variety of disparities in health and health care, but it may not be immediately clear how SES specifically influences communication patterns. But just as one's cohort and ascribed gender connote experiences that shape how they perceive and interact with the social world (including clinical encounters), our SES shapes contexts within which we are socialized, and through which we experience the world. Our expectations and perceptions of social life are shaped significantly by our class experiences (recall the concept of habitus from Chapter 6). Sociologist Max Weber (1946) long ago highlighted class as a social construct that expanded far beyond the boundaries of income and into the realm of social status, or one's level of prestige. Pierre Bourdieu (1990) goes further to highlight that class is associated with a particular way of seeing the world and transmitted particular behavioral tendencies across time and generations, including particular ways of speaking. Class comprises then, not only a material feature of social life, but also a cultural one. That is, insofar as we internalize particular ways of seeing and interacting with the world through our socialization and experiences, the things we encounter amidst particular socioeconomic contexts become part of our cultural worldview.[3] For the purposes of this chapter, this means that practitioners often contribute to patterns of clinical communication due to the influence of socioeconomic class.

A significant body of literature demonstrates the salience of class for understanding problems of clinical communication. A classic work by Waitzkin (1985) demonstrates that physicians utilized more multi-level explanations (i.e., re-explaining technical statements in everyday language) and spent more time overall with patients who had higher levels of education (i.e., a proxy measure of social class), even when controlling for a host of other variables, including prognosis and diagnostic certainty. He highlights that despite assumptions to the contrary, patients from all class levels desired the same amount of information, but those from the lower class strata received significantly less (Waitzkin 1985). A more recent systematic review uncovers similar results, including that

> patients from lower social classes receive less positive socio-emotional utterances and a more directive and less participatory consulting style, characterized by significantly less information giving, less directions, and less socio-emotional and partnership building utterances from their doctor. (Willems et al. 2005:139)

These authors also confirm Waitzkin's (1985) finding that physicians mistakenly believe that patients of lower SES desire less information.

Good communication may be particularly important for patients of low SES since research shows that they have more difficulty accessing good sources of information about their illnesses (which are more numerous to begin with, largely due to SES; see Chapter 4). One study of women struggling with infertility, for example, found that women in higher class strata tended to access information from support groups, their doctors, and the Internet (Bell 2014). In contrast, women in lower class strata tended not to access these sources of information, but rather were more dependent on media (e.g., television and magazines). This is especially problematic where media depictions of infertility not only tend to represent infertility as an upper class, white problem, but also over-represent success stories, despite the fact that assisted reproductive therapies only work about 30% of the time. Where these representations alienate poor women, they may exacerbate communication patterns in a clinical encounter, for example, by further suppressing the likelihood that a poor minority woman will advocate for treatment.

The Influence of Race/Ethnicity

In the United States, race and class are tightly bound social phenomena and they exhibit strong statistical associations with one another. African Americans, for example, are disproportionately more likely to be poor. In turn, it can be difficult

[3] This notion should not be oversimplified to suggest that those from lower SES brackets speak poorly or are necessarily uneducated. The phenomenon is more subtle and complex. Take, for example, two sets of students applying for medical school: one comprised of first-generation college students and the other comprised of children of physicians. Both groups have the same level of education and high GPAs. But one group was socialized in and among physician culture. Many medical school interviewers will attest that, *on average*, the children of physicians carry themselves differently. They are more likely to have a natural sense of comfort and fitting-in amidst the physicians and faculty that interview them (this doesn't mean they necessarily *will*, or that the other group *will not*, but it represents an overall tendency).

to separate the extent to which class and race/ethnicity, as social structures, independently shape the contours of clinical communication. Nonetheless, the effects of race/ethnicity as a sociocultural influence cannot be explained away by SES (Smedley et al. 2003). Indeed, numerous studies suggest that implicit race bias affects clinical communication. A study by van Ryn and Burke (2000), for example, found that physicians tended to perceive African American patients as less intelligent, having a greater propensity for risky behavior, and felt less affiliation toward them (i.e., they were less likely to see an African American patient as the kind of person with whom they could be friends). In a sample of registered nurses, Haider et al. (2015) reported that, while 71% did not believe they held any racial bias, about 85% demonstrated such bias in an implicit association test. Interestingly, while implicit race bias did not demonstrate any effect on acute clinical decision-making when various providers (including nurses, physicians, and medical students) were presented with hypothetical clinical vignettes (Haider et al. 2011, 2014, 2015), bias and discomfort surrounding race clearly influence clinical communication patterns in real-life encounters, which, in turn, affect care outcomes.

Just as the intimate moments of our personal lives contain in them larger social conditions (recall the sociological imagination from Chapter 1), clinical encounters are, at least in part, a microcosm of larger social arrangements. While the explicit functions of the clinical encounter center on resolving issues of health and illness, both the patient and the provider as human beings carry into it broader behavioral and psychological dispositions. With respect to race, the clinical encounter is not immune to the ubiquitous social forces surrounding racial stereotyping, racial inequalities of power, and pervasive social and residential segregation, among others. As such, African American patients experience more verbal dominance and less positive affect (Cooper et al. 2012; Penner et al. 2014). In their review of the literature, Penner et al. (2014) importantly note that these trends persist in different geographic locations and therefore cannot be reduced to the culture or history of a particular region. Moreover, they also highlight that implicit bias in clinical encounters is associated with shorter visits, as well as the provider speaking faster and using more anxious language. While the direct relationships between race-biased communication patterns and health outcomes is underexplored, African American patients experience significantly less patient-centered communication, which is associated with worse emotional health and fewer subsequent tests (Penner et al. 2014). Discomfort and racial bias are not only communicated through language, but also nonverbally. One study of differences in physician communication with white and black terminally ill patients found that even though verbal communication scores did not significantly differ in their sample, physicians utilized significantly more "closed postures," less physical contact, and less proximity (Elliott et al. 2016). Bias and discomfort surrounding race in the clinical encounter likely combines with a troubling historical relationship between minorities and medicine to exacerbate distrust in providers (Gamble 1997; Wasserman et al. 2007), which is linked to poor treatment adherence (Penner et al. 2014). In African American cancer patients, less patient-centered communication is associated with less patient confidence in recommended treatments, as well as patient perceptions that side effects will be worse and a propensity to estimate greater difficulty completing treatment (Gordon et al. 2006).

The reality that race bias and discomfort are associated with less-positive clinical communication suggests that the effects of race in clinical encounters can be combated with greater attention to communication skills. For example, Schoenthaler and colleagues (2012) demonstrated that collaborative communication styles were significantly associated with treatment adherence in encounters when physicians and patients were not of the same race. Similarly, Aruguete and Roberts (2002) had study participants watch simulated encounters where they were in the role of a patient, but where the physician's presentation was a prerecorded video. They found no differences in the resulting evaluations of same-race and different-race physicians. In real-life encounters, race differences between providers and patients may create communication problems. But this study by Aruguete and Roberts (2002) holds that variable constant by standardizing the responses of the physician irrespective of the race of the participant acting as the patient. This is particularly important because practitioners cannot unilaterally change the social forces of race in the wider society, but they may be able to adopt patient-centered perspectives and communication strategies that mitigate the extent to which these negatively affect patient care (Martin & Cooper 2013).

The Influence of Culture

The ways that culture can influence clinical communication are practically infinite. The term itself captures an immensely wide variety of worldviews and traditions, any one of which might affect the discourse of a clinical encounter in its own way. Moreover, culture is at once something given to us through socialization, and something that we act out in ways that reproduce and change it, at least incrementally (see Chapter 5). Just like the other factors discussed above, culture affects the meanings and values associated with health and the body, and therefore has the potential to separate providers and patients. Crossing the gap between a practitioner who is focused on certain dimensions of a disease and a patient whose cultural backgrounds lead them to focus on other facets of that experience certainly requires exceptional communication skills. But before we shift our discussion toward these skills, we need to explore some key ways that cultural differences can become problematic for clinical communication.

In a systematic review of the literature, Schouten and Meeuwesen (2006) identified five key predictors of problems in clinical communication caused by cultural differences between providers and patients, which we summarize here:

1. *Cultural differences in explanatory models of health and illness.* Particularly where patients have an understanding of health and illness influenced by various personal and cultural beliefs and traditions, whereas providers often operate from a biomedical explanatory model.
2. *Differences in cultural values.* For example, patients with more collectivist as opposed to individualist values tend to be more deferential in a clinical encounter.
3. *Cultural differences in patients' preferences for doctor–patient relationships.* For example, there are cultural differences in the amount and type of information a patient desires, with some favoring less disclosure and participation

in decision-making, while others may value conversation about psychosocial aspects of the illness to a greater or lesser extent.

4. *Racism/perceptual bias.* As discussed above, race-discordance creates a level of discomfort associated with less patient-centered communication.

5. *Linguistic barriers.* The inability to communicate because of linguistic barriers not only presents obvious obstacles to providing care, but is also associated with poorer compliance and reticence to seek treatment in the first place.

Most of the studies in this review highlight a number of communication problems that emerge from some combination of the above predictors. The majority found that white physicians demonstrated less-affective behavior and decreased empathy in encounters with patients from different cultural backgrounds. More specifically, one study reported that physicians used fewer open-ended questions (a strategy discussed below), allowed patients to ask questions less often, and gave less medical information when talking to Hispanic patients. Another found that *shared understanding* was not commonly achieved in encounters between Aboriginal patients and health care workers in Australia, speaking perhaps most clearly to differences in their respective explanatory models of illness and cultural values (Cass et al. 2002; see also Kleinman et al. 1978).

Another qualitative study of intercultural communication by physicians and patients in Canada similarly demonstrates the ways that cultural misunderstandings can become problematic for health care (Rosenberg et al. 2006). In one encounter, a physician who had counseled a young woman on the use of contraception reported that, like other young people, she failed to properly conceive of, and plan for, future events. In actuality, there were stronger cultural influences at play, particularly where the patient reported significant stigma attached to the use of contraception from friends and family in light of a prevailing belief that babies were gifts from God. In another example, a physician reported of a patient, "Her tears do not mean severe distress as they would for a local person; the whole family is the same. Mediterraneans are all like this" (Rosenberg et al. 2006:243). To the contrary, when the researchers followed up with the patient, they found she had high levels of psychological distress. This example highlights the critical problematic for providing culturally competent clinical care. Not only is it important that cultural knowledge is accurate, but there is also a difficult and delicate balance between utilizing knowledge about a patient's cultural background and stereotyping them. Put another way, knowledge about cultural values and perspectives on health and illness is a double-edged sword. It not only holds the potential to significantly enhance patient care, but it also remains dangerous if it is not accompanied by an understanding of the ways that any individual may deviate from those cultural norms. So while knowledge about culture and other social factors provides an important starting place for incorporating social science into clinical practice, good communication is the key to working from that baseline to the individual patient. One way to think about the roles that factors like age, gender, SES, race, and culture play in clinical encounters with individual patients is to conceive of them as *sensitizing concepts*. That is, the practitioner, in employing a good sociological imagination, can envision the ways that various social factors can influence health, but uses these as signals of what to investigate, rather as factors from which to directly draw conclusions. We elaborate on this in the next section.

Narrative and the Art of Clinical Practice

A good sociological imagination helps us understand the many ways that social influences shape the individual moments of our lives. Of particular concern in this chapter is how we carry those influences with us in our social habits and everyday practices, including our communication patterns. The above discussion demonstrates just some of the social factors that influence those individual interactions. But this does not mean that individuals are fated to act out larger sociological patterns. We *tend* to recreate and reproduce them, but doing so is not *inevitable*. In particular, working on good clinical communication skills can mitigate the effects that social influences—like age, class, gender, race, and culture—have on patient care.

Medicine has long been considered both an art and a science. The same can now be said of other health professions as they have evolved, particularly in recent decades, to include both a firm foundation in scientific literature and critical roles in patient care (including diagnostic and treatment processes). The great puzzle of clinical practice concerns how to connect the scientific evidence surrounding health and illness—which refers to the generalized knowledge and tendencies of groups (see Chapter 3)—to individual patients who may deviate from those aggregate trends in ways that are clinically significant. That is, how should generalized science inform individualized care? Figure 9.1 is a hypothetical scatterplot depicting the relationship between group-level constructs such as culture or class-based dispositions (see Chapters 5 and 6) (horizontal axis) and any number of outcomes including health beliefs and health behaviors (vertical axis). The line drawn through the individual data points represents the evidence base from which clinical practice draws heavily, and this evidence base provides a starting point for understanding how particular factors *tend* to be related in populations. This is the *science* of medicine. But clinical practitioners do not treat populations as a whole, and the particular individuals they do treat can deviate, sometimes a great deal, from the aggregate trends. As a result, clinical practice is about navigating from the baseline evidence to the individual patient, represented by the dotted line in Figure 9.1. This is the *art* of clinical practice.

The process of working from generalized evidence to individual patients fundamentally requires good communication skills. Often students utilize checklists of issues to cover with patients. These can be helpful reminders for budding professionals whose clinical habits may not be well developed. But such an approach also presents problems (see also Chapter 10). Checklists presuppose what constitutes important information in the clinical encounter and often guide the patient to produce a narrative that is strongly influenced by the presupposed concerns of practitioners—concerns prepopulated to the checklist, but not necessarily universally applicable to the individual patient. Patients often experience sickness in ways that significantly differ from the concerns of professional providers (see the discussion in Chapter 8 on disease and illness). So to understand the ways an individual patient experiences illness, including how it affects their life and how their broader goals may influence treatment plans, a practitioner needs to be able to work their way into the patient's way of seeing. This requires, at least in the early stages of an encounter, a more artful practice that solicits the patient's own narrative and encourages the patient to develop and elaborate the story of their

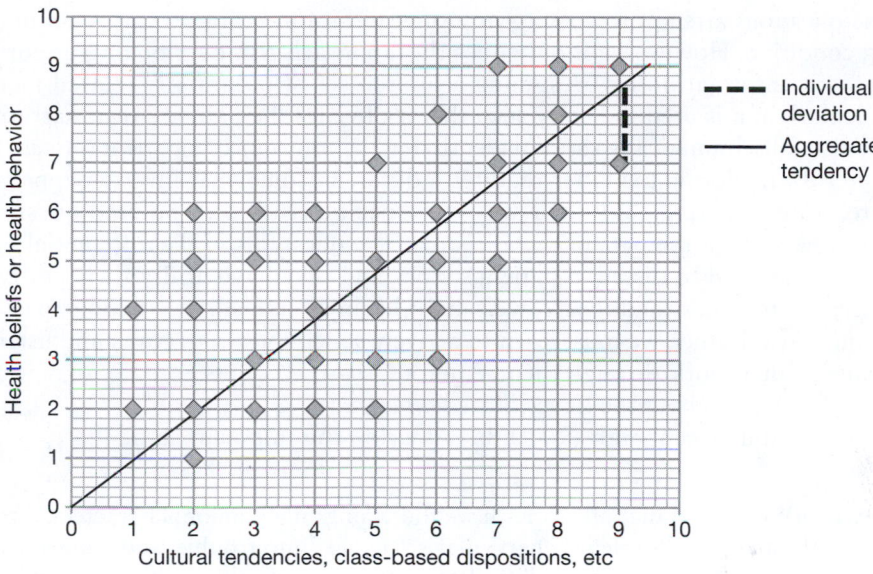

FIG. 9.1 Hypothetical scatterplot capturing the relationship between art and science in clinical practice.*

Note: *Not real data.

illness. The traditional process of differential diagnosis, where discriminating questions sort relevant biomedical information, undeniably plays an important role in the diagnostic process, but should be positioned later in clinical discourse so that it does not disrupt the earlier, foundational work of eliciting the patient's narrative. Similarly, checklists and standard questionnaires retain importance particularly at this later stage because they help ensure that key diagnostic information is not overlooked. If clinical dialogue begins with a focused interrogation of symptoms, however, it immediately places the patient on the practitioner's terrain and limits the extent to which the clinician can understand what is happening from the patient's own perspective.

Narrative approaches to patient care reframe the purpose and technique of a patient interview in ways that are especially important in the chronic illness era (see Chapter 2). The demands of long-term illness management (now more prevalent than ever) require a kind of relationship-building with patients that arguably was less important when treating acute infection and injury was the primary business of health care. Indeed, biomedical understandings of disease inherently involve processes of differentiation that sort and discriminate relevant and irrelevant factors (Wasserman 2014). That is, scientific approaches to disease inherently function by sorting the relevant physiological information from the rest, which is deemed less important from a strictly biomedical view. This perspective can shape clinical communication, especially from the patient's perspective, where it becomes a series of directed questions designed to produce a differential diagnosis. For example, a patient reporting a headache might be asked a series of discriminating questions like: "Where does it hurt? How long has it been hurting? Is the pain sharp or dull?"

These questions attempt to solicit symptoms and information to clarify an underlying condition. However, not only does this approach risk overlooking important diagnostic information by presuming a limited set of potentially related factors (particularly if it is used too early such that it obviates the patient's own narrative), but it also falls dramatically short in identifying the contours of a patient's *illness* (see Chapter 8). Exploring the latter requires a different, somewhat inverted approach, where, instead of tunneling their way to a specific issue with pointed questions, practitioners solicit the patient's whole story. The questions of the differential diagnosis are designed to dissect a patient's story and they have utility for identifying *disease*. But to understand *illness*, we cannot begin by immediately taking apart the patient's story. Rather, we must learn to actively solicit these narratives and listen to patients as they work through them. After all, these accounts contain a great deal more information about the larger *illness experience*.

Loftus and Greenhalgh (2010:85) describe the importance of the patients' stories:

> Aristotle observed that all stories have four things in common: characters, setting, trouble, and plot. People in a particular setting get into trouble, and work must be done to get them out of trouble or lessen its impact. In the health professions we sometimes talk about the illness narrative, where trouble is disease, disability, disfigurement, and so on—plus the accompanying loss of status and independence in society. Coping with diabetes, for example, and preventing its complications requires perseverance and the help of family, friends, religious leaders, health professionals, and others. No person's experience of diabetes is the same as any other person's. Every patient faces different biomedical events and complications, different day-to-day challenges, a different social context, different constraints of work or neighbourhood, different moral choices.

To avoid prematurely forcing the patient onto the narrower terrain of biomedical discourse, good clinical communication cannot begin with a directed, differentiating inquiry. Rather, practitioners must learn to actively encourage patient narrative. And because patients usually are not professional storytellers with neatly packaged narratives, providers should be able to assemble these narratives as patients verbally work through them. While we may naturally think of communication as fundamentally characterized by what we verbalize, the foundations of good clinical communication are built on encouraging the patient to tell their story, and not prematurely disrupting that narrative with one's own biomedical agenda.

Rita Charon's (2006) landmark work *Narrative Medicine* captures the power of employing narrative strategies in communicating with patients. Charon's insights about the importance of narrative emerged from her early clinical experiences working with a diverse patient population. "Most were poor, sick, elderly women of color—from the Dominican Republic, Puerto Rico, Central America, and the American South—who now lived in Manhattan's Washington Heights or Harlem," she describes (p. 4). Above we discussed the ways that social structural contexts can create divides between practitioner and patient, and thereby complicate and confound clinical communication. Similarly, Charon realized early in her clinical career that mitigating the myriad of ways that social factors and structural inequalities create problems in the clinical encounter required listening and understanding each patient's story about their illness experience, each with its own complexities and idiosyncrasies. She writes:

> I realized slowly that my task as an internist was to develop the skills required to absorb my patients' multiple, often contradictory, stories of illness. I came to understand that what my patients paid me to do was to listen expertly and attentively to extraordinarily complicated narratives—told in words, gestures, silences, tracings, images, laboratory test results, and changes in the body—and to cohere all these stories into something that made provisional sense, enough sense, that is, on which to act. (p. 4)

Notice how Charon (2006) acknowledges the importance of the biomedical aspects of disease and related information. But what also becomes clear is that clinical judgments, including both diagnosis and treatment, require bringing the biomedical information (both individual lab results and the larger body of evidence) into the singular narrative of an individual patient (the *art* of medicine, as described above). For individual stories of illness to make sense, they should include the patient's wider social and psychological experiences. After all, the patient's disease is always nested in larger social contexts. Narrative practices represent a way to push back against the social forces that can interfere with clinical trust and interpersonal rapport. Moreover, eliciting and actively listening to the patient's story is critical to working from the aggregate evidence to the individual patient. In the next section, we describe a few basic strategies for doing so.

Basic Interviewing Techniques

There are many good resources that explain how to conduct a good patient interview (e.g., Cole & Bird 2014). In this section, we will not detail all of the required, useful, or desirable techniques. Instead, we highlight key strategies for soliciting effective narrative. Doing so is the critical component involved in navigating the complex social terrain that stands between practitioners and patients. It entails cultivating a narrative understanding of the patient's experience, one that honors the patients' perspectives, their relationships to their illnesses, and their impacts on their lives and relationships, rather than assuming the priority of its biomedical aspects. The ability to procure a patient's story and to understand it as a holistic narrative is of singular importance in addressing "health care's divides," many of which we have discussed throughout this book (Charon 2006).

At its most basic level, what tends to be so difficult for practitioners involves actively listening without disrupting the flow of the patient's story. After all, providers often envision their role as fundamentally about solving the problems of disease. Indeed, that undoubtedly *is* one of their roles, if not the most important one. But there are times when the problem-solver role should recede, lest it become disruptive. This is especially true in the early stages of a patient interview. It is common to think of the interview as a cone (see Fig. 9.2), where the early portion represents a wide-ranging exploration of the patient's illness, which eventually, at the appropriate time, begins to narrow its focus through a process of differential diagnosis process (Cole & Bird 2014).

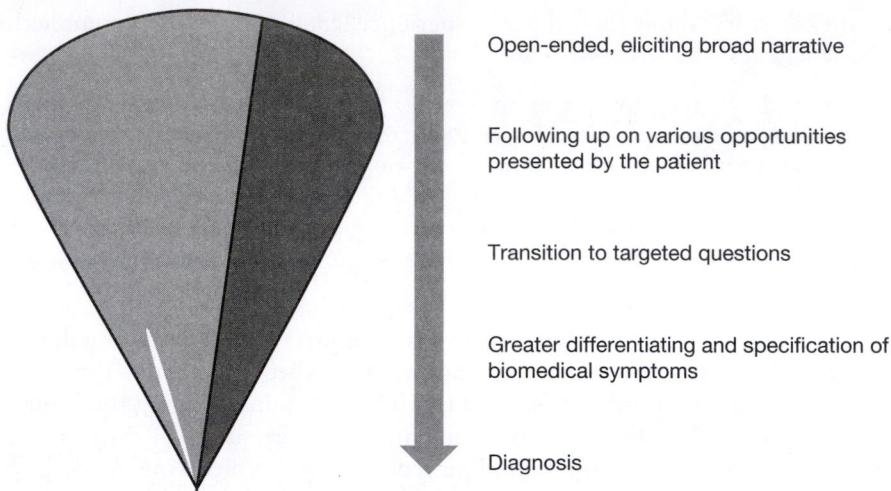

Open-ended, eliciting broad narrative

Following up on various opportunities presented by the patient

Transition to targeted questions

Greater differentiating and specification of biomedical symptoms

Diagnosis

FIG. 9.2 Eliciting narrative in the patient interview.

Loftus and Mackey (2012) identify three broad phases of the interview. The first is the *introductory phase*, which includes introducing yourself and clarifying what you are there to do. While relatively short and typically straightforward, it is a critically important part of the process. First, the introduction sets a foundation for the remainder of the encounter. This is the first impression you will make, and how you go about it will create for the patient a variety of impressions and expectations. For example, Loftus and Mackey (2012) recommend asking permission to interview the patient. This can be as simple as asking, "Is it okay if I ask you a few questions?" But this may well represent a powerful moment to the patient, insofar as it signals respect for the patient and specifically their autonomy (see also Chapter 11). This is critical to establishing trust and rapport, which are at the foundation of eliciting a robust patient narrative. Simply put, patients may be hesitant to open up to providers they do not trust. Second, clarifying your role in the patient's care provides the patient with critical information, particularly today where larger, multidisciplinary teams provide care, instead of lone practitioners (see Chapter 10). Just as health care has become more complex when we consider the nature, origins, and treatment of chronic disease, health care delivery is more complicated and confusing for patients trying to understand just who is providing their care. One striking research study found that 75% of general medicine inpatients "were not able to name anyone when asked to name a physician in charge of their care" and of the 25% that did answer the question with the name of one of their physicians, only 40% could do so correctly (Arora et al. 2009:199). The introductory phase therefore represents more than an exchange of pleasantries. It plays an important role in mitigating the confusion patients may experience in a complex health care setting, often at a time that they may be sick or suffering.

Loftus and Mackey (2012:190) describe the second phase of the interview as the *working phase*, which normally takes up the bulk of the time and is represented in Figure 9.2. In this phase, it is important (especially early in the encounter) to use open-ended questions to avoid leading the patient, which may divert them onto biomedical terrain but away from other things that are potentially important with regard to their illness experience. A question such as, "So, what brings you in today?" allows the patient to begin talking about their problem. As they speak, it is important to avoid interrupting. Failure to allow the patient to complete their narrative risks missing important information, since patients often do not lead with their most significant problem or symptoms, particularly if they are sensitive in nature. While most patients take between 90 and 120 seconds to complete their initial narrative about "what brought them in today," early research in doctor–patient communication found that physicians interrupted, on average, eighteen seconds into that description (Frankel & Beckman 1989; Stewart 1995). By most estimates, the time constraints of managed care have exacerbated this problem (see Chapter 12). This explains why, as Stewart (1995:1424) writes:

> Studies have shown that 50% of psychosocial and psychiatric problems are missed ... that 54% of patient problems and 45% of patient concerns are neither elicited by the physician nor disclosed by the patient, that patients and physicians do not agree on the main presenting problem in 50% of visits, and that patients are dissatisfied with the information provided to them by physicians.

Using open-ended questions, particularly early in the interview process, represents an important strategy to counter these tendencies.

While interrupting the patient will all but guarantee that they will not articulate their full narrative, asking an open-ended question at the start of the interview does not automatically guarantee that they will. It is therefore important to develop skills for extending or facilitating the narrative (Cole & Bird 2014). This presents a fine line to walk for any provider. The goal is to encourage more of the patient's own narrative, not (yet) to lead the patient in a specific direction. At the same time, providers sometimes must ask questions or make statements to draw more of that narrative out, and it is easy for these statements to lead the patient. The goal is to say enough to get them talking again, but to be as minimally disruptive to the patient's narrative as possible. The use of *minimal encouragers* (a concept widely utilized in counseling and therapy practices) can help strike the appropriate balance, though how minimally one can or should encourage will depend on the individual patient and how forthcoming they are with their narrative.

A minimal encourager may be as simple as saying "mm hmm" and waiting for the patient to continue talking. More directly, one might say, "Tell me more about that." It is critical to avoid "closing the cone" before a patient has a chance to elaborate his or her own narrative. Consider the provider–patient dialogue in Table 9.2. In the dialogue on the left, the nurse practitioner uses not only an initial open-ended question, but also continues to elicit the patient's own narrative. In the dialogue on the right, the nurse practitioner "closes the cone" too early by introducing closed-ended questions that lead the patient with a limited set of options with which to describe his complaint. Because the dialogue on the left uses minimal encouragers to allow the patient to put his illness experience into his own words, it succeeds at eliciting not only more information about his physical illness and its potential causes or exacerbating factors (i.e., the physical demands of his job), but also raises an *empathic opportunity* where the patient discusses his worry about how this illness might affect other important areas of his life (Avdi et al. 2008; recall from Chapter 8 that for patients, illnesses are inextricably linked to social roles and functions). This allows the nurse practitioner to build greater rapport with the patient because she is able to demonstrate empathy and legitimize his concerns (both physical and psychosocial; Cole & Bird 2014).

The dialogue on the right in Table 9.2 shows a far too common practice whereby the provider attempts a differential diagnosis too early in the encounter, thereby failing to get sufficient information, both physiological and psychosocial. This also impedes her ability to develop rapport with the patient, particularly where she does not allow for the emergence of empathic opportunities. As a result, she cannot capitalize on them. Put another way, eliciting patient narrative is like fishing for both evidence about the illness and opportunities to connect interpersonally with the patient. In the dialogue on the right, the practitioner presents the patient with a limited set of options (e.g., sharp or dull, line 17). When this happens, patients often assume that these are the only two meaningful choices in the diagnostic process and will not add information outside of them. In the dialogue on the left, the nurse elicits the same information and more (line 18) by simply encouraging the patient to put his experience into his own words. Notice that at one point (line 13) the nurse simply acknowledges that she is listening with an "mm hmm" and then waits for the patient to start talking again. Allowing silence can be difficult in an interview, particularly since many providers are predisposed to jumping in to solve problems. But silence, insofar as it is slightly awkward in an ongoing dialogue, represents a pressure on both parties to speak. One "trick" of sorts that is useful to practitioners attempting to encourage more patient narrative is to use silence as an encourager by *not* being the party in the conversation that breaks it. Of course, there is a point at which it can become awkward, but if used properly (as in Table 9.2, line 13), it can elicit more of the patient's story.

Another trick involves repeating the last few words that a patient says, which not only acknowledges that you've heard them, but also represents a sort of nondisruptive turn taken by the practitioner in the conversation, which therefore psychologically encourages the patient to continue. In the case of the patient in Table 9.2, the narrative on the left contains information about the pain that is not circumscribed by the sharp/dull dichotomy, including that it is intermittent, worse at night, and radiates up the rib cage, not just down the leg. All of these may be diagnostically useful. Moreover, patients often hold back emotions such as worry or fear. Allowing this patient to speak more appears to have given him time to come to the parts of his story where the illness intersects with psychology (he is worried) and social life (this illness is threatening his livelihood).

Of course, providers often resist the idea of open-ended questions and narrative interviewing techniques over concerns that they simply do not have enough time in their schedules. Indeed the interview on the left in Table 9.2 lasts a little longer than the one on the right. But of course, this frames the notion of time within very narrow parameters. That is, if one only compares the time spent in each of these interviews, the one on the left definitely takes more time. However, we might also reasonably conceive of that time as an investment. Consider that spending extra time eliciting patient narrative gives the provider better information to make a diagnosis (thereby reducing the number of misdiagnoses) and helps establish a rapport such that patients find it easier to disclose and discuss problems in the future. In this way, we can understand the extra time that narrative interviewing takes as an investment that pays dividends in time saved later on.

TABLE 9.2 Contrasting Examples of Provider–Patient Dialogue

Line	Open-Ended Questions and Minimal Encouragers	Close-Ended Questions
1	Nurse: Hi Mr. Paul. I'm Ms. Moore. I'm a nurse practitioner here at the hospital and I'm going to be taking care of you. Is it okay if I ask you a few questions?	Nurse: Hi Mr. Paul. I'm Ms. Moore. I'm a nurse practitioner here at the hospital and I'm going to be taking care of you. Is it okay if I ask you a few questions?
2		
3		
4	Patient: Sure.	Patient: Sure.
5		
6	Nurse: Can you tell me what brought you in today?	Nurse: Can you tell me what brought you in today?
7	Patient: I've been having pain in the left side of my body.	Patient: I've been having pain in the left side of my body.
8		
9	Nurse: Mm hmm…<waits a few seconds>	Nurse: When did it start?
10	Patient: It started about 4 weeks ago and it's gotten much worse over the last few days.	Patient: About 4 weeks ago.
11		
12		
13	Nurse: Hmm… can you tell me a little more about it?	Nurse: Is the pain sharp or dull?
14	Patient: It's most intense at my hip, and then it radiates down my leg and up my rib cage. It's this intermittent sharp, stabbing pain and it's gotten to the point that I just can't stand it. I can't sleep at night because of it and then I have a hard time keeping up at work and my boss is getting irritated with me.	Patient: Sharp.
15		
16		
17		
18		
19	Nurse: Tell me a little more about what you do?	Nurse: Does it radiate down your leg?
20	Patient: I work on a road crew installing concrete barriers.	Patient: Yes.
21		
22	Nurse: That sounds like it's pretty physically difficult …<drifts off to give the patient space for more narrative<	Nurse: Okay, I'm going to order a few tests to see what's happening and we'll go from there.
23		
24	Patient: Yeah, it is. We have lifts and other equipment, but in the end, sometimes you have to just put your back into it. I don't know how much longer I'll be able to do that.	Patient: Okay.
25		
26		
27		
28	Nurse: Hmm …it sounds like, in addition to the pain itself, you're worried about how this might affect your job?	
29		
30	Patient: Definitely. It's all I've ever done and I have to earn a living, you know?	
31		
32	Nurse: Sure … That must be very stressful. At this point, I'd like to do a couple of tests so we can see what's going on, is that okay?	
33		

There are many other important skills involved in interviewing patients. You will notice, for example, that at the end of the dialogue on the left in Table 9.2, the nurse offers supporting statements to the patient and uses "we" language to signal that they are a team working together on the problem (i.e., the patient's pain). Elaborating these many skills is beyond our focus here,[4] which concerns ways to bridge the gaps between the providers' understanding of disease and the patient's experience of illness. We began that discussion in Chapter 8, but in this chapter have identified a variety of potentially confounding factors. Narrative interviewing and the use of open-ended questions represent useful techniques to account for and respond to the social forces and experiential differences that can be problematic for clinical communication.

Moreover, learning these skills is not easy and isn't solely accomplished by reading about them in a book. From a resource like this, one can learn what these skills entail and why they are important, but learning how to utilize them is fundamentally a matter of practice. We liken it to learning to play an instrument. Striking the right notes is initially a tortured and stilted process where one has to think very consciously about finger positioning and which strings or keys to strike at which particular moments. But over time, we internalize the notes and rhythm of a musical piece and playing it becomes an embodied action that simply flows naturally from the performer. Interviewing patients works much the same way. The various skills and techniques are initially artificial and forced, but over time become a natural part of your habits of interaction.

Conclusion

The problems of communication highlighted in this chapter often have at their core a social distance creating discomfort between patient and provider. Often this can result from differences in race, gender, age, and the like. But no matter what the reason, a theme that emerges clearly from the literature is that discomfort is the enemy of good communication. Jeffrey Michael Clair's (1990) work on physician communication with patients at the end of life makes incredibly clear that practitioners are human beings whose social behaviors, even in the context of their professional work, are not immune to complicating and disruptive social forces and pressures. In Clair's (1990) seminal communication research, he finds physicians struggling to communicate well with terminally ill patients. They appear to feel out of control, somewhat defeated by the reality that, despite their best efforts, their patient is dying. In response to feeling a lack of control as they watch this process, they begin to utilize a variety of discursive strategies in which they unconsciously assert power and authority, to the detriment of their relationships with their patients (see also Wasserman 2014). Practitioners are not comfortable with death. That is generally a good thing; nearly the entirety of health care is designed to avoid it. But like other forms of discomfort that we have addressed in this chapter, this can negatively affect their ability to develop or maintain strong, trusting relationships with their patients.

[4] We recommend several resources that cover interviewing skills in far greater depth, including Cole and Bird (2014); Higgs et al. (2012); and Smith (1996).

There are many unique models of interaction and specific communication strategies relevant to various clinical situations. At the core of most of them, however, is being able to understand the patient's perspective and to work from within that perspective, and bring a diverse biomedical and humanistic skill-set with you. In this chapter we have focused on the ability to do just that, and offer a starting point for some communication strategies that are consistent with building a collaborative clinician–patient relationship. Except in certain cases (e.g., emergencies, trauma, etc.), the ability to take on the perspective of the patient and collaborate alongside them (on particular treatment plans and on broader health care goals) lies at the core of so many other more specific communication strategies that you can and should explore in much greater depth (including many of the resources we have referenced in this chapter).

Take, for example, the popular communication technique of Motivational Interviewing (see Miller & Rollnick 2013). This is a communication strategy designed to promote behavior change, an objective of particular importance today, when health behavior and lifestyles are among the most powerful predictors of chronic disease (see Chapter 6). Motivational interviewing emerged out of addiction treatment contexts with the idea that for significant lasting change to truly occur, the person/patient in question had to be ready to undertake that change themselves. Talking to an addict about abstaining from substance use when they do not believe they have an addiction problem, for example, is unlikely to encourage any meaningful change. In that case, the practitioners might direct a more meaningful conversation toward helping the client/patient uncover the problems that substance use has caused for them, which may engender recognition that they do indeed have a problem. This is sometimes referred to as "meeting the client where they are at."

Similarly, clinical practitioners should provide counseling about diet and exercise as part of delivering preventative medicine that helps not only to manage illness, but also to delay its onset or perhaps prevent it altogether. But, clinicians must "meet the patient where they are at" as well. Discussing the kind or amount of exercise required may be misplaced if a patient is not currently even contemplating increasing their physical activity (Rosen 2000).[5] In that case, a more effective conversation will revolve around stimulating the idea of exercise, not planning it out. Tailoring messages to the attitude and perspective of the person to whom you are speaking is one important component of this insight (Prochaska et al. 1992, 2008a). But motivational interviewing goes further, in that the practitioner assumes a role of facilitating ideas and change strategies that emerge from the patients themselves, rather than taking on the more traditional and authoritative

---

[5] In understanding where a patient is "at" with respect to behavior change, practitioners sometimes utilize what is called the "Transtheoretical" or "Stage of Change" model. This model suggests there are five general stages involved in changing a habit or practice: Precontemplation, Contemplation, Preparation, Action, and Maintenance (Rosen 2000). One would interact differently with someone who is at one stage than someone at another. For example, a person who is contemplating a dietary change may be ready for general information about healthy and unhealthy dietary practices, whereas someone who is preparing may be ready for help planning an actual menu and shopping list. As we discussed in Chapter 8 with the stages of grief, Rosen (2000) importantly cautions based on a large meta-analysis of interventions using the Transtheoretical Model, that the ordering and experience of these stages is variable such that while they have heuristic value, they are not absolute.

role of giving instruction. Of course, in order to do this, you must possess the core skills and dispositions to enable you to understand the patient and their perspective. In general, though perhaps this is rather obvious, any patient-centered communication strategy, no matter the variety or specific intention, must begin with being able to take on the role and perspective of the patient (see discussion of *verstehen* in Chapter 8), an integral element of the sociological imagination.

CHAPTER 9 ACTIVITY

Eliciting Patient Narrative: Role-play Activities

For the following scenarios, play the role of the practitioner while a friend or classmate plays the role of the patient. The scenarios each have a basic premise, but the person playing the patient will need to fill in details. The more creative they can be in the role, and the more details they can add to the backstory of the patient, the better these will turn out. As the practitioner, you should employ the best practices for provider–patient communication that we have discussed in the preceding chapter.

Remember to start with open-ended questions and try not to miss *empathic opportunities* (Avdi et al. 2008). *The goal here is **not** to diagnose the problem.* Rather, you should view this as a practice for the first four to seven minutes of the patient encounter, and your goal is to elicit as much narrative from the patient as you can. In other parts of your professional training you will learn more about the details of taking a history and physical, making a differential diagnosis, and so on. Here, your goal is to elicit as much of the patient's *story* as possible (i.e., social and psychological information). After finishing each role-play, work through reflection questions below. If you have the ability to film yourself and review the video, we highly recommend doing so.

You will notice that these situations are relatively simplistic. This is to allow the patient narrative to develop organically as the practitioner elicits it. This also means that you should feel free to make up your own scenarios. Some people find it easier to use experiences they have had themselves as the basis for the role-play. Additionally, many students find it easier to ask open-ended questions as the practitioner, when they have no information about the patient in the first place.

Situation 1

Patient: You are a 28-year-old married parent of three children. You have come to the clinic today because you've had several migraine headaches over the last two weeks. While you've had them intermittently since you were 16 years old, you are very worried because they seem to be getting more frequent and intense. (Add in more details of your life as needed.)

Practitioner: Your job is to conduct an interview in which you elicit as much narrative from the patient as possible and to acknowledge and legitimize his or her feelings and emotions.

Situation 2

Patient: You are a 17-year-old, all-county lacrosse athlete. During a game last night you got tangled up with an opponent and heard a loud pop. Your knee was swollen afterward and there's some pain, but you can still walk on it. You have come into the clinic to figure out exactly what type of injury you have. You're worried that you might not be able to compete in your senior season. (Add in more details of your life as needed.)

Practitioner: Your job is to conduct an interview in which you elicit as much narrative from the patient as possible and to acknowledge and legitimize his or her feelings and emotions.

Situation 3

Patient: You are a single parent of two children and have come into the clinic because you're having severe abdominal pain and have been feeling weak for the last two months. You also feel like your lower abdomen is distended. Your mother died of intestinal cancer four years ago, and you've delayed getting medical care for fear that you might have it too. (Add in more details of your life as needed.)

Practitioner: Your job is to conduct an interview in which you elicit as much narrative from the patient as possible and to acknowledge and legitimize his or her feelings and emotions.

Situation 4

Patient: You are a 74-year-old ex-factory worker presenting to the clinic for chronic coughing that has been going on for four months. In the last three weeks, you notice that you've been short of breath. You smoked for thirty years, but quit when your first granddaughter was born, when you were 69 years old. You're worried that you have lung cancer and won't live long enough to see your granddaughter graduate from kindergarten. (Add in more details of your life as needed.)

Practitioner: Your job is to conduct an interview in which you elicit as much narrative from the patient as possible and to acknowledge and legitimize his or her feelings and emotions.

Discussion Questions

After each role-play activity, spend some time considering the following questions:

1. Examine and discuss what you did well? (E.g., asking open-ended questions, using minimal encouragers to facilitate more narrative, etc.)

2. What do you need to work on for next time? (E.g., did you ask leading questions, interrupt the patient, miss opportunities to empathize with the patient, etc.?)

3. What did you learn about the patient's social life that might later affect either your diagnosis or treatment plan(s)?

4. What is the patient experiencing emotionally? How might this affect their treatment?

Health Professions and Interprofessional Teamwork

LEARNING OBJECTIVES

After reading this chapter, students should be able to

- Articulate how interprofessional teamwork is becoming more complex, challenging, and necessary as a result of shifts in the social landscape of health professions.

- Identify the characteristics of a profession and discuss the ways in which professionalization is expanding and contracting in different fields and disciplines.

- Discuss the challenges of interprofessional teamwork that stem from different professional and social identities.

- Describe various strategies for promoting positive interprofessional collaboration.

- Discuss types of medical error and reduction strategies, particularly from a systems perspective, highlighting the purpose facilitating a "just culture" in health care institutions.

- Characterize the fluidity of interprofessional teams, especially when accounting for the patient and family as team members.

Introduction: Specialization and Complexity

We have described the complexity of the health and health care landscape in several previous chapters. Not only are diseases themselves more complex, but the vast number of diagnostic tools and high-tech interventions leave the patient at the center of a swirling number of professionals, attendants, trainees, and technicians, each with a different role to play in complex care processes (see also Chapters 2 and 9). Writing of how mistakes, oversights, and suboptimal care emerge from the chaos and complexity of this system, Atul Gawande (2011) notes, "It's like no one's in charge—because no one is. The public's experience is that we have amazing clinicians and technologies but little consistent sense that they come together to provide an actual system of care, from start to finish, for people. We train, hire, and pay doctors to be cowboys. But it's pit crews people need." While Gawande was addressing physicians in particular,[1] his observations are similarly important

---

[1] The referenced *New Yorker* article originated as a commencement address to graduates of Harvard Medical School.

for other health care providers. Indeed, the educational accreditation bodies for a variety of health care professions require training in interprofessional teamwork. The complexity of the health care process today requires collaboration among a variety of specialists from multiple professions in order to provide the best possible care for patients. But effective collaboration across different disciplines, and even across subspecialties within disciplines, is not always easy to achieve.

In addition to the increasing complexity of health and disease, the growing demand for interprofessional teamwork also results from basic sociological processes of specialization that give birth to intricate divisions of labor in society. Emile Durkheim (1933 [1997]) classically articulated how the birth of economic systems emerged from basic environmental conditions. When populations grew, so too did the demand for more goods (e.g., food, clothes, etc.). In other words, specialization emerged from necessity as a more efficient means of production. For example, those with particular talents for farming might focus on agriculture, while those with talents for building shelters might focus their efforts on construction. While more efficient, this also introduces new problems, because when people specialize in their work, they no longer produce everything they need all on their own. Builders cannot eat their houses and farmers cannot live in their crops. As a result, individuals need one another to survive, and they trade the fruits of their own labor for things they need but do not produce on their own. As the demand for more goods and services grows and grows, work becomes more and more specialized. But this also means that individuals increasingly produce a smaller portion of the total goods they need and therefore have to exchange more often, and with more partners, to get the things they need. These processes illustrate, in a general way, how different occupations come into existence and how the landscape of occupations becomes more and more complex. In fact, health care professions have undergone similar processes of differentiation and specialization, and are therefore presented with the same challenges of coordination and cooperation that attend highly specialized, complex, interactive economic systems.

In the past, physicians practiced medicine in relative isolation. That is, an individual physician conducted the diagnostic and treatment work associated with caring for the patient. They often were assisted by nurses who attended largely to the convalescent needs of the patient, or with support staff who handled ancillary affairs associated with running a practice, but the single attending physician most often made all of the decisions about care alone. But as the technological capacities of medical practice grew, both in diagnostic and therapeutic terms, patient demand for more treatments for more conditions grew, as did the ability of physicians to provide them. Increasing demand for a much larger range of services, however, necessitated greater efficiency through specialization. Put simply, no one physician could know *everything*. And as these demands continued to grow—as more tests, treatments, and drugs emerged to treat more and more illnesses—the degree to which medical practitioners had to specialize correspondingly increased. But as each individual practitioner was providing care that covered a smaller and smaller proportion of the total care that the profession as a whole needed to provide, the practitioner faced a growing tacit obligation to coordinate care with other practitioners.

Today, professional medicine is so highly specialized that entire domains of its practice have opened up to other professions (see Budrys 2005). Nurse practitioners and physician assistants, for example, increasingly provide primary care services that were formerly the exclusive domain of physicians. Other areas of clinical care have branched out into stand-alone occupations or burgeoning professions, such as respiratory therapy and physical therapy. While some argue that physicians should rediscover a greater focus on primary care, this is unlikely to ever represent a complete solution to the complexity of an interprofessional landscape. Specialization arguably was less a "bad choice" on the part of professional medicine, and more the natural result of its growing capacities to treat disease. Since that landscape will only expand and become more complex (see Chapter 2), specialization appears inevitable now and into the future. What is needed then is a greater capacity for collaboration across professions and subspecialties. In this chapter, we describe the nature of professions themselves, and highlight a number of pressing challenges confronting interprofessional collaboration. We then articulate several best practices that are fundamental to establishing positive interprofessional interactions, and identify some common models of collaboration that draw in different ways on these core practices. The chapter concludes by exploring the inherent fluidity of the roles and identities that coalesce on health care teams, particularly exploring the role of patients and their families as team members.

Professions in Transition

While people often use the term *profession* loosely in everyday life, from a sociological perspective a profession is a very particular kind of work. Goode (1957:194) identified eight characteristics of a "community of professions." As you read these, think about the extent to which they apply to various health professions:

1. Its members are bound by a sense of identity.
2. Once in it, few leave, so that it is a terminal or continuing status for the most part.
3. Its members share values in common.
4. Its role definitions vis-à-vis both members and nonmembers are agreed upon and are the same for all members.
5. Within the areas of communal action there is a common language, which is only partially understood by outsiders.
6. The Community has power over its members.
7. Its limits are reasonably clear, though they are not physical and geographical, but social.
8. Though it does not produce the next generation biologically, it does so socially through its control over the selection of professional trainees, and through its training processes it sends these recruits through an adult socialization process.

Others add that professions inherently possess a service component and that professional societies are granted autonomy to set the standards for their field and to select and vet their members (Reed & Evans 1987). Additionally, professional practices are legally protected; for example, unlicensed individuals can be prosecuted for practicing medicine. However, these socially granted freedoms and protections come with a reciprocal obligation for professions to serve society in some way. As Reed and Evans (1987:3279) note, medicine, like other professions, is distinguished in part by a "service orientation [that] supersedes the proprietary interests of the professionals." Physicians are, for example, expected to put the health of their patients before traditional economic concerns about profitability. The *quid pro quo* arrangements between professions and society have often been described as a *social contract*. This concept was articulated in political philosophy in the 1600s, but has been applied to professions, especially medicine, to highlight the reciprocal obligations that society and those professions have with each other. Cruess (2006) provides a useful summary of the reciprocal expectations between society and professional medicine (see Table 10.1).

In the various criteria above we see a number of ways that professions are distinguished from other types of work. Many jobs, even those that are high paying, involve isolated individuals performing particular functions in exchange for pay. While these forms of work are no less valuable and may still be prestigious, they are not bound together by the characteristics of a professional community. We can characterize various health professional groups as small societies of individuals with a shared culture, though to greater and lesser extents depending where a particular field sits with respect to its professional development.

Physicians historically represent the most professionalized group of health providers, and in the past other practitioners were expected simply to follow their orders. But today we see new professional fields with greater degrees of independence and autonomy emerging in health care delivery, including the growing professionalization of nursing. Moreover, these shifts are occurring alongside what has been referred to as the *deprofessionalization* of medicine (Ritzer & Walczak 1988). These transitions complicate various elements of interprofessional teamwork because they subvert traditional hierarchies that in the past largely obviated the

TABLE 10.1 Social Contract between Medicine and Society

Society's Expectations of Medicine	Medicine's Expectations of Society
• Services of the healer	• Trust
• Assured competence	• Autonomy
• Altruistic service	• Self-regulation
• Morality and integrity	• Health care system
• Accountability	- Value-driven
• Transparency	- Adequately funded
• Source of objective advice	• Participation in public policy
• Promotion of the public good	• Shared (patients and society) responsibility for health
	• Monopoly
	• Status and rewards
	- Nonfinancial
	• Respect
	• Status
	- Financial

Source: Cruess, Sylvia R. (2006). "Professionalism and Medicine's Social Contract with Society." *Clinical Orthopaedics and Related Research* 449, 170–76.

need to develop more democratic procedures for working interprofessionally. To better understand these hierarchies and their broader historical contexts, we next describe the processes of professionalization and subsequent deprofessionalization in medicine, the latter of which effectively sets the stage for other professional groups to emerge in contemporary health care delivery.

The Emergence of Professional Medicine

Prior to the discovery of the germ, the landscape of healing was diverse and pluralistic (Kaptchuk & Eisenberg 2001). That is, there were many varieties of medical practice, with allopathic medicine being just one. *Allopathic* or *regular* practitioners often restricted their practices to the wealthy, and their methods (which included bleeding, purging, blistering, and the like) created a general wariness of physicians. Folk and other *irregular* practitioners therefore played a significant role in the diverse landscape of medical practice. Duffy (1993:80) notes that, "how much care was provided [by irregular and folk practitioners] is difficult to say, but it may well have exceeded that given by orthodox practitioners." Thomsonians, homeopaths, hydropaths, and botanical practitioners all utilized different practices that tended to be much less aggressive than the methods employed by allopathic physicians. These practitioners, particularly the Thomsonians, also often emphasized the ability of ordinary people to practice medicine on themselves. As a result, these traditions were particularly popular in the American colonies where a spirit of Jacksonian individualism resonated with the populist tendencies of many of these traditions (Flannery 2002). But ultimately this pluralism was made possible by the relatively ineffective nature of medicine at the time. None of these various traditions could promise much in terms of curing disease and therefore, each possessed as much of a legitimate claim to the practice of effective doctoring as any other. Paul Starr (1982:100), writes that, "Many saw diversity in medical practice as a counterpart to religious differences," highlighting how in the absence of conclusive scientific evidence validating the practices of any particular tradition, much was left to faith and preference.

This all changed, of course, with the discovery of the germ, because medicine gained, for the first time in history, the ability to reliably cure a range of diseases. The ability to cure was a valuable commodity that upended the pluralism of medical practice. Allopathic physicians moved to organize the profession in a way that excluded irregular practitioners and eventually limited their practices so severely that they eventually were largely left out of medicine altogether. These alternative practitioners (including homeopaths) remain largely at the periphery of health care today, though some exceptions (such as chiropractors) were more successful in establishing and protecting claims to their own professional terrain. Notably, even fields ultimately able to successfully coexist and even compete with allopathic medicine did so by largely accepting the general paradigm of medical practice and finding a niche within it (e.g., early osteopathy; Hinote & Wasserman 2012).

In some ways, these professional shifts naturally resulted from scientific advances and the emerging demands of patients in the health marketplace. But they also resulted from intentional sociopolitical movements. By organizing professional societies and developing their own training accreditation, allopathic physicians limited or actively prohibited involvement of (and collaboration with) other practitioners. In some cases, for example, allopaths were explicitly prohibited from consulting with homeopaths (Starr 1982). In fact, the American Medical Association (AMA), as medicine's earliest professional society, served as an effective barricade between orthodoxy and the irregulars at this time. Its antisectarian consultation clause and Committee on Quackery internally policed the profession for collaboration with outsiders (Kaptchuk & Eisenberg 2001). The contours of doctoring as we know it today resulted from just these kinds of boundaries—that is, from this process of *professionalization*.

If we look back at Goode's (1957) delineation of features of a profession, we see that they characterize the profession of medicine quite well. Physicians clearly share core values that are formally articulated in a variety of professional oaths (e.g., the Hippocratic Oath and the Oath of Geneva). Moreover, physicians control particular areas of practice like diagnosing disease and creating treatment plans, and these roles distinguish them from nonphysician health care providers (although arguably less today than in the past, as we will see below). Moreover, the community of physicians has the power to set practice and licensure standards through its professional bodies, giving it power over its present and future members. Similarly, while faculty from many disciplines participate in medical education (particularly in the first two years), it is primarily other physicians that set core competencies and establish content areas covered on gateway exams. Along with establishing admissions criteria to medical schools, this gives the profession of medicine control over the selection of future doctors and of the training processes themselves. Throughout training, medical students not only learn medical knowledge in the classroom, but also learn about the culture of medicine with clinical mentors and through the *hidden curriculum*, in which the unwritten rules and norms of the profession are modeled by more senior practitioners (Hafferty & Franks 1994). Finally, there certainly is a shared sense of culture and identity among physicians, which is perhaps best illustrated through the language of case presentation (Anspach 1988) and *medical slang*, which serves to create a "private means of communication" among professionals (Coombs et al. 1993:995).

The Deprofessionalization of Medicine

The development of doctoring as a profession emerged from historical conditions whereby the commodity of medical treatment became effective and sophisticated enough to require specialized training and expertise. Society therefore granted the rights and protections needed to govern that terrain to expert-physicians. But emerging conditions around the 1970s served to contract the professional autonomy of physicians in various ways (see also Chapter 2). Just as the emergence of doctoring as a profession can inform other emerging and developing health professions, the deprofessionalization of doctoring can inform other fields about potential challenges and transitions that may come later (Hinote & Wasserman 2012).

Perhaps one of the biggest changes signaling a contraction in the physician profession concerns the movement away from self-employment in private practices. Historically, the common model for medical practices cast physicians as entrepreneur-owners. Increasingly, however, physicians find it difficult to economically sustain smaller private practices and therefore secure employment within larger corporate hospital systems. Kane (2015:1) describes some of these trends:

> there has been a marked decrease in the percentage of physicians who are owners of their practices, falling from 76.1 percent in 1983 to 50.8 percent in 2014. This is related to the changes in practice size that occurred over that period. In 1983, 79.6 percent of physicians worked in practices with 10 or fewer physicians. In contrast, only 60.7 percent worked in practices of that size in 2014. Solo practice itself fell from more than 40 percent of physicians in 1983 to less than 20 percent in 2014.

There are a number of reasons for these shifts. The costs of private medical practice often can be prohibitive, particularly where new technologies are continually emerging. Additionally, bringing together larger groups of practitioners can help mitigate the considerable expense of malpractice insurance. Reimbursement for services also must be negotiated with insurance companies, which may be a burdensome process for an independent practice, whereas larger hospital systems can dedicate staff to those sorts of tasks and leverage their volume of care to get better deals. Smaller practices might struggle with maintaining the army of clerical staff often required to navigate the hundreds of insurance plans (along with the requisite workflows, procedures, and processes of each class of plan) operating in the United States. While generally (and perhaps accurately) portrayed as a negative shift toward decreased power, prestige, and autonomy, some physicians point out that employment within larger systems has benefits, including the ability to off-load work tasks on the periphery of patient care (e.g., administrative support, reimbursement, payroll, etc.) to support staff, and to redistribute the work associated with a large population of patients among several colleagues in the same geographic and specialist area of practice. Despite these conveniences, however, the deprofessionalization of doctoring has raised concerns (Ritzer & Walczak 1988).

Physicians' employment in the larger structure of corporate health systems has given rise to new evaluations of their work beyond simply whether they successfully help their patients, and an emphasis on efficiency and profit. "Relative Value Units (RVUs)," for example, attempt to measure the amount of time and training required for any given medical service provided (Midkiff & Cordaro 2012). Physician Work RVUs are used to quantify a physician's service and weigh it against various expenses. Physician RVUs also are used in many places to determine bonus pay, merit raises, and the like. This sort of performance evaluation, however, contradicts some basic premises of professional work. In particular, service and altruism are expected to supersede concerns about profitability in a profession. However, in an RVU or similar model of evaluation, the value on efficient productivity arguably encourages less time spent on nonbillable conversations with patients, which often includes attending to broader social–psychological needs that, ironically, are increasingly important in the chronic illness era (see Chapter 2). We discuss health care systems more fully in Chapter 12, but the critical point here is that the contemporary landscape of health care delivery makes private practice more difficult and less attractive to many physicians, who increasingly choose to become employees of larger corporate systems. While there are benefits, many argue that efficiency, profitability, and other concerns definitely run counter to the ideals of medicine as a profession in the fullest sense of the term.

Emerging Professions

Other health care disciplines find themselves at other points along the continuum of professional development. Nursing, for example, arguably emerged as a nascent profession, in some ways, alongside (but largely dependent upon) medicine in the late 1800s. In 1889, for example, at the inauguration of the new nursing school at Johns Hopkins led by Isabel Hampton, the hospital's superintendent Henry M. Hurd notes, "In the eyes of the Trustees, nursing the sick is not to be considered a trade but a learned profession" (quoted in James [1979] 2001:44):

> The speakers' emphasis on the word "profession" is striking, since the question of whether nursing is a profession in any strict sense of the word is still moot today. It is true that the term, then as now, was commonly applied to vocations which, if less exacting and autonomous than medicine, for example, could be considered equally altruistic. Hurd and Hampton could simply have been indulging in rhetoric intended to enhance the status of nursing. Nor did the term, in 1889, have today's sociological denotations; medicine itself had not become a profession in the full modern sense.

But the development of nursing as a profession, with regard to the criteria noted above, particularly those related to autonomy of practice, would not develop in the same way as medicine or with the same social protections (Tosh 2007). However, that appears to be changing some today.

Since the publication of James's analysis in 1979, it is clear that nursing has grown even more professional in the strict sociological sense. While a sense of service and altruism has always been inherent to nursing, before the field moved to codify, coordinate, and regulate nursing education, one could argue that nursing lacked a specific body of knowledge over which it claimed ownership as well as the autonomy to control its own terrain. Maggs (1993:1313) writes, "In some early nursing textbooks, the first role of the nurse became elevated to a science, the science of hygiene, while the second became translated as learning about scientific medicine in order to carry out orders better." Relatively recently, however, we have witnessed the development of a clear and specialized body of knowledge as well as greater autonomy in nursing practice. Nurses now participate more fully in the core functions of medical care, and nurse practitioners are licensed in many states to operate as solo practitioners who diagnose disease, prescribe treatments, and perform procedures without the oversight of physicians.[2] Still, some states require collaboration agreements between licensed physicians and nurse practitioners, thereby mitigating the latter's autonomous practice.

Even more recently, a sharp increase in the number of physician assistants (PAs) marks an important trend in the health care division of labor. Notably, the average predicted job growth rate for all occupations was 11% and was 20% for all health diagnosing and treating practitioners between 2012 and 2022. However, the U.S. Bureau of Labor Statistics predicted a growth rate of PA positions of 38% during that same time period. As of 2015, all states in the United States require some degree of physician supervision over PA practice, suggesting that the development

---

[2] As of 2014, twenty-four U.S. states allowed nurse practitioners to practice without physician oversight (Gadbois et al. 2014).

of the field with respect to the sociological criteria of professionalization may not be as advanced, particularly on those criteria that relate to autonomy of practice. However, it should be clear that professionalization is always in flux and we will likely witness increasing professionalization of nursing, PAs, and other fields in the future. Indeed, a study by Gadbois et al. (2014:200) finds that:

> most states loosened regulations, granting greater autonomy to nurse practitioners and physician assistants, particularly with respect to prescriptive authority and physician involvement in treatment and diagnosis. Many states also increased barriers to entry, requiring high levels of education before entering practice. Knowledge of state trends in nurse practitioner and physician assistant regulation should inform current efforts to standardize scope-of-practice nationally.

In these findings we can see multiple features of professionalization that are increasing, including (1) the codification of a specialized body of knowledge as evidenced by greater educational requirements, (2) the regulation of access to participation in the profession as evidenced by growing requirements for entry, and (3) the granting of greater autonomy to these professionals as evidenced by the loosening of restrictions on their rights and scopes of practice.

Despite occupying similar positions along the continuum of professionalization, advanced nursing specialties and PAs exhibit very different historical trajectories. PAs, as a relatively recent player in the health care division of labor, reached this point more quickly than nurses, for very specific historical reasons. The history of nursing stretches back nearly two centuries and eventually spawned the nurse practitioner as a specialized professional group. On the other hand, the first PA training program was established in 1965 for medics returning from Vietnam, as a way to transition into the civilian workforce. PA education developed as an expedited subset of medical (i.e., physician) education, designed to train quasi-independent clinicians to work under the loose supervision of physicians. In contrast, nursing education developed alongside and subordinate to medicine, fueled not only by efforts to protect professional terrain, but also by gendered notions of women and work. While more autonomous subspecialties have emerged in nursing education, many nurses still struggle with this historical legacy (i.e., the "handmaiden" image, see Tosh 2007). For many reasons, but primarily due to physicians' control over the work of nurses, nursing was slow to professionalize. Alternatively, medicine directly sponsored early PA professionalization, while forcing nursing to take a different path, thereby delaying the latter's development as a more autonomous group of practitioners (Cockerham & Hinote 2015).

Other fields like respiratory therapy, chiropractic, physical therapy and the like may find themselves at different points in the processes of professionalization, possessing greater or fewer of the qualities that distinguish professions from other occupations, and to greater or lesser degrees. But what remains clear is that all fields in health care are in transition, and that their professional structures can wax and wane within the larger landscape of health and illness, which is also in flux.[3]

---

[3] Coburn (1994) presents a more thorough and interesting analysis of the complexity of "professionalization and proletarianization" among various health professions, illustrating how these social shifts are interconnected.

The complex and dynamic nature of health professions, which we only briefly articulate here, presents a number of challenges for working across interprofessional boundaries. For example, the historical identity of nursing, particularly at the intersection of normative gender roles, is at odds with more contemporary shifts in the nursing terrain. But the views of other providers may be at odds with nursing team members, leading to significant conflict. In the next section we identify these and other challenges before discussing several approaches to promoting better interprofessional collaboration.

Problems within a Complex Professional Landscape

Insofar as health care is a social institution, it almost always manifests dynamics that are reflective of the broader social order. For example, in a gendered or race-stratified society (see Chapter 5), we can expect the same social and economic gradients to exist in one form or another within its social institutions (i.e., the economy, family, politics, etc.). Health care in the United States therefore exhibits various elements of stratification and related social biases, not only for patient care (see Chapter 9), but also within its workforce and divisions of labor. Above, we discussed how evolving and intersecting professional roles make interprofessional teamwork a complicated endeavor. Add to this picture the complicated features of working across age, gender, race/ethnic, and cultural lines, with all of the social complexities and biases that those entail for social interaction, and the challenges of interprofessional teamwork begin to come into full relief.

As with any social institution, race/ethnic, gender, and other sources of bias complicate professional relationships in the workforce. Recall from Chapters 4 and 9 that all of us are socialized within particular family and neighborhood contexts, and we learn the norms associated with our gender, race/ethnicity, and culture. That is, we internalize a particular sense of how to think, act, and make sense of the world. Recall also that society is also heavily stratified by socioeconomic status (SES) and race/ethnicity, such that (with some variation) people of different income levels or from different race/ethnic backgrounds *tend* not to live in the same neighborhoods or attend the same schools. The end result is that we learn to see those who are more like us as normal and typical, and those who are less like us as more abnormal or atypical. In short, because of the highly segregated society in which we are socialized, and because we share many of the same outlooks, dispositions, aspirations, interests, and experiences, we learn to prefer people who are like ourselves.

This manifests in health care not just where patient–provider communication in race- or gender-discordant scenarios results in suboptimal care (see Chapter 9), but also in a number of areas that complicate interprofessional collaboration. For example, within various institutional hierarchies in health care, underrepresented minorities and women report a lack of opportunity for promotion, consideration for leadership roles, and disparities in pay (Tolbert Coombs & King 2005). Foreign medical graduates report especially high rates of discrimination, while gender disparities in health care leadership are similarly striking and persistent. Surveys conducted by the American College of Healthcare Executives between 1990 and 2006 show that the number of women in leadership increased from 11% to only 12% in that time period (Lantz 2008). In 2006, female health care CEO pay was nearly $40,000 less than their male counterparts, even among those women who had not had any interruption in their careers.[4] In another more humorous study of leadership at the fifty American medical schools with the most NIH funding, researchers found that there were more moustaches in academic leadership positions than women (Wehner et al. 2015). That is, highlighting the dramatic disparities, women were outnumbered not only by men in general, but by men with moustaches. Bias perpetuates itself through the ranks of health care workforces because many of us are predisposed through socialization to favor individuals who are more similar to ourselves, something that has been demonstrated in numerous experiments on hiring practices (e.g., Bertrand & Mullainathan 2004; Dovidio & Gaertner 2000).

A lack of diversity at multiple levels of health care creates significant problems in the provision of health care, particularly where patient populations may be significantly different and not well understood by provider populations. Diversity requires we work through our own biases and predispositions, and collaborate with other people who may have different ideas, experiences, values, and habits than we do. To be clear, diversity among interprofessional health care teams can create an incredibly challenging work environment. As many diversity advocates are quick to point out: diversity is hard. It is much easier and more comfortable for us to work with people who already think and act like we do.

At the same time the evidence is clear that diverse teams (those diverse both in terms of professional experience and personal attributes and experiences) consistently outperform homogenous teams, particularly when there are challenging problems to be solved. It is not hard to understand why this is the case. Despite the challenges involved in working with others who may think and act in ways that appear foreign, diverse teams possess broader sets of experiences and ways of thinking to draw on when approaching a problem (see Paige 2007; Phillips 2014). For patient care, imagine that a patient with a particular cultural background is hesitant to agree to a variety of tests being recommended by the treating physician. A diverse health care team is simply, by virtue of simple probability theory, more likely to include someone that is equipped to communicate and build rapport with that patient than a less diverse team (see Vyt 2008). Thus, while diversity in the workforce complicates the process of interprofessional collaboration, it also is critically necessary for improving health care both in terms of patient care and at institutional and policy levels. Achieving diversity in the workforce, however, requires that we actively pursue it as a goal, and consciously work to overcome the social biases that, when unconsidered, create the homogeneity in the workforce that we still see in so many institutions.

From the above description, one might think that optimal health care outcomes are simply the result of greater diversity of opinions, that more diversity is always better. This is true to some extent, but only with a caveat. Diverse *teams* are better. From the patient's perspective, the range of specialties and professions that intermittently and chaotically come and go during the course of their care can be overwhelming. Recall from Chapter 9 that only about 12% of hospital inpatients

[4] A common, though inaccurate, explanation for the pay gap between men and women suggests that women lose earnings when they voluntarily exit the workforce to have and raise children. In many analyses, women that take time off have even greater disparities in pay, but even among those who do not, disparities persist.

could *correctly* name the physician in charge of their care. This highlights another important aspect of diversity and patient care: diverse *teams* are better, but they must function as a team. In fact, a case analysis by Stavert and Lott (2013) suggests that a greater number of specialists involved in a particularly complex and challenging case resulted in worse care, not because of the greater number of perspectives, but because each assumed another was taking the lead in the case, such that no one did. This is called the bystander effect. For our purposes, this highlights that more is not simply better, but that diverse interprofessional teams must coordinate their efforts to provide optimal care. In the next section, we explore some basic considerations of how to do just that.

Best Practices for Interprofessional Teamwork

Calls for interprofessional or interdisciplinary teamwork actually date back at least to the 1940s (Baldwin 1996), but it wasn't until the early 1970s that more structured efforts to conceptualize health care as a team-based practice, and to educate future professionals accordingly, began to take shape. Yet, interprofessional educational activities have remained challenging to implement. After all, programs are designed and coordinated within particular fields, meaning that training in interprofessional collaboration is often an afterthought to rather insular processes of curricular design. As Barr and Coyle (2013:185) point out:

> The barriers to closer collaboration erected during pre-licensure courses are formidable. Each profession engages in a process of "closure" through its own educational system with its own regulations, governance, corpus of knowledge and field of practice ... . Students are socialised into the values of their newfound profession, each with its different culture and its unique ways of thinking and acting ... . Distinctive semantics and discourses, modes of dress, demeanour and norms of behaviour associated with a profession perpetuate professional mores and beliefs.

Medical and nursing curricula, for example, are fundamentally designed and planned in isolation, so that even when the prospects for interprofessional activity are raised, they must fit into a typically inflexible set of curricula. Where cocurricular activities do exist, educators seldom invest sufficient time designing them, and in training students within different programs on best practices for interprofessional interaction. Moreover, since current faculty likely received little interprofessional training themselves, their attitudes toward interprofessional education also may hinder these efforts (Curran et al. 2007). For practitioners then, the difficulties of interprofessional teamwork emerge not only from the ways in which different disciplines coalesce around different identities, norms, and practices (Hall 2005), along with the complexities inherent to diversity more broadly defined, but also from the fact that few are well trained to work together in teams in the first place.

There are many different models of interprofessional teamwork that are making their way into medical education but most share several key characteristics. Vyt (2008:208) describes some of these:

> First of all, a team needs effective leadership from persons who have meeting management skills, and stimulate openness and self-reflection. A team should

consist of team members who complement each other's discipline and who take up complementary roles in the team. They should have knowledge of, and respect for, the competences, roles and contributions of other professionals in the team, without any prejudice or stereotyped perceptions. Effective teams can be characterized also by their search for and the definition of common and clear goals that everybody can agree upon. They have a common framework and working tools that stimulate the sharing of knowledge. Most likely, the administration is organized in such a way that it promotes interdisciplinary storage and consultation of patient records and data files. And finally, skills in communication and conflict management have to be present in every team member.

In this and other models, we can see both the need for diversity (professionally, socially, and personally) and the need for coordination of that diversity so that it can be channeled effectively into patient care. But what also begins to take shape are the more practical matters necessary to good team functioning. These first include leadership because it is the team leader who will spearhead most of the core functions of team organization described below. Leaders need not be the most senior, experienced members of the team, but they should, however, be vested with certain decision-making responsibilities. This is why physicians often take up leadership roles on patient care teams, but it also highlights that in other areas of health care, other practitioners may be well positioned to do the same (e.g., hospital policy committees that affect nursing or social work, for example, likely should to be led by individuals from those areas). As discussed above, other professionals are taking on greater ownership of various health care processes, and in the process are increasingly calling into question the default leadership of physicians in noncritical patient care settings, likely as a result of expanding responsibilities for the core functions of patient care (van Schaik et al. 2014).

The team leaders also should not position themselves as the foremost authority in the group, but rather should coordinate the team such that it can draw on the diverse expertise of its members most effectively. In particular, this requires mitigating the extent to which any one personality on the team is able to dominate discourse and decision-making processes, facilitating insights among the various participants. Research in social psychology has, since the 1950s, demonstrated convincingly that individuals have a tendency to conform to group influences surrounding decision-making, and that group membership itself exerts consistently observable effects on our behavior (e.g., social loafing, peer pressure, group polarization, and groupthink). Classic work by Morton Deutsch and Harold Gerard (1955) pointed out that individuals tend to conform in the face of group pressures, even when not intended to be coercive (such as a majority opinion) out of a desire to be right (informational social influence) and a desire to be liked (normative social influence). Many times, individuals will even subvert their own opinions about physical facts, let alone ambiguous judgments, out of deference to others in a group (see Tajfel 1979). The result is that dominant personalities, or even the unintended social pressures of majorities, can corrupt the judgment of individuals who are, for whatever reason, less secure in their perspectives and opinions. This obligates the team, and particularly the team leader, to manage the social psychology of the group accordingly, particularly by creating a comfortable environment for all team members to voice their concerns, ideas, and perspectives. Actively managing particularly effusive or dominant group members and intentionally soliciting the contributions of less assertive team members may be a necessary part of that process. This will help avoid the deficits introduced by group discourse and help the team capitalize on the diverse talents of its members as they navigate the decision-making process.

Importantly, understanding the team as a small society unto itself, along with the tendencies that emerge in such groups, will help you create and maintain positive interprofessional collaborations. A paradox of Western societies concerns how to promote cohesion and collaboration while at the same time promoting individualism. For health care teams, it is the diversity of individual perspectives and experiences that optimizes teamwork. But at the same time, avoiding the problems of uncoordinated care requires the group to cohere, something seeming antithetical to this individualism. As a result, mutual respect is always at the foundation of good teamwork (Vyt 2008). This may require educating the team about the benefits of coordinated diversity, or even of interprofessional teamwork itself, in order to obviate resentment and conflict when perspectives inevitably differ. That is, if we understand that different perspectives improve our teams, then we can simultaneously value our own individual position, but with enough humility to value the team's decision even when it differs.

Finally, on this foundation of mutual respect, and with an appreciation for diverse opinions spearheaded by the team leader, the communication processes of a team are critical to its success. As we know from Chapter 9, communication is a complicated process, infused with various social biases. Interprofessional communication in health care also can be incredibly complex, particularly where different professions have different training, identities, norms, concerns, and even ways of speaking. Good interprofessional communication has many things in common with best practices for patient-centered communication (Zwarenstein et al. 2007). For example, it is critical for each member of the group to clearly understand other members' roles in the team, just as it is important to clarify one's role to a patient (see Chapter 9).

It is also important for someone, often the team leader, to clarify the issues under consideration. Often, miscommunications and professional conflicts emerge not because there is fundamental values conflict—everyone on the team usually wants to do what is best for a patient—but because there is disagreement or misunderstanding about the facts of a situation or the definition of the problem. Take, for example, a patient who is at the end of life and who has requested that no further aggressive measures be taken to prolong his life. A physician may view this case from a more medicalized, treatment perspective, seeing the primary issue as concerning the transition of goals of care toward palliative measures, consulting with the palliative care team, and so on. However, the nursing staff may approach the situation from the perspective of dealing with a grieving family who has not accepted the inevitable death of their loved one. These standpoints do not necessarily invalidate one another. Rather, the complexity of cases like this means that both are reasonable, and even compassionate. But interprofessional discussions of cases, even relatively ordinary ones like this, can result in conflict when the particulars of the terrain are not well defined. Clarifying that terrain and dedicating time and space to discussing each aspect and incorporating multiple insights and perspectives set the stage for more productive dialogue.

Interprofessional communication also benefits from practices that elicit and respect the views of others on the health care team. Most of these include using "I" language and avoiding judgment of others. For example, imagine that a nurse, concerned about the grieving family of a dying patient described above, responded to a physician on the team by saying, "Well, you don't have to deal with the family, so you don't care about that. What should we do about that?" This not only expresses judgment about the physician's level of concern for a problem that may primarily affect the nursing staff, but it doesn't accomplish much by way of solving the problem itself. Additionally, these sorts of statements might be exacerbated by conflicting professional roles (e.g., if the physician's expectation frames nurses in a more passive role, or if the nurse in this scenario feels underappreciated for her expertise). Moreover, attempting to solve the problem will likely fail, because the question about what to do comes after the insinuation that the physician herself, rather than the family's needs, is the challenge. Instead, the nurse might say, "Because I have a lot of contact with the family, I see their reactions to all of this as particularly problematic. What should we do about that?" In this version, the problem is stated explicitly from the perspective of the nurse, and, moreover, the challenges presented by the family are placed at the center of the discussion. Rather than appearing as a challenge presented by a group member in opposition to other group members, the challenge becomes one that the entire team is asked to engage. This promises to be much more productive.

Finally, developing interprofessional teamwork skills requires a process of self-evaluation and peer feedback. Still popular work by Michaelsen and Schultheiss (1988) offers four criteria for making feedback helpful. In their recommendations they note that feedback should be (1) descriptive rather than evaluative, (2) specific, (3) sincere, and (4) usable. *Descriptive* feedback focuses on what someone did or said and the results of those actions, but without assigning value judgments such as "wrong" or "bad" to him or her. *Specific* feedback utilizes actual behavioral examples of when something occurred, which orients the recipient so that the feedback can be most helpful. Rather than saying, for example, "You tend to dominate the conversation," someone providing specific feedback might say, "When we were talking about Ms. Smith's prognosis last week, I felt like you dominated the conversation." This gives everyone a point of reference and keeps the focus on a behavior rather than a tendency of someone's personality, which can border on judgmental. *Sincere* feedback avoids sugar-coating such that the important message may be lost. A common manifestation of this concerns nesting a constructive critique within a compliment such that the true message can easily be lost. Michaelsen and Schultheiss (1988:109) write:

> we might say, "That's a good idea, but ..." in hopes that the receiver will be receptive to what follows the "but." Unfortunately, doing so creates the impression that things are OK when they really aren't and when the truth comes out (and it almost always will), the receiver: a) often loses confidence in the sender's credibility and, b) sometimes reacts even more negatively because he or she feels they have been misled.

Finally, *usable* feedback focuses on things over which the recipient has control and can therefore change. Saying something like, "It's difficult to understand you with your accent," for example, is unlikely to yield any positive transformations, since an accent is largely out of a person's control. The concepts embodied in these recommendations have become pervasive in medical and allied health education where it concerns giving feedback to students, but these are useful for interprofessional interactions in practice as well.

There are a number of models that are built upon the foundation shared by the best practices described above (Baker et al. 2005). Because particular heuristics for interprofessional teamwork tend to come and go, we focus on the types of best practices common to all of them. Additionally, various models seem to take root in different health care fields so that it is important to focus on the commonalities between them, as a way to bridge the training received by clinical practitioners from different disciplines. For example, the Crew Resource Management (CRM) strategy represents a popular approach in medicine that was adopted from aviation, particularly since the latter has an enviable safety record by comparison. CRM was advocated as an error reduction strategy by the Institute of Medicine (IOM 2000) and the Agency for Healthcare Research and Quality (AHRQ 2003). Its key strategies include *creating and managing a team*, *recognizing adverse situations*, *communication techniques*, and *applying a shared mental model for decision-making*. While each of these entails best practices specific to CRM itself, they also proceed on a foundation of mutual respect, clarity of roles, specification of challenges, and so on (see Baker et al. 2005). Its specific adaptations have been especially popular in emergent or intensive care settings, particularly because it emphasizes team-based strategies most useful in acute decision-making.

Another popular model, managed and disseminated by AHRQ, is called Team Strategies and Tools to Enhance Performance and Patient Safety (TeamSTEPPS 2013). TeamSTEPPS (2013) emphasizes establishing an effective team structure, along with four intrateam functions including *communication*, *leadership*, *situation monitoring*, and *mutual support*. Here again, one can see alignment with our discussion of fundamental best practices above, particularly where we note that diverse teams (i.e., structure) need to be coordinated (i.e., leadership) such that problems are clearly identified (i.e., situation-monitoring) and individuals feel safe in expressing their perspectives and positions (i.e., mutual support). Other models exist as well, and more will be developed in the future to meet the evolving demands of the increasingly complex health care landscape. However, as Goetz Goldberg and colleagues (2013:152) note:

> Team-based practices all exhibit similar cultural characteristics including: shared responsibility, respect for diversity of skills and knowledge of team members, an open environment in which to raise concerns and make suggestions, an emphasis on comprehensive patient care and quality improvement, and team member willingness to take on additional roles and responsibilities.

In the end, what matters for good interprofessional teamwork is that the team brings a variety of perspectives to coordinating their engagement with a particularly task or challenge, so that they can engage in effective dialogue as they search for ways to respond.

Just Culture and Medical Error

In the preceding section, we characterize interprofessional teams as small societies of actors figuring out how to function together in the most optimal way. Of course, these small health care societies are nested in larger organizational systems that represent even larger social systems. The organizational culture within one's professional institution can facilitate or impede the functioning of individual professionals and health care teams. One clear example of this concerns the way institutions approach medical error. While we often think of error as a mistake made by an individual person (and that is indeed a factor involved in many errors), more recent work on medical error, following the lead of the aviation industry, wisely focuses on systemic precursors of medical error. This endeavor to make health care safer has raised awareness about the importance of organizational culture in how professionals function in their roles, and how well they work together within the complex health care system.[5] In this section we highlight common types of medical errors to illustrate the role of organizational culture not only in minimizing error, but in dealing with errors that occur in a just and humanistic fashion, both with respect to the patients to whom the error occurs and the practitioner who causes it.

The IOM issued a landmark report in 2000 on medical error, where, extrapolating the results of multiple studies to the total number of hospital admissions, the data suggest that "at least 44,000 Americans die in hospitals each year as a result of preventable medical errors" (2000:31). This sobering number highlights the need to improve systems to reduce the number of medical errors, many of which result in adverse events that could be prevented. Citing Leape et al. (1993), the IOM report specifies three types of errors. *Diagnostic errors* occur when diagnosis is unreasonably delayed or diagnostic information is overlooked or misinterpreted. *Treatment error* includes mistakes made in selecting or delivering a particular treatment (e.g., giving a patient the wrong medication). *Preventative errors* include the "failure to provide prophylactic treatment" or to follow-up or appropriate monitor a patient (IOM, 2000:36). However, in terms of thinking about preventing error, we must juxtapose its various causes into the different arenas in which error can occur.

Graber and colleagues (2002) articulate a useful typology of diagnostic error, by distinguishing *no-fault errors* from *system errors*, and *cognitive errors*. In short, some medical errors are inevitable (e.g., a disease may have very unusual or difficult-to-detect symptoms that delay diagnosis), while others result from problems within health care systems, or because the practitioners involved either lack knowledge or fail to utilize it properly in providing care (e.g., mental mistakes). For a particular institution, preventing no-fault errors appears nearly impossible because they largely emerge from the broader limitations of medical science. Intervening upon cognitive errors is somewhat more promising, because practitioners can improve

---

[5] Also, medical error is an example of how, despite the partitions we make in this book, the nature of health care and the social and psychological factors one must utilize within it are seamlessly woven together. Medical error highlights the interdependent nature of health care systems, various professionals, human judgment and ethical decision-making, and interpersonal communication.

their knowledge and work habits in ways that make them more mindful and less error-prone, but ultimately any human endeavor will witness some degree of error. Medical errors that result from the suboptimal functioning of a system, however, represent an area where intervention can be most successful (Graber et al. 2002).

Human error has been further specified into three types, which require different approaches to remediation. Following Reason's (1990) broader framework for understanding human error, David Marx (2009) has highlighted the qualitative differences between *inadvertent human medical error*, *at-risk behavior*, and *reckless behavior* (see also Boysen 2013). At-risk behavior constitutes a behavior where one knowingly deviates from a protocol, but has a genuine belief that such behavior does not put others at greater risk, or they genuinely believe the increased risk is justified. Reckless behavior constitutes a conscious disregard for safety (Marx 2009).

Each type of human error articulated above is best approached with a different strategy. Rates of inadvertent human error may be modifiable through training and systems improvements, but because some degree is inevitable, focus should be on consoling those involved (Marx 2009). After all, practitioners usually feel incredible amounts of remorse and guilt when they make a mistake causing an adverse event for a patient. At-risk behavior, insofar as it constitutes a conscious choice, but without full recognition of the corresponding risk, entails coaching the practitioner, especially making sure they become aware of the potential dangers of a particular behavior. Reckless behavior, however, because it is engaged in consciously, likely is, "grounds for disciplinary action, and civil or criminal charges may be filed against the individual" (Boysen 2013:405).

Generally speaking, and echoing our discussion of health disparities from earlier chapters, error reduction strategies that focus on modifiable features of health care delivery tend to be the most successful (Singh et al. 2006). Put another way, rather than being focused on individual behavior, which easily becomes an environment of blaming individual practitioners, questions about preventing medical error are best framed as "What can we (as an organization) do better?" Importantly, except in cases of callous disregard for safety (i.e., reckless behavior), punishing individuals for making mistakes actually impedes the goal of improving safety because it does nothing to alter the modifiable factors that preceded the error. Moreover, an organizational culture that punishes inadvertent mistakes or even those made in "good faith" (i.e., at-risk behaviors) suppresses the willingness of practitioners to report errors. Less reporting means less knowledge about how well a system is performing and less ability to make it better. Additionally, coaching individuals may improve their performance, particularly if an error is the result of lack of knowledge or skill that can be gained through education and training. But the inevitability of human error suggests that the most effective error reduction strategies are those that minimize the opportunities for such mistakes.

Forcing functions, for example, constitute a systems change that precludes individuals from making an erroneous choice in the first place. A classic example from health care concerns the anesthesia machine that delivers both oxygen and anesthetic gasses to patients. In the past, hanging the wrong gas cylinder in the wrong yoke would result in delivery of the wrong gas to the patient, a potentially deadly mistake (Eisenkroft 2008). As a result, a pin index system was created such that, each gas has a specific pin configuration and cannot therefore be inserted into the wrong hanger yoke (unless pins are broken or missing). This circumvents the potential error that could result from human judgment and has promoted a significant reduction in adverse events. Simply addressing errors idiosyncratically when they occur has limited effect (Khatri et al. 2009), while a focus on how to improve systems rather than punish individuals (except under specific sets of circumstances) emerges from a broader institutional orientation toward performance.

Promoting a *just culture* across an institution is an important means for reducing error, optimizing professional and interprofessional collaboration, and ultimately improving patient care. In contrast to the *blame culture* that they argue permeated health care for many decades, Khatri et al. (2009:315) define a just culture (or a *culture of psychological safety*) as a "supportive work unit in which members believe that they can question existing practices, express concerns or dissent, and admit mistakes without suffering ridicule or punishment." While fear of blame and punishment can suppress error reporting, a just culture encourages it as part of a quality improvement process. While best done broadly across an institution itself, just culture best practices can be informative and lead to quality improvement at any level of health care, including within departments or among specific interprofessional care teams. In doing so, it is important to recognize that persistent fear of blame and punishment, as well as concerns about the potential of error reporting to increase the administrative regulation of practitioners, can function as barriers to the implementation of just culture practices (Waring 2005).

Just culture practices are critical to health care systems (at the institutional level) and health care teams (at the clinical level). Not only does a culture of psychological safety promote error reporting and lead to quality improvement, but it also holds the potential to reduce stress and burnout in practitioners (Iedema et al. 2006). One also might argue that creating such a climate is an imperative of professional ethics, particularly since the probability of disclosing errors to patients is significantly increased in a just culture climate (Fein et al. 2014). When preventable adverse events occur, patients want to know "what happened, why the error happened, how the error's consequences will be mitigated, and how recurrences will be prevented" (Gallagher et al. 2003:1001). Moreover, in the shifting landscape of the health professions, responsibility for disclosing errors is increasingly delegated to different health care providers. While formerly the exclusive domain of physicians, recent studies show that nurses want to be involved in discussions of medical error and disclosure to patients (Shannon et al. 2009). When nurses or other team members are not included in such discussions, it can place them in a difficult, sometimes ethically compromised, position as they continue to care for patients after the error has occurred. Policies that promote a safe environment in which these issues can be raised, discussed, and addressed are critical to creating not only the best functioning systems, but also health interprofessional collaborations.

Conclusion: Beyond Checklists

While any number of teamwork models may be helpful for codifying the basic processes inherent to interprofessional collaboration, all of them require a basic understanding of how groups of people with various individual roles function. That is, all articulated models of interprofessional teamwork rest on basic psychological and sociological understandings of how individuals bring diverse, professional, personal, and social identities to bear on a particular event. This includes being cognizant of the ways in which those different perspectives and identities, both personal and historical, can disrupt positive collaborations between health care practitioners. While there are some common best practices for promoting good, effective collaboration between clinical practitioners from various disciplines, in the end, diverse groups of individuals will defy the rigidity of all prefabricated models. Instead, practitioners need to be prepared to utilize good collaborative methodologies, such as those briefly described above, in order to harmonize the variety of social, personal, and professional identities that comprise any given team.

Of course, part of the goal of the bureaucratization of health care is to mitigate the complexity of collaboration between individuals, by instead focusing on collaboration between role-actors. One core feature of bureaucracies, including those in health care, centers on replacing individuals, who are complex and have a variety of personal idiosyncrasies, with well-defined roles, such that anyone who is appropriately trained can fill a given role and the rest of us know what to expect from them (see Weber [1922] 1978). The idea is that if, for example, one understands the role of the social worker on the health care team, then which individual is filling that role becomes decidedly less important than the performance of the role functions themselves. More simply, individuals in bureaucracies are expected to function as agents of their professional roles.

However, this is neither possible nor desirable in contemporary health care settings, where complexity pervades across multiple domains of practice and patient care. The origins of disease may be very different for similar diagnoses, and patients might experience and evaluate those illnesses differently in the context of their individual private lives. To be sure, the provision of health care today involves a great deal of judgment in the midst of uncertainty. In complex situations, personal values, preferences, and perspectives matter so much that we often retreat into these entrenched ways of seeing the world when we encounter perplexing uncertainty. The bureaucratic model presumes that the goals of the actors in an institution are clearly defined and measurable, but the most challenging situations in health care defy this assumption. Think again about an end-of-life example where a patient or their proxy must decide whether to pursue further aggressive treatments in attempt to prolong life, or transition the goals of care toward comfort and palliation. There often is no definitively "correct" answer to these sorts of conundrums, and these more complex challenges are growing more and more common. Rather, the diverse and often-contradictory opinions of the health care team are critical for producing the best judgments in these fields of uncertainty. But this also means that it is impossible to disaggregate the roles of practitioners from their personal identities (including their personal perspectives and values). Part of what distinguishes a profession from other occupations is that professions require a greater investment of one's self-identity. The work of professions usually requires conscientious, morally important decisions such that one cannot leave one's *self* aside and merely perform a prefabricated role. In turn, this means that interprofessional teamwork in health care, while it can benefit from codified models of collaborative interaction, will always require attention to the deeper interplay of teams with regard to the individual values and identities of its members.

Finally, despite the rhetoric about the value of patient-centered communication, most models of interprofessional collaboration undervalue the role of the patient and their family as members of the health care team. As noted, in the chronic illness era, patients are more often responsible for a greater share of their own health care. That is, health is something typically managed outside of the clinic, by patients themselves or their families, who have to dispense their medications, manage their treatments, diets, physical activities, and the like. Additionally, when complex decision-making scenarios emerge, for which there are no right answers (e.g., to continue aggressive treatment or shift toward palliative care and hospice), the patient's values matter a great deal in choosing the best course of action. The result is that working with patients and families as members of the team is critical, even though it presents an entirely new layer of complexity.

Patients and their families do not have pre-defined roles for participation, at least not to the same degree as health care providers. In fact, historically, patient roles were defined as particularly passive and nonparticipatory. With the advent of patient autonomy and various efforts to promote shared decision-making, we must now understand patients and families as full-fledged members of the team. They are, if nothing else, experts in their own values and perspectives, and these will significantly affect treatment decisions. How patients and their families participate in the health care team will vary. Some educate themselves and take leadership roles in directing their care. Others outsource care nearly entirely, not just in technical terms (e.g., medication selection and dosing), but also with respect to value-laden decisions such as when to transition toward hospice and palliative care (and these may also vary by relationship, SES, age, race/ethnicity, cultural background, etc.). Thus, working with patients as team members requires adapting basic teamwork methodologies to harmonize with the various roles they might choose on any given day. That is, members should establish and recognize common ground with respect to the situation or challenge the team is facing, the role of the team members including the patient or their family should be clarified (i.e., how do they see themselves and how specifically do they want to be involved), and there should be mutual respect and ample opportunity for discussing everyone's perspectives.

The variety of interprofessional collaboration models certainly are useful in practice. In particular, when adopted at the institutional level, they can provide a common language and training platform that can facilitate improvements in teamwork. At the same time, effective teamwork requires acknowledging the fundamental social–psychological processes that emerge from diverse professional histories, the stratified nature of the societies and groups in which we were socialized, the institutional culture of a practice setting, the individual identities of the team members, and the group behavioral tendencies that commonly emerge during the course of social interaction. By bringing together an understanding of various professions and their historical development, broader social biases that can affect communication, and some best practices for interpersonal communication among team members, clinical practitioners can improve their interprofessional collaboration no matter which specific strategy they utilize.

CHAPTER 10 ACTIVITY

Teamwork and Just Culture: The Case of "Psycho Mike"

Part 1

A male patient who is known around the neighborhood as "Psycho Mike" is brought to the emergency department (ED) early on Friday morning. He presents with severe, uncontrolled bleeding from severe gastritis and esophageal varices (enlarged veins in the lower esophagus that sometimes leak blood and are at risk of rupturing), secondary to alcohol abuse. Mike is well known to the staff in the ED as a "frequent flyer" (someone who presents to the ED often). The ED resident administers a medication called octreotide, which reduces the bleeding, but does not stop it entirely. Mike is admitted to the critical care unit and after a consultation with a radiologist, it is determined that he needs to undergo an endoscopic procedure where bands will be placed to constrict the blood flow from the varices.

Mike is homeless and in the past has been resistant to interventions from various social workers who have tried to connect him with resources and services, but he seems fond of one particular social worker named Tisha, who happened to grow up in the same small town as Mike. When the attending physician and the radiologist tell him that he needs the banding procedure, Mike refuses and says he'll "take his chances on the street." "I got God-love, and God loves me," Mike tells them. When they ask if he understands that he will likely die and very soon without the procedure, Mike tells them, "I'll pray on it, but only God can tell me when I'll die."

The next day at morning rounds, the floor nurse Salwa tells the team that Mike has been belligerent with the night shift, including spitting at one nurse assistant. "I can't tell if he's legitimately religious or just out of his mind ... they probably call him 'Psycho Mike' for a reason," she says. The charge nurse, Mary Ann, replies, "Maybe, but a lot of people in my congregation talk the same way about disease and God's role in life and death. I wouldn't call them crazy."

Discussion Questions

1. How should the team approach Mike and what should their goals be?

2. What strengths can you identify among the various team members and how might they be useful in achieving the goals of care?

Part 2

Because you worked well as a team, utilizing the diverse strengths of each team member, Mike agreed to undergo the banding procedure, which successfully stopped the bleeding from his varices. However, about thirty-six hours later, Mike began running a fever and breathing rapidly. A blood test showed that he had septicemia (systemic inflammation caused by bacteria in the blood). While he was successfully treated with antibiotics, a procedural review at a team meeting the next morning uncovered that the endoscope used in the procedure had not been properly sterilized. The surgical assistant responsible for sterilizing the equipment admitted that she did not complete a leaking test of the endoscope after its previous use because she was very rushed that day. She feels very guilty and begins to cry in the meeting.

Discussion Questions

1. What kind of error is this? Discuss different approaches to preventing this kind of error in the future.

   Helpful Hint: Think about the variety of different approaches that address not only staff behavior, but also systemic processes.

2. How would you classify the behavior of the surgical assistant and how would you respond to her from the standpoint of the principles of *just culture*? How might it change your classification and response if this was a recurring problem?

Bioethics, Social Science, and Clinical Practice

LEARNING OBJECTIVES

After reading this chapter, students should be able to

- Articulate how shifting social contexts and medical advances in concert with key historical events in research and clinical medicine have raised important bioethical questions.

- Identify and define the four principles of bioethics, how are they each related to different forms of ethical reasoning (deontology and consequentialism) or are focused at different levels of scale (individual and social), and apply this framework to clinical cases.

- Identify and define the limitations of the four principles of bioethics, discuss alternative ways of framing ethical situations (e.g., virtue ethics and ethics of care), and apply these alternative ways of thinking about ethics to clinical cases.

- Describe the social and psychological forces that can complicate or confound our ability to think and act ethically in the clinical context.

Introduction

Bioethics is a field that addresses moral concerns in the life sciences, including, or perhaps primarily, in health and medicine. Of course, ethical issues have been discussed since the origins of medical practice itself. For example, the Hippocratic Oath lists a number of moral obligations of physicians. However, bioethics emerged as a field unto itself in the late 1960s, when it began to crystallize around cultural trends toward autonomy that were emerging from civil rights and countercultural movements, in concert with poignant events that galvanized public consciousness around patient rights, as well as technological developments in medicine that, for the first time, gave practitioners the ability to dramatically extend life.

The intersection of bioethics and the social sciences has not always been entirely clear. After all, bioethics discourses emerged primarily from philosophers who were turning their attention toward the issues of health and medicine. They tended to address normative questions more than empirical ones. That is, they tended to focus on articulating theoretically based positions on the rightness or wrongness of various courses of action, such as removing life support or hastening the death of a terminally ill patient. Social scientists, on the other hand, have traditionally limited their inquiries into what *is* happening in the social world, rather than what they believe *ought* to happen.[1] In keeping with this, social scientists working in health and medicine have traditionally relegated their work to describing structures and relationships within that terrain. However, work in bioethics has become increasingly empirical, with more attention being paid to the social contexts in which ethical decisions are made and the social factors that influence those decisions.

While normative discussions of ethical action in health and health care are increasingly incorporating social–psychological contexts, we can also recognize that social science deals with inevitably moral terrain. It is difficult, in fact, to argue that any scientific activity, let alone any social science, is *value free*. After all, inherent in most scientific activity is a drive to solve some kind of human problem. Implicit in that activity, therefore, is a judgment about how things *ought to be*. The connection of social science to moral questions is at the heart of what Mills (1959) referred to as the *promise* of the sociological imagination. Recall from Chapter 1 that the sociological imagination is the ability to understand the connections between social structures and private, individual experiences. However, foreshadowing the role of social science in bioethics, Mills wrote that this capacity was essential in the moral activities of social life as well: "in factual and moral concerns, in literary work and political analysis, the qualities of [the sociological] imagination are regularly demanded" (Mills 1959:14). Indeed, understanding how social and psychological factors influence decision-making among both patients and practitioners, how cultural notions shape public policy around the provision of health care, or how institutional frameworks and professional roles affect patient care, are all social science questions with significant moral weight.

In this chapter, we describe the emergence of bioethics from key events in research and clinical practice that disturbed the public consciousness and disrupted the historically paternalistic practice of medicine. We then review key normative or philosophical frameworks, which may guide ethical decisions in health and medicine. In the next section, however, we discuss how ethical decision-making in practice rarely is organized neatly around particular philosophical commitments, but rather is complicated by the social and psychological features that attend ethics in practice. This will inform our concluding discussion about the *bioethical imagination* (De Vries et al. 2007), the skill of a practitioner to bring an understanding of various social contexts and psychological factors together with normative considerations in the process of coming to an ethical decision.

---

[1] There has long been a recognized divide between *ought* and *is*, most famously articulated by philosopher David Hume (1739 [1978]). Hume argued that one cannot derive *ought* from *is*, meaning that nothing about the way things are tells us anything about their moral character. In the premodern period, moral notions were endemic to the world, that is, concepts of morality were real and lived within the universe. Recall from Chapter 2 that the notion of "man as the measure" is definitive of the modern period. Similarly, in modernity, concepts of morality transformed into something superimposed on the empirical world by human beings.

The Emergence of Bioethics

Issues of moral judgment in health care practice involve decidedly empirical phenomena. For example, changes in prognosis can significantly alter our ethical perspective on a particular case. But the field of bioethics itself also must be understood as having emerged from a particular set of social conditions, punctuated and activated by watershed historical events such as the Tuskegee Syphilis study in the case of research, or the clinical cases of Karen Ann Quinlan and Nancy Cruzan.

Ethics has been a component of medicine since ancient times. Most famously, the Hippocratic Oath delineates "do no harm" as the first ethical obligation of the practitioner. At the same time, ethics does not exist in a vacuum and even where its prescriptions and meanings seem simplistic, they must be understood in a broader social context. This basic ethical precept from the Hippocratic tradition, for example, appears to be a simple proclamation against hurting a patient, a specific extension of a more general moral rule against hurting another individual. However, recall from Chapter 2 that the premodern consciousness was dominated by a sense of the power of nature and the dominance of the larger universal cosmos. In view of the social and cultural ethos of the times, we can understand the basic ethical precept to "do no harm" as having an additional, alternate meaning where it expresses concern about aggressive treatments that might attempt to usurp the power of the cosmos. Right action for ancient Greeks had less to do with the rights of individuals (a largely modernist notion), and more to do with maintaining appropriate humility and proper balance in the face of a powerful universe. The critical point is that our underlying epistemological orientation and cultural dispositions strongly influence how we think about ethics. In short, morality itself is a social enterprise.

While ethical questions, generally speaking, have attended health care since ancient times, bioethics is a comparatively new discipline that emerged when Enlightenment-influenced philosophical perspectives were applied to advances in medical science. After all, from an historical perspective, the ability of medicine to extend life is a relatively new phenomenon. While the advent of antibiotics and antisepsis procedures radically extended life expectancies, with few side effects, subsequent gains in the ability to sustain life have raised more troubling moral questions. In particular, the ability to prolong life using mechanical ventilation and feeding tubes raised questions about whether life under such conditions *ought* to be extended. The abilities of medical science represented a factual condition, but the moral questions attached to that condition require sound analysis of professional responsibility, as well as personal and social values.

Bioethics itself is representative of the late-modern landscape of health and illness. As noted in Chapter 2, reflexive modernity refers to a situation where the particular kind of thinking characteristic of the modern period (means-ends rationality) produces solutions to problems (the ability of science and technology to extend life), but where those solutions raise new problems (the ethical question about whether it is *always* the right thing to do to keep someone alive) that may require new types of thinking.

Just as advances in science and technology promoted ethical questions in medicine and health care, other social conditions also galvanized the field of bioethics. In particular the Civil Rights Movement of the 1950s and 1960s and countercultural revolution of the 1960s and early 1970s emphasized individual freedom and autonomy, which, as it leaked into the area of health care, manifested as resistance to a long history of medical paternalism and a move toward patients' rights and autonomous decision-making. As these cultural undercurrents were sweeping through health care, they were punctuated by key historical events that helped frame various ethical dilemmas. Sociologist Charles Bosk (2010) has referred to these kinds of events as "essentially contested total social conflicts," because they are so destabilizing to social institutions that wrestling with them produces a new language and procedures for dealing with similar situations in the future. That is, these watershed events have transformed how we think about and practice ethics in health care. Specifically, we will see that a principlist approach that favors patient autonomy tempered with notions about what is best for the patient has emerged from a variety of events that have been framed as conflicts over medical authority and individual patient rights and freedom.

In the area of research, a number of events helped crystallize tensions surrounding health care and ethics. The revelation of Nazi medical experiments that came to light at the end of World War II darkened the heroic image that had been enjoyed by medical science throughout the first half of the twentieth century.[2] Following the war crimes trials of Nazi officials, the 1947 Nuremburg Code established ethical standards for the conduct of research, but it held no force of law, and in light of several experiments that would come to light over the next several decades, it was largely unsuccessful at ensuring ethical research conduct. Then, in the 1960s there was intense public outcry over experiments performed at the Willowbrook State School in New York, a residential facility for children with intellectual disabilities. While it was designed to house 4,000 residents, by the mid-1960s it had approximately 6,000 (Rothman & Rothman 1984). With overcrowding and understaffing came severe neglect and frequent disease transmission. These general conditions were first exposed in 1965 when Senator Robert Kennedy visited Willowbrook and famously referred to it as a "snake pit." Yet by 1972, the institution was still dramatically overcrowded and its residents continued to suffer. In this year, a relatively unknown New York reporter named Geraldo Rivera was invited by a staff member to film an exposé. The grotesque conditions shocked both Rivera and his viewership. Amidst this abhorrent state of affairs, it was uncovered that two researchers had intentionally infected residents with hepatitis A in order to investigate the effect of protective antibodies in mitigating the effects of the disease.

The Willowbrook study was one of twenty-two listed in a now infamous 1966 article by Henry K. Beecher, describing research that he believed violated basic ethical principles, including failure to obtain informed consent (Beecher 1966). Beecher's goal was to prove such studies were not rare, nor conducted in secret, but rather the products of systemic failures (including lack of oversight). As a testament to this, many of these studies persisted after Beecher highlighted their ethical problems. Another of the twenty-two research protocols highlighted in Beecher's report was the Tuskegee Syphilis study.

In 1972, the same year that Geraldo Rivera exposed the conditions at Willowbrook to the wider public, a story broke in the Associated Press about a Public

---

[2] It is important to remember, however, that Nazi eugenics programs were inspired by eugenics programs underway in the 1920s and 1930s throughout the United States.

Health Service (PHS) study of untreated syphilis being conducted on African American men in Tuskegee, Alabama. The Tuskegee Syphilis study had originated in 1932 to investigate the natural course of syphilis in African American men, with the goal of assessing whether the long-term effects of the disease were in fact less harmful than the relatively toxic treatments available at the time. The men enrolled in the study were not informed of their diagnoses (instead being told they had "bad blood," a colloquialism that referred to a range of nonspecific conditions) and while they were provided routine medical care, none of the 399 men in the experimental group was treated for their syphilis across the forty-year duration of the study, even after penicillin became the widely available standard of care for syphilis in the mid-1940s. Public outcry was deafening and congressional review called by Senator Edward Kennedy, along with a review panel convened by the Centers for Disease Control and Prevention (CDC) and PHS, lead to the expeditious termination of the study only months after it was first reported in the popular press.

Social context is important for understanding both the origins of these experiments and the eventual backlash against them. Both originated in a period of medical paternalism and fervor over the promise of medical science (recall from Chapter 2 the discussion of the heroification of physicians in this period; Loewen 1995). Both were terminated during a time when a sociocultural emphasis on civil rights and individual freedoms had emerged in U.S. society. And both, along with other watershed moments in the history of health, medicine, and ethics, constitute "essentially contested total social conflicts" because they destabilized long-held dispositions with respect to race and disability stigma and reshaped the terrain of research ethics (Bosk 2010). In particular, these studies led to the creation of the National Commission for the Protection of Human Subjects of Biomedical and Behavioral Research. This commission eventually produced the Belmont Report (United States 1978), which provided an ethical framework for human subjects research and led to the creation of oversight committees now known as Institutional Review Boards (IRBs). Informed consent and the rights of individual research participants stand at the center of research ethics in the United States today, emerging from the discourse that erupted when key events such as Tuskegee and Willowbrook punctuated a sociocultural landscape that was arcing toward greater emphasis on individual freedom. Paradigm cases such as those of Karen Ann Quinlan and Nancy Cruzan affected clinical ethics in a similar way.

Karen Ann Quinlan lapsed into a persistent vegetative state in 1975 after taking a combination of pills (barbiturates, benzodiazepines, or both) and alcohol. She lost brain function, and was admitted to a Catholic hospital in New Jersey where she was kept alive on a ventilator. The Quinlan case was emblematic of the need for redefinition and clarification of long-standing precepts of medical decision-making in light of advancing technology, particularly where the criteria of death at the time included a variety of bodily functions that for Quinlan were being provided or supplemented by a ventilator. Given that these functions could now be sustained mechanically, questions about whether it was ethically permissible to remove that technology and allow her die now had to be confronted. After several months, Quinlan's parents asked that her ventilator be removed and stated that doing so would be consistent with her expressed wishes. However, her physician refused for fear of legal and professional reprisal and a court initially ruled that ventilator support must be continued, largely as an effort to uphold the physician's professional standards. The New Jersey Supreme Court later issued a landmark ruling that both upheld the right to refuse medical treatment as an extension of individual privacy and allowed for next-of-kin to make substituted judgments for incapacitated patients. The criteria for the latter, however, would be contested again some fifteen years later in the case of Nancy Cruzan. Quinlan was removed from the ventilator in 1976, but did not die until 1985 from pneumonia.

Nancy Cruzan sustained significant brain injury after a car accident in 1983. She never regained consciousness and a feeding tube was inserted to keep her alive. While Quinlan's parents had sought removal of her ventilator, but not her feeding tube, Cruzan's parents requested that artificial nutrition be stopped, stating that their daughter would not want to be kept alive in such a state. In this case, however, the Missouri Supreme Court ruled that there was not clear and convincing evidence in the case that Cruzan herself would have wanted hydration and nutrition discontinued. Despite the way they ruled on the facts of the case itself, the court upheld a number of important precepts. First, the court equated removal of nutritional support with removal of other medical care, such as a ventilator. Additionally, the court upheld the right of competent patients to refuse medical care. Finally, the court affirmed the right of states to require clear and convincing evidence that a surrogate's judgment, in the case of an incompetent patient, is aligned with that patient's own wishes. The notion of clear and convincing evidence would again be at the heart of high-profile cases, notably that of Terri Schiavo (discussed below), where family conflicts over what the patient would have wanted present ethical dilemmas about how to proceed with the patient's care.

Like Willowbrook and Tuskegee, the Quinlan and Cruzan cases fundamentally disrupted long-standing practices and attitudes about end-of-life care and the professional duties of practitioners. Those events brought about a reflexive moment for practitioners who traditionally conceived of their role as aggressively curing disease and promoted a shift in conceptualization, whereby the ethical limits of aggressive treatment had to be considered and worked into professional practice. In concert with the wider sociopolitical context of the time, these landmark cases destabilized and caused thorough reevaluation of long-standing research and clinical practices. Bioethics as a discipline crystallized around the results of these social developments, bringing moral philosophy to bear on the very practical questions being confronted in health care. In particular, the Belmont Report (United States 1978) outlined three principles to guide ethical research (respect for persons, beneficence, and justice). Later, similar principles would be adapted for the clinical context (Beauchamp & Childress 2001).

Principles of Biomedical Ethics and Beyond

The dominant discourse of bioethics is grounded on modernist moral philosophies that developed in the 1700s and 1800s. Recall from Chapter 2 that as premodern cosmologies, which gave preference to more intuitive forms of thinking, began to erode, Western thought became dominated by rationalism. This also was true of moral philosophy, where notions of right and wrong could no longer be based straightforwardly on appeal to religious sources, but had to employ secular justifications (though religious notions still played significant functions for Locke, Kant, and many others). That is, philosophers could no longer simply refer to the traditional authority of religious texts, but now were compelled, by the spirit of the Enlightenment, to ground philosophies of ethics on reason, such that they could, in theory, be widely agreed upon by humanity without appeal to cosmic powers.

In the 1600s John Locke, by rationally justifying the entitlement of all men[3] to life, liberty, and property, laid a foundation for individual rights in Western culture that had eventual import for the development of notions of patient's rights and freedoms. However, the discipline and practice of bioethics are primarily dominated by a tension between deontological and teleological ways of thinking that were developed later. Deontological approaches emphasize principle-based reasoning. That is, they suggest that the right thing to do is that which follows from a universal moral principle. Consequentialist reasoning, on the other hand, focuses on the outcomes of an action (i.e., whether it produces more good than harm).

Deontological reasoning traces to a number of thinkers, but Immanuel Kant is among the most influential. Kant posited a moral philosophy grounded in what he called the *categorical imperative*, which represented "a [moral] action as being objectively necessary in itself without regard to any other end." That is, for Kant, we ought to follow moral rules simply because they are moral rules, regardless of the consequences those actions produce. We ought not to lie simply because it is wrong to do so, because a lie fails to treat the person, or more generally humanity, as "an end in itself." Where bioethics in both the research and clinical context demands that patient rights and freedoms be respected, it does so primarily on the grounds that patients (as human beings) ought to be respected as ends in themselves, and therefore given the dignity of self-determination.

On its face, deontological reasoning has particular appeal, especially where we often conceive of moral action as a matter of following our ideals and values (principles) even when the consequences are not particularly easy to experience. However, ignoring the consequences of actions entirely leads to situations that many find morally questionable. While certainly it is wrong to tell a lie in most situations, what if telling a comparatively small lie would produce significantly positive consequences? For example, suppose a gunman asks where to find his ex-boss who fired him and you tell him that you do not know, even though you do. Most people would not find such a lie to be morally problematic, because the positive consequences significantly outweigh the negative ones. The failure of deontological reasoning to be able to weigh outcomes in this way was addressed by John Stuart Mill and other thinkers with a more pragmatic approach to moral reasoning called utilitarianism that gained popularity in the 1800s.

Utilitarianism, generally speaking, relies on teleological or consequentialist reasoning, which is the polar opposite of deontological reasoning. That is, teleological approaches focus on the consequences of actions. Utilitarianism can be broadly characterized as suggesting that an action is right when it produces the

[3] Showing that traditional thinking was not completely eclipsed by rationality, traditional gender views persisted in philosophical writing for several centuries (and gendered philosophical perspectives arguably still dominate today, see discussion of feminist ethics below).

greatest good for the greatest number. Utilitarianism emerged in an era of urbanization as Western societies tackled a variety of social problems in the process of moving from agrarian to industrial economies. As such, utilitarian approaches have often underpinned work on social problems. In medicine, issues of rationing scarce medical resources often appeal to those sorts of consequentialist arguments. For example, in the case of limited blood supply, we might easily say that those patients who will benefit most from the blood should receive it.

Consequentialist approaches also have tremendous appeal, particularly because they are so pragmatic and grounded in our tangible experiences of the world (they seek to minimize suffering, for example). However, the *rationality* of doing what produces the best outcomes can easily become a matter of *rationalizing* what one desires to do by supposing future consequences that may or may not be accurate or important. For example, the proxy decision-maker for a seriously ill patient might request aggressive care ostensibly on the grounds that they believe the patient can recover, when in reality they are assuaging or avoiding their own potential feelings of guilt about making a decision to terminate life support. There often is no way to verify future consequences, or that decisions being made based on those future consequences are genuine. Thus, while it appears very pragmatic, consequentialist approaches can demand a lot of us in making moral decisions, by effectively requiring that we know the future consequences of our actions and that we have fidelity to those outcomes. In reality, especially in the complex and unpredictable world of health and illness, consequences are not always easy to predict and any number of influences may affect our decision-making.

The Four Principles of Biomedical Ethics

As noted, the Belmont Report (United States 1978) articulated three ethical principles to guide ethical conduct in human subjects research. *Respect for persons* represented the idea that every human being has inherent dignity and the right to self-determination (to make choices that are related to their own life and their own body). In addition to the ability to make choices for oneself, respect for persons entails the inherent dignity of human beings, which must be respected. For example, privacy protections for health information are not only justified based on the consequences that might befall a patient if that information is disclosed, but also, and perhaps primarily by a sense that one's health information is their own, something intimate and private, and that, except in certain circumstances, each patient should decide for themselves who gets to know such private things about them.[4] *Beneficence* recognizes that research must, overall, produce benefits for patients (at least for patient populations, though not necessarily for individual patients enrolled in particular studies). Finally, *justice* recognizes that the burdens of research, where participants submit to some level of risk in order to benefit humanity, had to be fairly distributed. That is, no one particular population should disproportionately

---

[4] See Department of Health and Human Services (2003), particularly pages 3 and 4, for a summary of the Health Insurance Portability and Accountability Act, outlining what types of information is protected and the rules under which such information can be accessed and disclosed. For our purposes in this chapter, it is important to know that these protections emerge from considerations of the rights and dignity owed to individuals.

be recruited for research simply because they are easy to access or more easily coerced. Recall that the Tuskegee Syphilis study (arguably) failed on all three of these principles, insofar as (1) patients were not informed about their condition or the true intentions of the study (violates respect for persons); (2) particularly after penicillin became widely available, the study had little potential benefit (violates the principle of beneficence); and (3) because the participants were poor, lived in a rural environment with limited access to health care, and were African American in the segregated South, they arguably were unfairly targeted to bear the burdens of the research (violates the principle of justice).[5]

The principles articulated in the Belmont Report reflect long-standing Enlightenment notions of morality, particularly where respect for persons represents a deontological approach to moral reasoning while beneficence and justice tend to draw on teleological considerations. Thomas Beauchamp and James Childress (2001) adapted these to the clinical context, articulating four principles of bioethics: (1) autonomy; (2) nonmaleficence; (3) beneficence; and (4) justice.

Autonomy refers to the right of persons to make decisions that relate to their own life and body. It is effectively a right of self-determination. As Beauchamp and Childress (2001:100) note, "Virtually all theories of autonomy view two conditions as essential for autonomy: *liberty* (independence from controlling influences) and *agency* (capacity for intentional action)." Additionally, they note that autonomy can be read as both a negative and positive obligation. It is a negative obligation where we have the duty *not* to interfere with a competent person's decisions. It is a positive obligation where we have duties to assist with individuals' attempts to fulfill their own autonomous decisions. In the former, for example, we ought not force continued treatment on a competent patient who decides to forgo aggressive care in favor of hospice. With respect to the latter, we may have obligations, not only to refrain from forcing unwanted treatment, but also to provide palliative measures that help the patient remain comfortable through the end of his or her life.

Informed consent is a critical component of fulfilling our obligations with respect to the autonomy of patients. That is, in order to make decisions that accord with their own values and wishes, patients must be fully informed of their diagnosis, prognosis, the variety of available treatment options, and so on. Additionally, in order to make autonomous decisions, individuals must possess the capacity to make reasonable decisions. That is, they must be able to demonstrate an understanding of the situation, consistently communicate a decision, and show that they recognize the likely consequences of that decision. Put simply, in health care we must inform patients so that they may make good, autonomous decisions, but those patients also must be able to be informed, possessing the cognitive ability to understand and utilize the information they are given.

Nonmaleficence refers to an obligation not to harm a patient, or not to put them at undue risk of harm. It represents a negative obligation specifically by telling us we ought *not* cause harm to others. While the idea that health care practitioners ought not harm their patients seems incredibly obvious and simplistic, in practice there are complex scenarios that appeal to this principle. For example, suppose a

[5] Some argue that the sample selection was not unjust because the study site was chosen because of high prevalence of syphilis in the area of Tuskegee. Others contend that the effects of syphilis certainly reached beyond that enclave and the burdens of the research could have been more fairly distributed.

patient has a terminal illness, is in severe pain, and disoriented with no ability to communicate his wishes regarding his care and no proxy decision-maker to do so for him (e.g., no next-of-kin). One practitioner argues that the man needs a tracheotomy and mechanical ventilation. Another might object, on the grounds of nonmaleficence, that such a procedure would be causing undue suffering to the patient, both in terms of the operation itself and because it might prolong his suffering. While the principle of nonmaleficence is straightforward in theory, its application often is demanded in highly contested empirical situations such as this.

As a principle, beneficence is closely related to nonmaleficence, but it represents a positive obligation to do things that promote the welfare of others. Here again, the idea that health care practitioners have an obligation to promote the welfare of patients may seem obvious and simplistic. Most practitioners enter their fields because they want to help others. However, as with nonmaleficence, in practice, considerations of beneficence can be difficult to navigate. Beneficence focuses on producing good outcomes, but it is not always easy to determine the best course of action, particularly when disease trajectories and various interventions can be so unpredictable. Moreover, the duty to do what is best for the patient can often conflict with competing obligations. Patients, for example, can exercise their autonomy in ways that, objectively speaking, are not good for them. Additionally, institutional influences can exert pressure to treat patients in ways that might not always maximize the promotion of their interests. For example, hospital policies may pressure the discharge of a particular patient who would have benefited from continued hospital care. Finally, the principle of beneficence often emerges in situations where medical care is futile, that is, where there is "no benefit." For example, a family may want continued ventilation and nutritional support for a patient who is already neurologically deceased. The current ethical consensus is that such treatment is of "no benefit" and therefore practitioners are not obligated to provide it, even when removing those treatments conflict with the demands made by the patient's proxy decision-maker.

Recall that justice refers to the fair distribution of burdens in the research context. Similarly, in the clinical context, justice refers to the fair and equitable treatment of patients. Of particular import in the area of health care, distributive justice concerns the fair and equitable allocation of medical resources and treatments. Importantly, while the first three principles focus squarely on the individual patient, justice considers the wider social landscape in which patients will be treated, the obligations we have to a particular patient are considered in the context of our obligations to our other patients. For example, if a hospital was running low on a particularly potent and effective drug, a physician might reserve use of that drug for more serious cases and utilize a slightly less efficacious treatment for less serious cases. So long as this decision was made genuinely on medical criteria (e.g., efficacy relative to patients' conditions), and not on the basis of race/ethnicity, religion, sexual orientation, ability to pay, and the like, then it would conform to the principle of justice.

Figure 11.1 demonstrates, in admittedly broad terms, how the principles of biomedical ethics fit together with the classic modern paradigms of moral reasoning. While some have argued that Beauchamp and Childress's four-principle framework is inherently deontological (they are all referred to as "principles"), when we

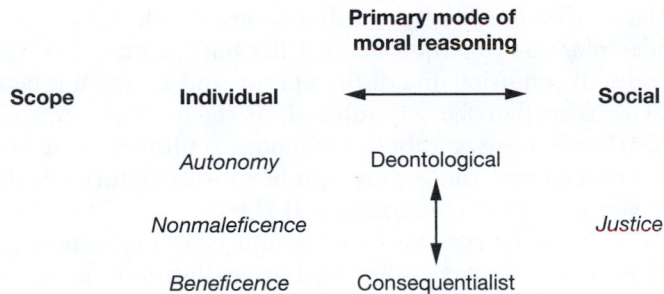

FIG. 11.1 Moral reasoning, social scope, and the principles of biomedical ethics.

examine the logics underlying each principle, we can see that together they reflect tensions between deontological and consequentialist reasoning, on one hand, and a tension between our obligations to individual patients and our obligations to the wider community of patients, on the other.

While autonomy *can be* grounded on consequentialist notions (see Beauchamp & Childress 2001), it primarily manifests as an inherent right of persons, and therefore an obligation to respect it typically follows from a moral rule, rather than consideration of its consequences. Simply put, it is widely held that people with the capacity for self-determination have the right to make their own decisions with regard to their health and health care, even if it results in bad consequences for them.

Nonmaleficence can be read as alternatively deontological and consequentialist. Obviously causing harm represents a bad consequence, and we might invoke the principle of nonmaleficence on those grounds alone. But also, where harm represents a violation of the inherent dignity or personhood of a patient, it invokes more deontological considerations. Beneficence, where it requires the promotion of the welfare of others, rests nearly exclusively on consequentialist considerations.

Justice often is seen as primarily consequentialist in orientation, particularly within the health care setting. After all, core considerations of justice, as in the example above, rely on determinations about where to invest scarce resources so that they are most efficacious. This is clearly focused on promoting the best outcomes. However, violations of justice can also concern attacks on the inherent dignity or humanity of a group of people. Using a racial slur, for example, is not only wrong because it offends and humiliates the specific individual at whom it was directed, but because it dehumanizes an entire group of people. Where its scope transcends the individual to violate the humanity of a larger social group, even if that larger group experiences no direct harms from the act, we can see how justice can be grounded on more inherent (i.e., deontological) concerns.

Understanding how these principles work in concert is critically important for navigating ethical decision-making in health care contexts. Rarely are ethical dilemmas so simple that we can choose just one principle and follow it to its conclusion. Rather, ethical dilemmas in health care force us to weigh multiple considerations against each other. Take for example a situation where an 85-year-old woman is transferred from the emergency department to the intensive care unit with advanced chronic obstructive pulmonary disease (COPD) and severe difficulty breathing. Unless she is intubated, she will not survive. She refuses intubation and appears to understand the consequences, but her husband tells you that she sometimes has episodes of confusion and disorientation and should not be able to make that decision. He insists that she be intubated. As the practitioner, you believe that given the patient's prognosis, intubation would not ultimately be beneficial and, in fact, that the procedure would cause significant discomfort and distress to the woman. However, you also recognize that if she does not have the capacity for decision-making, removing the ventilator would be going against the expressed wishes of her husband, who likely is her legal proxy decision-maker.

Situations such as this are not uncommon and certainly not so simple that we can just select from among the principles in a way that tells us what to do. In this case, we have to decide who is the autonomous decision-maker in this case, that is, who has the right to exercise judgment on behalf of the patient (either the patient herself or her husband). If we decide that the woman lacks capacity to make a decision, things get even more complicated. Depending on the degree to which intubation may or may not be beneficial (another complicated matter in itself), we must decide whether the principles of nonmaleficence (the harm that would be caused by intubation) and beneficence (the fact that intubation will produce no significant benefit for the patient) outweigh the husband's right to make decisions regarding the treatment of his wife. In the end, ethical decision-making for health care practitioners is rarely a matter of following the prescription of bioethical principles and often a matter of professional judgment where the facts of a situation must be navigated with respect to competing ethical principles.

Other Forms of Ethical Reasoning and Decision-Making

Insofar as the four principles approach is grounded on modernist notions of morality and rationalism, it has been criticized as incomplete. For one, it does not fit well in many non-Western cultures, where a more collectivist sense of social organization and morality is utilized to resolve moral dilemmas. Particularly where autonomy, nonmaleficence, and beneficence are squarely focused on the individual patient, they can be difficult to reconcile with patients for whom health care decisions are made by entire families and with regard for the larger family dynamic, rather than simply the wishes or experiences of that individual patient. Thus, while the four principles approach forms a significant part of the formal discourse on ethical decision-making in health care in Western cultures, it is in reality supplemented by a number of other approaches (and, as we will discuss in the next section, a variety of approaches are simultaneously and often unconsciously utilized by providers in the decision-making process).

Casuistry

Unlike the categorical imperative or utilitarianism, casuistry is not so much a moral theory as it is a method for answering moral questions by appealing to similar cases. That is, casuistry utilizes case-based reasoning in an effort to resolve ethical dilemmas. It is particularly useful for parsing complex cases to uncover the core moral issues involved. A casuist approach looks for relevant similarities between a particularly troubling issue and one in the past that has already been resolved (preferably around which there exists less disagreement). By suggesting that the core issues of a troubling case are similar in kind to those of a less-troubling, already-resolved case, one can use the latter as a guide for what to do in the present. This process of reasoning, of course, is popular in the legal realm where an issue will be approached by appeal to precedent decisions and where judicial opinions are commonly based on, or justified by, those precedents. Casuistry is sometimes considered a weak form of reasoning because it relies on the relevance of past cases, which often do not parallel all of the nuances of the issue at hand, thereby potentially ignoring nuances and novelties arising from moral dilemmas with which we are confronted in the present.

Virtue Ethics

Virtue ethics is an approach that appeals to the character of the actor rather than their actions. While the connection between virtue ethics and medicine dates back to the Hippocratic tradition (see Chapter 2), its meaning has become more modernized as it has been woven into contemporary bioethics discourse. Recall from Chapter 2 that the premodern way of thinking focused on balance within the cosmos. Premodern ethics, to state it broadly, was similarly about the individual's proper relationship to the larger universe (the part's relation to the whole). In the premodern era, good character was less a starting point for ethical action and doing good works than it was important on its own for maintaining balance. However, today, we tend to have a very behaviorist orientation. That is, we largely speak of virtuous character in terms of its role in moral behavior. Nonetheless, virtue ethics adds an important perspective to bioethics discourse. Where deontological and consequentialist approaches are focused primarily on whether something we do is right or wrong, virtue ethics turns inward to ask whether a particular action emerges from a right or good character. This fills an important gap in modernist ethics in two ways.

First, intuitively it seems that the notion of morality, at least to some degree, includes features of character. Someone, for example, who donates money to charity, but for the wrong reasons (e.g., self-gratification), or with a malicious spirit, would not be judged as the moral equivalent of someone who performs that same action, but for altruistic reasons or with a caring or compassionate attitude. The character of the actor clearly matters for how we think about morality, but this is not well accounted for in consequentialism or deontology.[6]

Second, while deontological and consequentialist approaches give variable guidance about the right and wrong thing to do, they offer little guidance or means of determining the right or wrong way to go about executing moral judgments. For example, if we decide that ventilator support is no longer beneficial to a patient who is in a persistent vegetative state, and who's next-of-kin is requesting its removal, both deontological and consequentialist approaches tell us that removing the ventilator is morally acceptable (because it accords with the substituted autonomy of the patient and because the ventilator is of no benefit). But how should we go about the process? How should we talk to the family? How should we communicate this

---

[6] Kant suggests that the intentions of an actor are of significant moral weight, but stops short of developing a deeper notion of moral character.

decision to other care providers? Virtue ethics asks us to examine not only what a person of strong moral character would do, but also how they would carry themselves in the process. In this case, we might look toward a religious leader or a seasoned health care provider whom we respect as a role model for how we ought to behave in the course of carrying out our decision. Virtue ethics therefore is at once a very esoteric and very practical way of thinking about ethics. It is esoteric in that it concerns good character, something difficult to fully define, though perhaps we know it when we see it. But it is practical in that it gives us guidance not just for navigating major decision points, but for carrying ourselves with integrity throughout the process of providing care.

Ethics of Care

Ethics of care approaches emerged from a feminist critique of moral rationalism represented in the four-principles approach, in particular where these implicitly position the individual patient as a rational moral agent existing in a vacuum, or, in the case of justice, in a rational competition for resources with other moral agents. Just as virtue ethics highlights how deontological and consequentialist approaches say little about how we ought to behave in the execution of an ethical decision, care-based ethics highlights how such a modernist paradigm takes little account of the social context and relationships surrounding ethical decisions. Feminist scholars such as Carol Gilligan point out that moral reasoning tends to be gendered. While boys and men tend to employ hyperrationalist forms of reasoning, girls and women tend to focus on how particular decisions affect their relationships with others. This is informative for health care ethics in two key ways.

First, ethics of care approaches give an important perspective for ethical decision-making that is missing from traditional deontological and consequentialist approaches, which, again, focus on the rational thinking of relatively isolated "moral agents." In our case of a patient in a persistent vegetative state, for example, removing the ventilator conforms to a rationalist calculation that such care is no long beneficial. However, care-based ethics calls us to ask about the relationships among the patient's family and how removing the ventilator might affect those relationships. Ultimately, we likely will still choose to remove it, but as often is done in clinical practice, we may adjust the timeline for removal to allow the family time to grieve and come to terms with the decision, based on our understanding of that particular family, their particular relationships to the patient and each other, their personal beliefs and values, and so on. When we allow our actions to be guided by those sorts of considerations, we are drawing on care-based approaches.

Second, care-based ethics is informative because it accords with how people think about ethics and make decisions in the real world. As we know from our discussion of health lifestyles in Chapter 6, health behavior is not determined by purely rational thought, but by nonrational ways of thinking, including habits. A mix of rational and nonrational thoughts similarly guides ethics decision-making, for most people, most of the time. That is, beyond simply calculating the costs and benefits of a decision or following a principle, people draw on a variety of considerations such as religious beliefs, superstitions, other intuitive convictions, how they feel, how they think others might feel, and so on. Ethics of care approaches fill this gap in the calculative modernist paradigm of deontology and consequentialism, and therefore in the four principles approach. Care-based ethics, therefore, not only improves our decisions, actions, and relationships as we interact with patients, but helps us understand how our patients may be working through ethical situations in legitimate, though nonrational, ways.

Narrative Ethics

Recall from Chapters 7 and 8 that connecting interpersonally with patients requires the use of active listening strategies to solicit their full narrative and that many problems of practitioner–patient communication arise when that narrative is cut short (e.g., through exertions of power in attempts to control the clinical discourse). Narrative ethics refers to the way in which storytelling can capture poignant ethical moments, particularly by promoting connections between the teller and the listener.

In particular, narrative approaches recognize that stories capture experiences in a holistic way that protects their characters from the reductionist approaches of modernist ethics (and modernist medicine). For example, for both deontology and consequentialism, moral actors are simply rational decision-makers with a capacity to suffer. Those who do not display the ability to think rationally, to weigh outcomes, and so on are no longer considered autonomous and are no longer allowed to make their own decisions. Additionally, both deontology and consequentialism fundamentally are concerned with the ability of individuals to be harmed (either by having their inherent humanity stripped or, more practically, by being caused to suffer). Based on these two conditions—the individual's ability to make rational decisions and to suffer—we have, according to the modernist account, everything we need to know in order to make an ethical decision.

Narrative ethics rejects the idea that in moral decision-making we can reduce human beings to these two qualities alone. Rather, narrative ethics approaches suggest that the whole biographies of individuals, their whole stories, are part of an account that ethics must take into consideration. This is particularly true where ethical action, especially in health care, must be motivated and guided by empathy for the patient (and others). It is difficult to empathically connect patients if we see them simply as rational agents with generalized capacities for suffering. Rather, empathy, at least of sufficient depth, comes from knowing who patients are, what they value, how they have lived, what they have experienced, and the like.

From these different approaches to ethical decision-making a number of things should be clear. First, ethical situations are complex and difficult to navigate, such that we often must rely on a number of decision-making strategies. Ethics decisions are rarely well-guided simply by appealing to a single approach. In health care, ethics decisions often present core dilemmas where a patient's autonomy might conflict with what is medically in his or her own best interests, and where navigating such tensions requires an in-depth understanding of not only the medical facts, but also the patient and his or her family, as well as hospital policy and case-precedent. Second, it should be clear that ethics decisions in health care are not made in a philosophical vacuum, but rather where normative philosophies are brought into the complex terrain of biomedical and sociocultural phenomena. More simply, bioethics is as much a social–psychological enterprise as a philosophical one. This will become even clearer as we examine practical bioethics in the next section. While the theoretical approaches discussed above clearly require, to varying degrees, an understanding of the social terrain of a given case, ethical practice in real-world situations even more thoroughly requires a strong ability to bring together social structural conditions, normative principles, and the facts (social and biomedical) of an individual case. That is, practical ethics requires a strong sociological imagination.

From Theory to Practice

Navigating ethical situations involves bringing theories of ethics together with complex empirical situations. After all, ethical dilemmas usually do not arise when situations are simple. But while the philosophical and factual complexity of ethical dilemmas in health care are challenging in their own right, sociocultural considerations and human behavioral psychology further complicate ethics in the real-world health care setting. In this section, we examine some features of practical bioethics in clinical contexts.

A Framework for Practical Bioethics

In their book *Clinical Ethics*, Jonsen et al. (2010) approach clinical ethical decision-making from a practical standpoint. Table 11.1 shows their *four topics* approach, which takes more thorough account of the factual landscape than the more philosophically oriented four principles approach. What Jonsen et al. (2010) propose is that ethical dilemmas must first be approached as a matter of gathering all of the facts and considerations, before philosophical ethics frameworks can be brought to bear on those situations. Additionally, they map how the four principles fit with various kinds of empirical concerns including medical indications, patient preferences, quality of life, and contextual features of a particular scenario.

To examine how the practical (social and biomedical) features of a case come together with normative ethical concerns in real-world situations, consider the case of Jahi McMath. McMath was a 13-year-old girl in California in 2013 when she went into a hospital for surgery related to sleep apnea. While her initial recovery appeared normal, she began to have significant bleeding from the surgical site through her nose and mouth, suffered cardiac arrest, and her brain was deprived of blood flow for a significant period of time. She was subsequently declared brain dead, and the medical team recommended she be removed from the ventilator that was keeping her alive. The family disputed, on religious grounds, the declaration of her death based on neurological criteria and have referred to her as being "asleep." They argued that disconnecting ventilator support would be killing her. Additionally, while the hospital has referred to these procedures as complicated, her family, in subsequent interviews, referred to them as routine, signaling a potential breakdown in communication about the risks and complexity of the initial operation. Moreover, a lawsuit by the family would later allege that the surgeon noticed a congenital condition that predisposed the girl to hemorrhage but failed to disclose it to the family, while the family got mixed postoperative advice from nurses that the initial bleeding was normal. McMath was later transferred to an undisclosed facility, which performed a tracheostomy and inserted a feeding tube to allow for long-term mechanical support.

In the McMath case we clearly have a tension between autonomy and beneficence. The parents, as the proxy decision-makers, have the right to make decisions on behalf of their daughter. At the same time, autonomy does not mean that patients (or their proxies) are entitled to receive everything that they demand. Because McMath met the neurological criteria for death, the ventilator support was, according to the medical team (and by virtue of wide agreement in the field of bioethics), nonbeneficial care and, by virtue of the principle of beneficence, ethically could be discontinued. While the tension here between the inherent rights of the patient and her parents and the consequentialist analysis of the benefits and harms of continued mechanical support is complicated in its own right, there are numerous other issues present here. Referring back to the four topics approach (see Table 11.1), we can ask a number of additional questions.

For example, were McMath's parents fully informed about the risks of the procedures? After all, they appeared to represent what was, by the doctor's account, a complex surgery, as nothing more than a simple tonsillectomy. Additionally, the medical facts are incredibly consequential. Does McMath have any brain activity or capacity to have experiences? Her family, lawyers, and hired experts claimed that she did, but multiple other medical professionals have rejected those findings and repeatedly determined her to be neurologically dead. Moreover, while ability to pay for long-term care ideally does not factor into how we treat patients from an ethical perspective, it would be naïve not to question how financial concerns might influence decision-making in cases such as this. Finally, how might we need to accommodate the medically informed decisions of the health care team to the patient's religious beliefs? All of these questions are social in character, but have tremendous bearing on our ethical assessment of the case.

Many of the biomedical and social facts of the McMath case, in addition to informing what is perhaps the core decision about removal of mechanical ventilation, inform how we might interact with the family in the process. For example, ethics of care or narrative perspectives might inform our dialogues with the family or the need to listen fully to their story, understand their perspective on the meanings of life and death, and work with their religious convictions, even if the ultimate conclusion of the hospital is to remove the ventilator. Additionally, virtue ethics can inform how care providers carry themselves through the process, and in particular how they deal with any medical errors or insufficiencies in care or communication that may have occurred.

Indeed, clinical ethics consultations, where designated providers, often in teams, consult with the variety of stakeholders involved with an ethics case (the care team, the patient and family, etc.), necessitate drawing on complex sets of biomedical and social facts and bringing to bear on them a range of different theories of ethics. Sitting down with a patient or family in such delicate circumstances requires more than making an acute decision about care. It also requires active listening, narrative assessment, empathy, and appreciation for diverse perspectives that may arise from providers, patients, and families. Religious and cultural differences, for example, may lead to situations that simply do not conform to the calculative model of ethics represented by the four principles approach. Clinical interactions with patients before, during, and after also matter. For example, good communication increases the chances that patients or their proxies fully understand the risks of a procedure,

TABLE 11.1 Four Topics Approach

Medical Indications

The Principles of Beneficence and Nonmaleficence

- What is the patient's medical problem? Is the problem acute? Chronic? Critical? Reversible? Emergent? Terminal?
- What are the goals of treatment?
- In what circumstances are medical treatments not indicated?
- What are the probabilities of success of various treatment options?
- In sum, how can this patient be benefited by medical and nursing care, and how can harm be avoided?

Patient Preferences

The Principle of Respect for Autonomy

- Has the patient been informed of benefits and risks, understood this information, and given consent?
- Is the patient mentally capable and legally competent, and is there evidence of capacity?
- If mentally capable, what preferences about treatment is the patient stating?
- If incapacitated, has the patient expressed prior preferences?
- Who is the appropriate surrogate to make decisions for the incapacitated patient?
- Is the patient unwilling or unable to cooperate with medical treatment? If so, why?

Quality of Life

The Principles of Beneficence, Nonmaleficence, and Respect for Autonomy

- What are the prospects, with or without treatment, for a return to normal life and what physical, mental, and social deficits is the patient likely to experience if treatment succeeds?
- On what grounds can anyone judge that some quality of life would be undesirable for a patient who cannot make or express such a judgment?
- Are there biases that might prejudice the provider's evaluation of the patient's quality of life?
- What ethical issues arise concerning improving or enhancing a patient's quality of life?
- Do quality-of-life assessments raise any questions regarding changes in treatment plans, such as forgoing life-sustaining treatment?
- What are the plans and rationale to forgo treatment?
- What is the legal and ethical status of suicide?

Contextual Features

The Principles of Justice and Fairness

- Are there professional, interprofessional, or business interests that might create conflicts of interest in the clinical treatment of patients?
- Are there parties other than clinicians and patients, such as family members, who have an interest in clinical decisions?
- What are the limits imposed on patient confidentiality by the legitimate interest of third parties?
- Are there financial factors that create conflicts of interest in clinical decisions?
- Are there problems of allocation of scarce health resources that might affect clinical decisions?
- Are there religious issues that might influence clinical decisions?
- Are there considerations of clinical research and education that might affect clinical decisions?
- Are there issues of public health and safety that affect clinical decisions?
- Are there conflicts of interest within institutions and organizations (e.g., hospitals) that may affect clinical decisions and patient welfare?

Source: Adapted from Jonsen, Albert R., Mark Siegler, & William J. Winslade. (2010). *Clinical Ethics: A Practical Approach to Ethical Decision-making in Clinical Medicine*, 2nd edition. New York: McGraw Hill.

which can help avoid ethical dilemmas later on. Additionally, preventative ethics, where various contingency plans are articulated and discussed well in advance of crisis, can help avoid situations where patients or families feel at odds with providers and allow them to make decisions during a time of relative calm, rather than in the midst of an overwhelming and chaotic event. All of these social skills are critical to shared decision-making (Chapter 8), ethical resolutions, and patient-centered care.

No one theory can be applied to such complex terrain in order to successfully navigate these situations. Jonsen (2007) suggests instead that ethics in health care may be less a matter of following our theoretical commitments to a particular philosophy than a matter of "appropriating appropriately." That is, in its complexity, clinical ethics may be less concerned with following particular principles or theories, and more concerned with knowing when and how to utilize a range of ethics strategies. In clinical ethics we find ourselves in situations where it is necessary to draw simultaneously on the four principles, virtue ethics, the ethics of care, and so on. A good bioethical imagination (De Vries et al. 2007) helps us parse the complex terrain so that we can match these various philosophical tools to various situations in a sound and robust way.

The Social Psychology of Clinical Ethics

Preventative ethics is intriguing because of the way it can preempt ethical dilemmas and help us avoid them. This is always preferable to winding up in a situation where one party or another will feel slighted. But the notion of preventative ethics also implicitly recognizes something deeper about the limits of our own psychology when it comes to ethical decision-making that is important to understand. Put simply, our decision-making tends to be weaker when we are under stress and, in particular, in quick, complicated situations. The social psychology of decision-making, therefore, informs us not only about the challenges of decision-making for patients in the midst of crisis, but about our own abilities (or limitations) for processing complicated ethical dilemmas.

In the wake of notable cases in clinical ethics, like Quinlan and Cruzan, hospital ethics committees began to form at institutions across the United States, and in 1992, the Joint Commission mandated that all hospitals subject to its oversight have formalized methods for resolving ethical disputes. But there has been limited clarity about how these committees should function, if and how they should be accredited, what their membership should look like, and what sort of training members should have. Most HECs have settled into serving three primary functions: (1) education to the institution; (2) clinical case review and making recommendations (though sometimes a clinical ethics consult service performs this function as a subcommittee of the larger HEC); and (3) policy review and revision. However, where HECs or their subcommittees function to make recommendations to practitioners, patients, and families, how well they approach ethics cases is critically important.

There have been numerous calls for increased training of HEC members (see, e.g., Bishop et al. 2009; Hoffman et al. 2000; Tarzian 2013). However, some have questioned whether ethics training, particularly of the sort that focuses on understanding theories of ethics, will be effective (Bardon 2003). A deeper exploration of how individuals tend to think about ethics is informative for answering this question.

Two core psychological concepts are important to understand here. The first is that cognitive load affects decision-making. That is, when people are under stress (i.e., when their ability to process information is overtaxed), they often miss important considerations. Moreover, we are naturally resistant to situations that are cognitively taxing. That is, human beings, for the most part, have a propensity for avoiding situations that are complex, and therefore a propensity for accepting more simplistic versions of complex scenarios. The second related concept for understanding critical challenges facing clinical ethics practice is cognitive dissonance, which is the notion that we become mentally stressed when confronted with conflicting beliefs or evidence that is contradictory to what we believe to be true. Because of our deep-seated psychological aversion to these contradictions (which represent a form of complexity), we tend to revise our perceptions of contradicting evidence in ways that recast it as consistent with our prior beliefs. These two natural psychological tendencies create important challenges for doing clinical ethics work because such work is naturally and inevitably complex, while at the same time humans have an innate aversion to complexity. This manifests in two key patterns.

First, practitioners often are unreflexive about the ethical foundations that inform their decision-making (Wasserman & Dure 2008). This happens in a number of ways. Practitioners often look to various frameworks, such as the four principles, as decision-making algorithms rather than tools for reflexive consideration of a dilemma. The authors of these frameworks, including Beauchamp and Childress (2001) in their concept of *reflective equilibrium*, eschew any idea that they can be used in some straightforward way to determine ethical decisions. Still, practitioners often assume ethics is a matter of discovering *the* right course of action based deductively on evidence, rather than a complex negotiation of contested facts and conflicting values for which there may be multiple ways to proceed ethically. Add to this a basic human propensity for simplicity, and it is not difficult to see how doing ethics in clinical settings can become a rote activity of applying an ethics algorithm to complex cases. This propensity, and the way it confounds clinical ethics decision-making, is important for practitioners to understand. In recognizing the inherent complexity of ethics and the need to be reflexive in ethical decision-making, practitioners can step back from ethics as a rote activity and instead promote the indulgence of all the real complexities that attend ethical dilemmas.

Second, as discussed above, navigating clinical ethics situations often means appropriating elements from a variety of ethical frameworks that can inform various aspects of a complicated case. While there is nothing inherently wrong with this, as Jonsen (2007) notes, we must be able to "appropriate appropriately." In contrast, those involved in dilemmas of clinical ethics often make intuitive decisions about cases and then marshal all available justifications around that decision. That is, they appropriate from various ethics theories and frameworks not because of a genuine fit with a given scenario, but in a way that rationalizes support for a position on which they have already decided (Wasserman et al. 2015).

For example, in one study, HEC members were given clinical vignettes and asked to make a decision about the appropriate course of action (Wasserman et al. 2015). They were then asked to rank their agreement with a number of justifications for their decision, half of which fit a deontological framework and half of which fit a consequentialist framework. Remember that, in theory, deontological and consequentialist positions are opposed. The former specifically ignores the moral relevance of consequences, while the latter specifically avoids moral principles in favor of promoting the best consequences. Yet in the above study, scores for deontological and consequentialist justifications *were significantly positively correlated*, regardless of what decision the respondent selected for each vignette. That is, the more strongly respondents justified their decision from a deontological framework, the more strongly they also tended to draw on consequentialist justifications.

In keeping with work in behavioral economics, which has shown that individuals tend to make decisions in all sorts of nonrational ways, the above-described study suggests that individuals tended to not utilize prior philosophical and ethical commitments and follow the logic of those toward a decision. If they had, they would have selected justifications accordingly. Doing so arguably would have required more cognitive energy in that it would have required individuals to recognize that there were justifications that were either irrelevant to their decision or even opposed to it. Conflicting evidence such as this represents a cognitive burden. Thus, the HEC members in this study made a decision and then viewed all possible justifications as supporting that decision. As with the above tendency to seek simplicity, recognizing our propensity to dismiss or minimize conflicting evidence weakens our ability give thorough and fair review to complex ethical cases. In particular, we are especially susceptible to digging our heels in once we have made a decision, even when we are presented with conflicting evidence that may warrant a thorough reconsideration of our position.

By understanding not only the complex landscape of ethical philosophy and the broad range of biomedical and social considerations that might be relevant to a particular case, but also our own psychological tendencies that may limit our ability to do clinical ethics well, practitioners ought to be able to approach ethics dilemmas with due diligence, reflexivity, and with appropriate respect for their complexity.

Conclusion: The Bioethical Imagination

In addition to introducing basic principles and considerations of clinical ethics decision-making, the purpose of this chapter was to illustrate the complexity that arises from biomedical and social terrain where different values, held by a variety of differently positioned stakeholders, are in conflict. The ability to make sense of how the empirical and the ethical terrain come together in clinical practice represents another manifestation of a strong sociological imagination (or, in this case, a strong *bioethical imagination*; De Vries et al. 2007). While we often think of clinical practice as a matter of providing the best care based on the best evidence, our personal values and social positions color how we interpret such evidence.

The value-laden nature of "facts" in clinical ethics situations is perhaps made most clear by the relatively recent case of Terri Schiavo, a woman who went into a coma after her brain was significantly deprived of oxygen, likely due to an imbalance of potassium in her body due to prolonged anorexia (Pence 2011). While the Schiavo case reprised many of the issues wrestled with in the Cruzan decision, including contested or unclear accounts of what the patient would have wanted, it also highlighted how issues of clinical ethics reflect deep-seated moral conflicts in our society over the meaning and value of life. The Schiavo case witnessed not only conflict within her family about removing her ventilator, but the intervention of activists and politicians representing various "right to life" and "right to die" organizations. Early in this chapter we described Bosk's (2010) notion of "essentially contested total social conflicts." Clinical ethics cases such as that of Terri Schiavo, even when they do not receive the same amount of press coverage, are microcosms of larger philosophical and religious debates in our culture. That is, we can understand clinical ethics cases as instances of the complex and clashing cultural values of our society. As such, navigating ethical situations in clinical practice requires "the capacity to range from the most impersonal and remote transformations to the most intimate features of the human self" (Mills 1959:7). That is, doing bioethics well in clinical practice requires a well-developed sociological imagination.

CHAPTER 11 ACTIVITY

Navigating Bioethical Decisions

Case 1

Lamech Taamira arrived at his father Abbott's house one day to find he had collapsed on the floor. He called an ambulance and Abbott was transported to the hospital where he was admitted to the medical intensive care unit (MICU). After stabilizing Abbott on a ventilator, clinicians gave him a diffusion-weighted MRI and determined that he had an embolic stroke. Over the next five weeks, Lamech begins to see that his father is improving. For nearly a month after the stroke, Abbott's eyes were closed, but now he was beginning to open them for periods of time and it appeared that he was waking up and going back to sleep throughout the day.

The neurologist Dr. Moore, however, tells Lamech that his father is in a persistent vegetative state (PVS) and that recovery from PVS in adults after three months was exceedingly rare. "Given your father's age, my recommendation is for us to remove the nutritional support, refer him to hospice, and shift the goals toward making him comfortable as he passes." Lamech informs the physician that both he and his father deeply oppose "suicide" and that his father would never have consented to "giving up." He tells Dr. Moore that their religion prohibits terminating life support. Dr. Moore says, "at this point, the feeding tube offers little to no long-term benefit." Lamech, however, responds by saying, "Who are you to say what is a benefit " it's keeping him alive isn't it?"

Dr. Moore asks for an ethics consult and you are sent to gather the facts and write a recommendation. It's clear that Dr. Moore believes that from a medical standpoint, removing the nutritional support and providing hospice care is the right thing to do. At the same time, he tells you, "I'm a religious man myself so I don't want to go against anyone's faith. But there's another concern here too. The patient is uninsured so the money for his care is coming from our charity care budget for the year."

Discussion Questions

1. Use the four principles to articulate the various ways you could approach this situation. How might autonomy, nonmaleficence, beneficence, and justice each lead to different considerations and possible conclusions?

2. Thinking about the principles of ethics together, how would you balance them in this case? Which would take precedence and why? In other words, articulate a recommendation for this situation and justify your decision using the four principles of bioethics.

3. How might you approach this from a virtue ethics or ethics of care perspective? What role does good communication play in this process?

4. From a social–psychological standpoint, what sorts of factors (including your own biases) might confound your own decision-making process?

Case 2

You're a physician in Prairie Village, Kansas, seeing a 5-year-old patient named August. He attends a day care that the mother describes as a "community co-op." Yesterday, his parents found out that two other children from the day care were diagnosed with whooping cough and this morning August woke up with a fever and runny nose. "We usually stick with less toxic, natural treatments," they tell you, "but since he's been around those other kids who got sick, we decided to bring him in."

You notice on the chart that the child has had no vaccinations. As you conduct the physical exam and take a history from the parents you find out that August has a 6-month-old sister who also is unvaccinated.

The throat exam showed no exudate and there were no obvious decreased breath sounds on chest auscultation. An immediate complete blood count (CBC) showed lymphocytosis and nasal and throat swabs were sent for culture. Your presumptive diagnosis was *Bordetella pertussis* infection (whooping cough). You recommend standard antibiotic treatment for August and also that preventive antibiotics be started in the rest of the family, especially their infant daughter. You also recommend that both children be brought up-to-date on their vaccines.

The parents, however, refuse all treatment recommendations, claiming that antibiotics "do more harm than good."

Discussion Questions

1. From an ethical standpoint, can you compel the parents to treat their son, August? Why or why not? (Use the four-principle framework described in the chapter to justify your answer).

2. From an ethical standpoint, can you compel the parents to get treatment? Why or why not? (Use the four-principle framework described in the chapter to justify your answer.)

    Helpful Hint: You may want to review the American Academy of Pediatrics statement on parental rights and the limits of informed refusal (AAP 2013).

3. From an ethical standpoint, can you compel the parents to treat their daughter preventively? Why or why not? (Use the four-principle framework described in the chapter to justify your answer.)

4. How might you approach this from a virtue ethics or ethics of care perspective? What role does good communication play in this process?

5. Is it ethical to "fire" these patients (kick them out of your practice)? Why or why not?

6. From a social–psychological standpoint, what sorts of factors (including your own biases) might confound your decision-making process?

PART IV

Health Systems and Policy

Health Care Systems and Policy

LEARNING OBJECTIVES

After reading this chapter, students should be able to

- Describe the various paradoxes of U.S. health care delivery.

- Discuss three health care system goals and American trends in each of these three important areas.

- Explain the emergence and the development of health care systems as institutions, and how these processes are influenced by social and cultural values.

- Distinguish the four models of health care systems and identify the model to which American health care delivery most closely adheres, and why.

- Describe multiple scenarios where system-level arrangements directly affect the behavior and experiences of providers, patients, and families in American health care delivery.

Introduction

American health care delivery is different from any other system worldwide, most obviously because nearly all other major industrialized nations have national health insurance programs financed largely through general tax revenues. In turn, they have universal or near-universal access for citizens (Okma 2014) and a limited private health insurance sector with strong government oversight (Frogner et al. 2011). In contrast, U.S. health care delivery is a patchwork of providers, facilities, systems, and insurers of various sorts, both private and public, with limited centralized planning or government intervention. Access is far from universal, and private insurance is largely tied to full-time employment, or depends upon the individual's ability to secure it in the marketplace. The result is a loosely organized set of quasi-systems that are "fragmented, with higher costs than any other industrialized nation since the early 1970s, uneven access to care, and unfair distributive consequences" (Okma 2014:913).

Some might also find the intense focus and extensive public discussion on health care somewhat curious because so many Americans (including health care professionals and policymakers) know so little about how our health care system actually works, and recent reforms to the system seem to have added additional layers of complexity (Budrys 2015; Sultz & Young 2014). Many factors converge to complicate this understanding. First, the American health care system is not really a system at all, at least in the common sense of the term, which implies some sort of structure resulting from centralized planning and organization. American health care is largely the result of historical circumstances, limited government intervention, professional values, and market dynamics. Next, it is also massive, constituting a $2.7 trillion industry that encompasses thousands of independent providers, practices, partnerships, and organizations; public and not-for-profit institutions like hospitals and other specialized care facilities; large and powerful corporations that manufacture drugs, supplies, and devices; and massive health care corporations responsible for insurance and many hospitals and other facilities as well. Health care is the largest service industry in the United States, and alone is the world's eighth largest economy, even larger than the total economy of Italy. But more imposing than its size, however, is its complexity. It is also in flux, and this is especially true today because of recently implemented reforms (Budrys 2015; Kovner & Knickman 2011; Light 2011; Sultz & Young 2014).

The complexity and frequent misunderstanding that surrounds health care in the United States also brings into focus a number of important paradoxes (see also the brief discussion of Bradley & Taylor 2013 in Chapter 1). First, as just mentioned, our system is by all accounts quite unsystematic. It is more aptly described as multiple parallel systems working alongside and throughout one another, and it is largely fragmented because so many people and groups seek health care services from very different sources and through various means (Okma 2014; Shi & Singh 2012). Second, when thinking about either individual or public health, we often look to health care, when in reality it has little to do with why we get sick. If we have access to care, it can hopefully help us deal with disease and illness, and may even restore many of us to some degree of health following an acute episode (although to a lesser extent in the contemporary chronic disease era). But a *lack of health care* is not the cause of disease and illness and thereby is not likely the key to pursuing health.[1] That would be like saying: since aspirin often helps resolve a fever, the *lack of aspirin* must be the cause of the fever (Adelman 2008). Surely, expanding access to care, ideally to everyone, is a laudable goal, but doing so would not eliminate disease, because today its origins are largely social and environmental in nature (see Chapter 4). Indeed, other nations have expanded care to all citizens, yet, of course, disease and health disparities persist.

Third, we spend more on health care in the United States than most of our industrialized peers, but we exhibit aggregate health indicators that lag behind those peers. Fourth, we have one of the largest and technologically rich health care systems in the world, but nonetheless seem unable to address many of the health and disease issues that typically confront most Americans today. As Sultz and Young (2014:19) explain:

> The priorities of America's heath care system— the emphasis on dramatic tertiary care, the costly and intensive efforts to fend off death of terminal patients for a

[1] Vaccines might appear to be the exception here, but these are largely *public health* measures, rather than key features of the *health care system* as most define it in the United States (Kovner & Knickman 2011). Even so, some have documented the influential roles of social, political, and environmental transformations in historically declining morbidity and mortality trends in the United States, alongside (and even prior to) the introduction of widespread vaccination (e.g., McKinlay & McKinlay 1977).

few more days or weeks, and the heroic efforts to save extremely low birth-weight infants at huge expense while thousands of women go without the prenatal care that would decrease prematurity—contribute to the obvious mismatch between the costs of health care and the failure to improve the measures of health status in the United States.

Finally, most Americans think that ours is the best health care system worldwide (and it very well may be), but many of those same Americans also express a great deal of dissatisfaction with that system (Bradley & Taylor 2013; Budrys 2015). In fact, most citizens around the world are not completely satisfied with their own health care systems (Frogner et al. 2011), while the "leaders of virtually every industrialized nation think that the cost of medical care is spiraling out of control" (Light 2013:543). Among Americans surveyed by the Commonwealth Fund in 2013, 48% claimed that the system requires fundamental changes, while only 25% reported that things work reasonably well. Additionally, 27% reported that the system should be rebuilt, which is highest among the other Western, industrialized nations surveyed and more than double the percentage of respondents reporting similar views in Norway (12%), the next highest figure in this category. On the other hand, the 25% of surveyed Americans reporting that the system works reasonably well was the lowest of all nations surveyed and a little over half than that of France (40%), which was our closest peer in this category (Mossialos et al. 2015).

Despite the distinctive and often enigmatic features of U.S. health care, in this chapter we do not offer a complete explanation of the American system, or attempt to resolve these many contradictions. In keeping with our thematic focus on the sociological imagination, we are most concerned with promoting the ability to see that health care systems (like other social institutions) largely originate with one set of very important ideas: the social and political *values* of their respective populations. Health care thereby reflects the culture and dominant ideology of its population, so much so that "medical care and health services are acts of political philosophy" (Light & Schuller 1986:9). Drawing on the "building block" metaphor from Chapter 1 highlights that American health care was constructed like a house erected over multiple generations, with each set of inhabitants building upon, remodeling, or altering the bricks of those coming before them. The builders used the bricks at their disposal that they wanted to see included in the finished product. But the social construction of institutions is never complete because we are constantly reproducing or reworking the form and function of social institutions. This creates perhaps the biggest paradox of all: the system that poses so many problems for patients, providers, and policymakers today actually originates with deeply held values among many of those same individuals and groups.

Accordingly, in this chapter we first introduce the basic goals of health care before describing four *comparative models* of health care delivery systems (articulated by Light 2013). Next, we explain how American health care delivery fits within this broader typology. We conclude by examining the broad contours of health care in the United States, not as a way to provide a comprehensive, top-down description or analysis of the system itself, but instead as a way to begin to visualize what this means for the individual experiences of patients and providers within it.

System Goals

The "three major cornerstones of health care delivery" concern *cost*, *access*, and *quality* (Shi & Singh 2012:472, see also Budrys 2014, 2015; Cockerham 2016). Each goal is important in its own right, but it is impossible to maximize all three simultaneously, because at some point, they come into conflict with one another. For example, we might encourage system-wide increases in quality by spending more and ordering more expensive tests and treatments, or embracing more advanced technology. But these measures increase costs, which, in turn, may affect access to care, if, for example, resources are diverted from primary care or from subsidizing care for high-risk groups. On the other hand, we might set our sights on reducing costs, but the trick lies in doing so without compromising quality or otherwise inhibiting access to care. In short, manipulating one or more of these factors often impacts the other two.

Budrys (2015:6–7) elaborates that these goals are ambiguously defined and can be measured in a variety of different ways:

> What does "quality" mean? Who should define it?—doctors, patients, or some group of experts authorized (by whom?) to monitor quality? How much "access"? Does access mean that patients are entitled to have all the health care services they want? Or that they can pay for? Or that someone else, say politicians, decides that they need? How do we measure "cost containment"? Do we want costs to drop or just not go up so fast? Are we prepared to cut anything the health system provides?

All of these considerations are culturally dependent in many respects, because they are defined to a large degree by group norms and values.

Historically, quality of care was probably the principal concern in the United States until the Great Depression, at which time access to care surpassed quality as the most important consideration. The rise of health insurance, however, expanded access to care during the middle decades of the twentieth century. With the increased utilization of health care services and the growth of expensive technology as a part of those services, costs gradually began to rise. Consequently, cost containment became the highest health care priority by the late twentieth century, and balancing these three considerations remains problematic today as costs continue to rise, access remains limited despite some improvements, and assessments of quality depend on how it is measured (Budrys 2014).

Costs

There are a variety of costs associated with health care delivery. Shi and Singh (2012:472) point out the following:

1. When consumers and financiers speak of the "cost" of health care, they usually mean the "price" of health care. This could refer to the physician's bill, the price of a prescription, or the premiums employers pay to purchase health insurance for their employees.
2. From a national perspective, health care costs refer to how much a nation spends on health care, that is, national health expenditures (NHE), or health care spending.

In the United States, we can assess the former with, among other things, out-of pocket costs, while we may evaluate the latter with health care expenditures as a percentage of gross domestic product (GDP) or health care expenditures per capita. Table 12.1 provides national comparisons across three measures of health care costs from the World Health Organization's *Global Health Expenditure Database.* These nations represent a subset of industrialized nations from the Organization for Economic Cooperation and Development (OECD) and therefore provide interesting points of comparison for the corresponding American data.

When it comes to out-of-pocket health care costs per capita (i.e., per person in the population), the United States is one among four nations that spend the most. The citizens of Switzerland, Norway, and Australia on average spend a bit more out-of-pocket per capita than Americans, but not by much. Importantly, calculating these figures involves dividing the total out-of-pocket expenditures by the total populations of these countries. That is, the United States typically has far higher *total* out-of-pocket expenditures than Switzerland, Norway, and Australia, but with a population well over 300 million people (compared to about 8 million, 5 million, and 23 million people, respectively), *per capita* costs in the United States tend to approximate those of its smaller peers.

We can also assess costs as a percentage of a nation's total GDP, which is a standard measure of the value of goods and services produced by a country during a period of time, typically one year (OECD.org). If we compare the United States to the nations included in Table 12.1, we can see that the United States spends 17.1% of its GDP on health care, by far the highest among industrialized nations, and in recent decades, the costs of health care have outpaced the growth in national GDP. The Netherlands, France, Switzerland, and Germany are more than 4% points behind the United States, and nations like Norway, Sweden, Australia, and the United Kingdom are in single digits as a percentage of GDP. Importantly, this

TABLE 12.1   Health Care Costs by Country, 2013

Country	Out-of-Pocket per Capita*	Health Care as %GDP	Total Health Expenditure per Capita*
Australia	1,165	9.4	6,110
Canada	865	10.9	5,718
France	360	11.7	4,864
Germany	645	11.3	5.006
Netherlands	331	12.9	6,145
New Zealand	434	9.7	4,063
Norway	1,355	9.6	9,715
Sweden	927	9.7	5,680
Switzerland	2,401	11.5	9,276
United Kingdom	334	9.1	3,598
United States	1,081	17.1	9,146

Source: World Health Organization. (2016). *Global Health Expenditure Database.* http://apps.who.int/nha/database. Accessed January 16, 2016.

Note: * In 2016, U.S. dollar equivalent.

constitutes 17.1% of the largest economy in the world, and all goods and services produced in the United States in the GDP for 2013 total to 100%. In other words, 17 cents of every dollar of goods and services produced in 2013 was in some way related to health care. As White (2011:258) explains, "although the GDP was increasing [in recent decades], creating a much bigger national economic pie, health care spending was an ever-larger slice of that pie. It also means that less of the pie is available for spending on all other goods and services." If we divide these massive total expenditures across their respective national populations, the United States is again among those nations spending the most money on health care.

In summary, the total health care spending in the United States has been the highest in the world for a long time. The responsible factors frequently identified in the health economic literature include (Frogner et al. 2011:78):

1. *Growth of the private health insurance* market with increasing administrative complexity;
2. *Supplier-induced demand*, or the ability for physicians to recommend services that may or may not be medically necessary;
3. *Defensive medicine*, or services ordered by health providers primarily to reduce the risk of malpractice lawsuits;
4. *Factor productivity*, or the ability for health care workers to complete more tasks in the same amount of time; and,
5. *Medical technology*, or expensive, advanced capital investments.

Still, costs tell only part of the story. A person who spends a great deal of money on, say, education or groceries should rightly expect value from those expenses. Likewise, as a nation we may spend a lot of money on health care, but that would be less problematic if there were returns on this investment in the areas of access and quality. Instead, as we will see, the United States struggles to maximize value from its investment in this area.

Access

Access essentially refers to a person's ability to obtain necessary, affordable, convenient, and effective care in a timely manner. This corresponds to a number of factors, including whether an individual has a usual source of health care (like a primary care physician) and whether the individual has the ability to use such services (which, among other factors, is related to the quality of insurance coverage). Access is an important reflection of the health care system because it informs assessments of overall effectiveness, particularly whether health care resources are equitably distributed and, more generally, whether those resources are getting to where they are needed (Shi & Singh 2012). Billings and colleagues (2011:152–53) explain that:

> The potential health impact of lack of insurance on patients is well documented, as are the benefits of health insurance coverage. For instance, both children and adults with Medicaid or private insurance are more likely to have a usual source of care than people who are uninsured. Having a large number of uninsured patients also has deleterious effects on the health care delivery system, as providers struggle to shift costs to other payers who can subsidize the expenses incurred by patients without coverage.[2]

---

[2] The latter phenomenon is called *cost-shifting*.

There are many ways to measure access, but exploring rates of insurance and having a source of usual care are particularly illustrative.

Table 12.2 presents the rates of *uninsurance* for the entire United States and for individual states for children (<18) and for the general population (≤65).[3] In these data, an individual is uninsured if he or she is not covered by private insurance, Medicare, Medicaid, or any other type of civilian, military, or

TABLE 12.2 Percent of Persons without Health Insurance Coverage by Age and State; United States, 2013

	<18 years	<65 years		<18 years	<65 years
United States	7.1	16.7	Missouri	7.3	15.2
Alabama	4.5	15.9	Montana	10.4	19.7
Alaska	11.7	20.3	Nebraska	5.9	12.2
Arizona	12.1	20.3	Nevada	13.9	23.4
Arkansas	5.7	18.8	New Hampshire	3.5	12.6
California	7.3	19.3	New Jersey	5.7	15.3
Colorado	8.4	15.7	New Mexico	9.0	22.2
Connecticut	4.1	10.8	New York	4.1	12.4
Delaware	5.1	11.7	North Carolina	5.9	18.0
District of Columbia	2.2*	7.1	North Dakota	7.7	11.9
Florida	11.0	24.2	Ohio	5.1	12.8
Georgia	9.5	21.1	Oklahoma	10.5	20.4
Hawaii	3.2	8.3	Oregon	6.3	17.4
Idaho	8.3	18.5	Pennsylvania	5.0	11.3
Illinois	4.3	14.4	Rhode Island	6.0	13.9
Indiana	8.4	16.2	South Carolina	7.0	18.4
Iowa	4.8	10.2	South Dakota	7.2	14.3
Kansas	6.6	14.3	Tennessee	5.7	16.2
Kentucky	5.9	16.8	Texas	12.5	24.5
Louisiana	5.6	19.2	Utah	9.0	14.7
Maine	5.1	13.3	Vermont	*	8.1
Maryland	4.3	11.4	Virginia	5.7	14.1
Massachusetts	1.5	4.4	Washington	6.3	16.1
Michigan	4.2	12.8	West Virginia	4.0	16.1
Minnesota	6.1	9.5	Wisconsin	4.4	10.4
Mississippi	7.3	19.6	Wyoming	6.3	14.6

Source: National Center for Health Statistics (NCHS). (2015). *Health, United States, 2014: With Special Feature on Adults Aged 55–64.* Hyattsville, MD: U.S. Department of Health & Human Services, Centers for Disease Control & Prevention.

* Denotes that data are considered unreliable and are therefore excluded.

[3] At 65 years of age, U.S. citizens qualify for insurance coverage under Medicare, making the rate of uninsurance at or near zero for those older than 65. Because other industrialized nations offer universal or near-universal access, we can assume that they have uninsurance rates at or near zero.

government health care coverage. About 7% of children under age 18 are uninsured in the United States, compared to nearly 17% across the total population less than 65 years old. Of course, state-level figures vary widely, with several states reporting greater than 20%, or one in five, of its residents uninsured, and two states approach 25%. Similarly, in multiple states more than one in ten children experience uninsurance, while some states like Vermont offer particularly accessible low- or no-cost coverage to qualifying children, lowering these rates tremendously. These numbers point to a problematic lack of access to the health care system, particularly when we remember the high percentage of GDP and the absolute value of money and resources that the United States invests in that system. Underscoring the scale of the problem, these figures do not reflect those who are *underinsured*, meaning their insurance does not give them access to all necessary or required services, or fails to protect them from incurring significant financial debt if they do access those services (Billings et al. 2011; Sanger-Katz 2016; Weiss 2013). Exacerbating these problems, Light (2011:129–30) points out that private health insurance in the United States reflects the *inverse coverage law*, where "the greater the risk of a group or individual, the less coverage will be offered and the more it will cost."

Tables 12.3 and 12.4 present a similar picture in depicting the percentage of adults and children without a usual source of care. Nearly half (46.4%) of children with no insurance coverage in 2012–13 had no usual source of health care (like a primary care physician), including about one-third (33.6%) of children under age 6 and about half aged 6–17. More than nine out of ten uninsured adults during the same period did not have a usual source of care for their health needs. Here again, the data suggest significant gaps in access to care. Moreover, access is not equitably distributed, but rather those in the lower SES strata, particularly the working poor[4], tend to be the most disadvantaged (Light 2011; NCHS 2015; Weiss 2013).

Quality

In the United States, health care is obviously very expensive and many citizens are unable to access health care services routinely and affordably. But the return on our collective investment in the health care system may still demonstrate value if it manifests levels of quality that are proportional to that investment. Indeed, in many ways medical care in the United States is the best in the world. As Budrys (2015) notes, many people travel from abroad to use the American health care system and we have some of the best medical technology worldwide. However, while some people do travel to the United States for care, those people also tend to be able to pay for that care, and most typically come to the United States to avoid the lines or waiting periods associated with nonemergency care or procedures in other nations, or to receive care not yet available in other countries. First, if you need knee

---

[4] Uninsured Americans tend to be employed, white, and subsisting at or around the federal poverty level, although in recent years members of the American middle class are at an increasing risk of uninsurance and underinsurance. The term *working poor* refers to people that are "working full-time or part-time, are on temporary layoff or are unemployed and actively looking for work *and* whose families earn less than 200 percent of the federal poverty level" (Weiss 2013:344).

TABLE 12.3 Percent of Children under 18 with No Usual Source of Health Care, United States, Average Annual, Selected Years 1993–1994 through 2012–2013

Percent of Children without a Usual Source of Health Care

	<18 years			<6 years			6-17 years		
	1993–1994	1999–2000	2012–2013	1993–1994	1999–2000	2012–2013	1993–1994	1999–2000	2012–2013
Insured continuously all 12 months	4.6	3.6	2.3	3.1	2.3	1.5	5.5	4.2	2.7
Uninsured for any period up to 12 months	15.3	15.0	12.7	10.9	12.5	10.1	18.1	16.4	14.1
Uninsured for more than 12 months	27.6	35.8	33.7	21.4	26.8	23.5	30.0	39.1	36.3

Source: National Center for Health Statistics (NCHS). (2015). *Health, United States, 2014: With Special Feature on Adults Aged 55–64.* Hyattsville, MD: U.S. Department of Health & Human Services, Centers for Disease Control & Prevention.

TABLE 12.4 Percent of Adults (18–64 years) with No Usual Source of Health Care, United States, Average Annual, Selected Years 1993–1994 through 2012–2013

Percent of Adults without a Usual Source of Health Care

	1993–1994	1999–2000	2001–2002	2003–2004	2005–2006	2007–2008	2009–2010	2012–2013
Insured continuously all 12 months	12.7	10.3	8.3	8.7	8.9	9.1	9.8	10.0
Uninsured for any period up to 12 months	30.9	31.2	33.3	32.1	33.4	35.1	36.5	34.1
Uninsured for more than 12 months	46.9	54.8	54.6	55.0	58.0	56.1	59.5	57.9

Source: National Center for Health Statistics (NCHS). (2015). *Health, United States, 2014: With Special Feature on Adults Aged 55–64.* Hyattsville, MD: U.S. Department of Health & Human Services, Centers for Disease Control & Prevention.

surgery in many other industrialized nations, you may have to wait a few weeks or months depending on the severity of the condition. However, if you have the means to pay for it and access to a qualified physician in the United States, it is more likely that you will wait only a few days. Next, the United States is often where major medical breakthroughs frequently originate[5], involving procedures not yet available in most or all other countries, thereby attracting patients from around the world. There are many examples to cite here, but one involves the British National Health Service (NHS), who for many years sent most cases of retinopathy of prematurity to Beaumont Hospital in Royal Oak, Michigan, where patients received timely, state-of-the art treatment from American health professionals who are recognized as among the best in the world.[6] While technology can also be another important element of quality care (and of rising costs), other nations have similar technology,[7] and more medical technology may not correspond to greater health care quality overall, particularly in the chronic illness era where low-tech preventative measures may be more effective for actually preventing disease.

As noted, quality in health care is quite difficult to define and measure. Containing costs in the United States was the major health care priority in the 1990s, and while it remains important today, there has been greater emphasis on assessing quality due to concerns that cost controls may degrade the quality of care that people receive (Shi & Singh 2012). In addition, many public and private organizations have emerged in recent years to measure and oversee health care quality and they use wildly different methodologies. There are now so many different hospital ratings, for example, that more than 1,600 medical centers can claim to be on a "top 100," "honor roll," grade "A," or "best" hospitals list (Rau 2013; Wachter 2016). Despite measurement issues and the shifting tides of quality assessment, two widely used proxies of population health provide a good illustration of quality outcomes of the U.S. health care system as a whole—*infant mortality* and *life expectancy*. While life expectancy has obvious import as an aggregate health quality measure, infant mortality may be the "most accurate indicator of a country's health status" (Budrys 2015:3) and reflects many dimensions of health, like a society's ability (or commitment) to protecting its most vulnerable members, or general socio-economic development.

Data in Tables 12.5 and 12.6 come from the National Center for Health Statistics and depict infant mortality rates and life expectancy at birth for OECD countries. At 6.1 infant deaths before one year of age (per 1,000 live births), infant mortality in the United States is double and sometimes nearly triple that of some OECD partners. In 1960, the United States ranked eleventh internationally in infant mortality; by 2011, that ranking dropped to twenty-seventh. In 2011, the United States ranked only above Turkey, Mexico, and Chile among other OECD nations. It is also worth remembering that these figures represent national aggregates. By state, infant mortality ranges from a high of 9.6 per 1,000 live births in Mississippi to a low

---

[5] Likely because of the level of medical expertise in the United States, and because in the United States we readily accept very high costs as the price of medical innovation.

[6] Thanks to Mark Haimann, MD, for this example, and for his thoughtful comments on this chapter.

[7] The United States possesses more total technology, probably because of its larger population, while some nations report more per capita (Budrys 2015).

TABLE 12.5 Infant Mortality Rates and International Rankings: Organization for Economic Cooperation and Development Countries, Selected Years, 1960–2011

Country	1960	1980	2000	2010	2011	International Ranking 1960	International Ranking 2011
Australia	20.2	10.7	5.2	4.1	3.8	5	19
Austria	37.5	14.3	4.8	3.9	3.6	19	16
Belgium	31.4	12.1	4.8	3.6	3.4	17	10
Canada	27.3	10.4	5.3	5.0	4.8	12	23
Chile	120.3	33.0	8.9	7.4	7.7	27	28
Czech Republic	20.0	16.9	4.1	2.7	2.7	4	5
Denmark	21.5	8.4	5.3	3.4	3.5	8	12
Finland	21.0	7.6	3.8	2.3	2.4	6	3
France	27.7	10.0	4.5	3.6	3.5	13	12
Germany	35.0	12.4	4.4	3.4	3.6	18	16
Greece	40.1	17.9	5.9	3.8	3.4	20	10
Hungary	47.6	23.2	9.2	5.3	4.9	23	24
Ireland	29.3	11.1	6.2	3.6	3.5	15	12
Israel	—	15.6	5.5	3.7	3.5	—	12
Italy	43.9	14.6	4.3	3.2	2.9	22	6
Japan	30.7	7.5	3.2	2.3	2.3	16	2
Korea	—	—	—	3.2	3.0	—	7
Mexico	92.3	52.6	20.8	14.1	13.7	26	30
Netherlands	22.6	8.6	5.1	3.8	3.6	2	16
New Zealand	22.6	13.0	6.3	5.5	5.2	10	26
Norway	16.0	8.1	3.8	2.8	2.4	1	3
Poland	56.1	25.4	8.1	5.0	4.7	24	22
Portugal	77.5	24.3	5.5	2.5	3.1	25	8
Slovak Republic	28.6	20.9	8.6	5.7	4.9	14	24
Spain	43.7	12.3	4.3	3.2	3.2	21	9
Sweden	16.6	6.9	3.4	2.5	2.1	3	1
Switzerland	21.1	9.1	4.9	3.8	3.8	7	19
Turkey	189.5	117.5	31.6	7.8	7.7	28	28
United Kingdom	22.5	12.1	5.6	4.2	4.3	8	21
United States	26.0	12.6	6.9	6.1	6.1	11	27

Source: National Center for Health Statistics (NCHS). (2015). *Health, United States, 2014: With Special Feature on Adults Aged 55–64*. Hyattsville, MD: U.S. Department of Health & Human Services, Centers for Disease Control & Prevention.

Note: — Data not available.

TABLE 12.6 Life Expectancy at Birth, by Sex: Organization for Economic Cooperation and Development (OECD) Countries, Selected Years, 1980–2012

Country (at birth)	Males				Females			
	1980	1990	2000	2012	1980	1990	2000	2012
Australia	71.0	73.9	76.6	79.9	78.1	80.1	82.0	84.3
Austria	69.0	72.3	75.2	78.4	76.1	79.0	81.2	83.6
Belgium	69.9	72.7	74.6	77.8	76.7	79.5	81.0	83.1
Canada	71.7	74.4	76.3	79.3*	78.9	80.8	81.7	83.6*
Chile	—	69.4	73.7	76.3	—	76.5	80.0	81.4
Czech Republic	66.9	67.6	71.6	75.1	74.0	75.5	78.5	81.2
Denmark	71.2	72.0	74.5	78.1	77.3	77.8	79.2	82.1
Estonia	64.2	64.7	65.6	71.4	74.3	74.9	76.4	81.5
Finland	69.2	71.0	74.2	77.7	78.0	79.0	81.2	83.7
France	70.2	72.8	75.3	78.7	78.4	80.9	83.0	85.4
Germany	69.6	72.0	75.1	78.6	76.2	78.5	81.2	83.3
Greece	73.0	74.7	75.5	78.0	77.5	79.5	80.9	83.4
Hungary	65.5	65.2	67.5	71.6	72.8	73.8	76.2	78.7
Iceland	73.5	75.5	77.8	81.6	80.4	80.7	81.6	84.3
Ireland	70.1	72.1	74.0	78.7	75.6	77.7	79.2	83.2
Israel	72.1	74.9	76.7	79.9	75.7	78.4	80.9	83.6
Italy	70.6	73.8	76.9	79.8	77.4	80.3	82.8	84.8
Japan	73.4	75.9	77.7	79.9	78.8	81.9	84.6	86.4
Korea	61.8	67.3	72.3	77.9	70.0	75.5	79.6	84.6
Luxembourg	70.0	72.4	74.6	79.1	75.6	78.7	81.3	83.8
Mexico	64.1	67.0	70.5	71.4	70.2	74.0	76.1	77.3
Netherlands	72.5	73.8	75.6	79.3	79.2	80.2	80.7	83.0
New Zealand	70.1	72.5	75.9	79.7	76.2	78.4	80.8	83.2
Norway	72.4	73.4	76.0	79.5	79.3	79.9	81.5	83.5
Poland	66.0	66.3	69.6	72.7	74.4	75.3	78.0	81.1
Portugal	67.9	70.6	73.3	77.3	74.9	77.5	80.4	83.6
Slovak Republic	66.7	66.7	69/2	72.5	74.4	75.7	77.5	79.9
Slovenia	—	69.8	72.2	77.1	—	77.8	79.9	83.3
Spain	72.3	73.4	75.8	79.5	78.4	80.6	82.9	85.5
Sweden	72.8	74.8	77.4	79.9	79.0	80.5	82.0	83.6
Switzerland	72.3	74.0	77.0	80.6	79.0	80.9	82.8	84.9
Turkey	55.8	65.4	69.0	72.0	60.3	69.5	73.1	77.2
United Kingdom	70.2	72.9	75.5	79.1	76.2	78.5	80.3	82.8
United States	70.0	71.8	74.1	76.4	77.4	78.8	79.3	81.2

Source: National Center for Health Statistics (NCHS). (2015). *Health, United States, 2014: With Special Feature on Adults Aged 55–64.* Hyattsville, MD: U.S. Department of Health & Human Services, Centers for Disease Control & Prevention.

Note: * 2011 data; 2012 estimates unavailable. — Data not available.

of 4.2 in Massachusetts[8] (Matthews et al. 2015), while there are even more dramatic disparities in infant mortality across neighborhoods, city blocks, and census tracts.

Life expectancy exhibits similar patterns. For female life expectancy in 2012, the United States and the Czech Republic are just outside of the top two-dozen OECD nations (81.2 years), trailing slightly behind Estonia (81.5 years) and Slovenia (83.3 years) and just ahead of Poland (81.1 years), but well behind France (85.4 years) and Spain (85.5 years). Longevity among American males, on the other hand, is about 76.4 years, just behind Slovenia (77.1 years) and Korea (77.9 years) but well behind Iceland (81.6 years), Switzerland (80.6 years), Sweden (79.9 years), and Canada (79.3 years). The data suggest that on both life expectancy and infant mortality indicators, the United States ranks nowhere near the top among industrialized nations, and over recent decades, has lost ground.

The data and discussion up to this point reflect the unique character of American health care delivery. On the whole, we spend more yet have less favorable access and quality outcomes. But these trends do not illustrate the full story, particularly where there is a very unequal distribution of advantages and disadvantages in the U.S. system. Caronna and Ong (2011:181–82) go on to explain:

> People with relatively few health issues, generous health insurance coverage, and a regular primary care provider might see the [U.S.] system as acceptable and even ideal. But for many others—often the ones who need medical care most—the system can be frustrating and even dangerous. Patients with several conditions, especially chronic ones, are likely to receive conflicting treatment plans from different specialists and prescriptions for drugs that adversely interact. Patients with low health literacy can be overwhelmed and bewildered by complex instructions, making treatment plans difficult to follow. And, for uninsured patients, most of the medical care system is simply out-of-reach.

But if health care systems reflect the values of the populations that they serve, what values does the American system reflect? In the next section, we explore different health care archetypes, each of which reflects different values and goals that shape efforts to respond to various epidemiological conditions while balancing cost, quality, and access.

Health Care System Models

It is important to remember that all health systems have shortcomings because issues related to cost, quality, and access often exist in tension with one another. Efforts to enhance one or more of these often produce unintended effects in the others. One way that many scholars, professionals, and policymakers try to anticipate the effects of this or that system or intervention involves comparing the various ways that countries (or subsystems within countries) deliver health care services. This type of comparative analysis often opens up our thinking to novel ways of doing things by providing new insights on our own approaches to health care delivery. The experiences and outcomes of other systems offer lessons that can

---

[8] As comparative data, Mississippi's infant mortality is in the range of Romania (9.89), Thailand (9.63), Bahrain (9.35), and Botswana (8.93), while Massachusetts is in the range of the United Kingdom (4.38), Australia (4.37), Denmark (4.05), and Slovenia (4.00) (*CIA World Factbook* 2016).

be applied to our own problems, like those related to cost, access, and quality, or inefficiency, duplication, or ineffectiveness of some services (Frogner et al. 2011). Often, however, these problems have more to do with a society itself rather than the nature of its health care delivery, since "Medicine is largely a repair service that patches up people or rescues them *after* they get in trouble" (Light 2013:543). Inequities in health care reflect socioeconomic status, geography, system-level economic and political policies, and so on, just like various social determinants affect health itself. Accordingly, comparative discussions should consider the elemental aspects of the societies and cultures in which respective systems and institutions operate, and the core element of all these systems are the values upon which they are built and the interests they serve (Light 2013).

One way to conceive of health care systems describes how three types of actors—the state (or government), non-governmental actors, and the market—engage in three types of action—financing, health service provision, and regulation (Wendt et al. 2009). While this yields a typology of twenty-seven theoretical systems, Donald Light (2013) provides a more useful set of comparative models that illuminate similarities and differences in health care systems across several key domains (see Table 12.7). This includes how states, non-governmental actors, and markets variously engage in financing, service provisions, and regulation, but importantly, Light's (2013) models highlight that these systems are coordinated around key societal values and the interests of particular stakeholders. These four models do not correspond to actual health care systems. Rather, they are *ideal types* that characterize "the essential and coherent relationships that inform them" (Light 2013:546), and provide unambiguous constructs to use in comparative and historical analysis (see Weber [1922] 1978; Wendt et al. 2009). They are not *ideal* in terms of being the most desirable or perfect manifestations of health care, but instead, they emphasize particular *ideas* (i.e., values) that underpin different health systems. In reality, most health care systems actually blend elements of several of these models, often creating contradictions like those described earlier in this chapter. In the next several sections, we draw heavily from Light (2013) to show how and why systems originate and function as they do, and to provide a basis upon which we can comparatively evaluate the U.S. health care system. Later we return to analyze how the values and structures underpinning American health care shape the behavior and experiences of providers and patients within it.

The Mutual Aid Model

The world's first national health insurance law was passed in Germany in 1883, and that system was firmly based on sickness funds that emerged from the mutual support systems originating in medieval miners' associations and guilds (Bärning-hausen & Sauerborn 2002; Brockmann & Schulz 2014). As far back as the sixteenth and seventeenth centuries, relief funds were developed among various groups, often around labor guilds, designed to collectively deal with the inevitable impacts of accidents, illness, and death. These associations quickly spread across Europe, continuing well into the nineteenth century (Garrioch 2011). Members regularly contributed small amounts of money and local councils administered funds and services (Light 2000). These funds provided money to those that became ill, or to their families if they died, including sick pay, compensation for lost wages, medical services, and medications. Beyond simply providing financial support in times of need, many of these associations were politically active, particularly in advocating for workers' rights and workplace safety (Di Cimbrini 2015; Light 2013).

The ideal type of the *mutual aid model* of health care is principally structured by the key values of (1) supporting fellow members and families when struck by illness; (2) minimizing accidents, illness, and unhealthy conditions; (3) promoting ties and mutual support among members; and (4) minimizing the financial impact of sickness (Light 2013:540). Solidarity is thus an important value in such systems (Light 2000). In countries adopting a mutual aid model, health consumer groups often organized themselves well before physicians were able to do so. As a result, they were able to dictate the terms of service to physicians, instead of vice versa (Abel-Smith 1976). In terms of the actors and actions of this system, we would say that non-governmental actors (the aid societies themselves) take on the primary role in financing and regulation, contracting with local doctors for the provision of services. Power within this system is both local and democratic so that the state and health care professions play secondary roles, and health services focus on low-technology primary care (Light 2000). This model characterizes the early Prussian and German approaches to health care delivery (Light 2013; Light & Schuller 1986), which closely align with what others (e.g., Frogner et al. 2011) call the Bismarck model. However, Jost (2012) has argued that the value of solidarity in the face of sickness at the heart of the mutual aid model also has informed state-governed systems, even including Medicare and Medicaid in the United States. Still, state models reflect a number of significant differences from these locally organized and administered collectives.

The State Model

In the state model of health care, governments develop national health insurance programs with the goal of protecting the interests of the state or larger society. Here the government displaces and assumes the activities originally undertaken by mutual aid groups. This includes the role of promoting social welfare by caring for the sick, but the state is also interested in minimizing the costs of health care services (for which it typically pays). This leads to a greater effort placed on minimizing illness through prevention and health promotion (which tends to be more cost-effective). In the ideal type of the state model, however, the state controls financing (usually through general taxes, though sometimes subsidized by insurance premiums), regulation (including price-setting for health care goods and services), and service provision (including employment of most or all health care providers) (Wendt et al. 2009). However, the way that state models take shape and execute health care delivery depends significantly on whether the state is democratic or autocratic in character (Light 2000, 2013).

Autocratic states might employ health care as a vital tool for indoctrinating its citizens or for shoring up its own political ideology. Hinote and colleagues (2009b:1256) describe such a phenomenon in Soviet society:

> the Soviet experiment was first and foremost an ideocratic regime ... [T]he primary social unit under Soviet-style communism was the collective, which served to ensure conformity while discouraging any sense of individualism. The implementation and provision of state services in economic sectors like housing and health care also reinforced the paternalistic character of Soviet leadership and social life.

TABLE 12.7 Comparison of Light's (2013) Four Health Care Models

	Mutual Aid Model	State/Societal Model	Professional Model	Corporatist Model
Key Values and Goals[1]	• *To support fellow members and their families when ill.* • To minimize accidents, illness, and unhealthy conditions. • To promote ties and mutual support among members. • To minimize the financial impact of illness.	• *To strengthen the state via a healthy, vigorous population.* • To minimize illness and maximize self-care. • To minimize the cost of medical services to the state. • To provide good, accessible care to all sectors of the population. • To indoctrinate or control through health care.[2]	• *To provide the best possible clinical care to every sick patient (who can pay and who lives near where a doctor has chosen to practice).* • To develop scientific medicine to its highest level. • To protect the autonomy of physicians and services. • To increase the power and wealth of the profession. • To increase the prestige of the profession.	• *To join together buyers and sellers, providers, and patients in deciding the range and costs of services.* • To minimize conflict through mandatory negotiation and consensus. • To balance costs against provider interests.
Power	• Local control. Mutual decision-making. • State and profession relatively weak.	• Centered on the governance structure of the society, either democratic or autocratic, or a cross-mixture.	• Centers on the medical profession, and uses state powers to enhance its own.	• Countervailing power structure. Subject to imbalance by one party or another. • Statutory powers to determine range and costs in the corporatist body itself. • State as the ultimate setter of rules and referee.
Finance and Costs	• Members contribute to an insurance fund which contracts with doctors and facilities for service. • Costs low compared to Professional model.	• All care free or nearly free. • Taxes, premiums, or a mix. • Costs relatively low. Doctor's share relatively low.	• Private payments by individual or through passive reimbursement by insurance plans. • Costs about twice the % GNP of the Societal model. • Doctor's share greater than the Societal model.	• Depends on the organization of the underlying health care system and resulting terms of countervailing negotiations." In German model, employers and employees contribute premiums. • Costs depend on results of negotiations and on society's sense of limits. • Doctors' share has tended to be high because they run services and dominate negotiations, but not inherent in the model.

Source: Abstracted and condensed from Light, Donald. (2013). "Comparative Models of 'Health Care' Systems." Pp. 543–57 in *The Sociology of Health & Illness: Critical Perspectives*, 9th edition. Peter Conrad & Valerie Leiter, eds. New York: Worth.

Notes: [1]Main/overarching goal is italicized. [2]Goal of the autocratic state variation only.

Cockerham and colleagues (2006) further explain that Soviet health care thus affected citizens by discouraging a sense of individual accountability when it came to their health lifestyles, since the state would assume responsibility for citizens if and when they became ill.

But not all systems reflecting the *state model* do so beneath autocratic regimes. Based on what Frogner and colleagues (2011) call the Beveridge model, the British National Health Service (NHS), for example, mitigates decision-making on the part of citizens, but most agree that the British government does not use the NHS as an instrument of indoctrination. The crucial distinction between the state and mutual aid models pertains to power and control over managing the system. While decision-making might flow out of a highly centralized government or regime in autocratic states to maintain stringent control over various aspects of social life (see the Soviet example above), democratic states tend to delegate more decision-making to the district or local levels (Ahgren 2014; Berwick et al. 2008; Light 2000). In the British NHS, the government provides and finances health care, and this single-payer system is what most Americans think of as socialized medicine. However, Wendt et al. (2009:84) note that in Britain, "the introduction of an internal market… has not led to the replacement of the state as the main regulator; however, it has created some space for self-regulation by NHS trusts." This highlights how most health systems blend various elements of public and private financing, regulation, and service provisions. The purest forms of the state or Beveridge model are actually found in Cuba and the U.S. Department of Veterans Affairs, since government oversees the total administration and delivery of health care in these systems (Reid 2009).

The state model reflects key values like (1) strengthening the state through a healthy and vigorous population; (2) minimizing illness and maximizing self-care; (3) minimizing health costs to the state; (4) providing good, accessible care to citizens; and (5) enhancing loyalty to the state (Light 2013:543). Because the government is often the single payer, costs in theory are kept relatively low, but, like other models, state health care systems struggle with cost containment (Maynard & Street 2006). The share of expenditures kept by providers is also low and primary care represents a core focus in health care delivery. When expenditures approach an upper acceptable limit, governments raise investment and expenditures, ideally in a somewhat controlled manner. Doing so requires maintaining an awareness of the potential ways that quality of care may be adversely affected, while access in this model is typically less affected (or not affected at all) since citizens are insured by the state itself. For instance, in 2000 the British government began a new NHS investment program, whereby health care spending increased by 7% per year for seven years, and toward the end of these reforms, it was clear that increased costs had improved some services, including decreased wait times, greater use of acute and primary care facilities, and newer and updated infrastructure. However, this spending increase did not result in improvements in every respect. Technologies were approved despite marginal cost-effectiveness, there was overlap of technology across the system, and some reforms were unevenly implemented due to local cost constraints (Maynard & Street 2006). Still, because the state retains controlling interest in financing, regulation, and service provision, it theoretically has the ability to contain costs in various ways (Wendt 2009). In the United States, on the other hand, there is no consensus on what the upper bounds of acceptable spending might be, and costs continue to rise past 17% of GDP with thousands of dollars of per capita out-of-pocket health spending (see Table 12.1 above), despite the access and quality issues discussed above.

The Professional Model

The professional model finds the medical professionals, historically physicians, at the center of health care financing, regulation, and service provision. Here health care professions leverage their expertise, citing the need for professional autonomy, particularly in clinical decision-making, in order to provide the best care for patients. The *professional model* emphasizes the key values of (1) providing the best possible clinical care to every sick patient that can pay for such care; (2) developing scientific medicine to its highest level; and (3) promoting and protecting the autonomy, power, wealth, and prestige of the medical profession (Light 2013:546).

The centrality of the medical profession means that other parts of the system, including financing and reimbursement structures, are arranged in ways that prioritize the role of medical practice and the interaction between the provider and the patient, with providers occupying dominant roles in these relationships. Regulation is also dominated by providers, particularly through professional associations that wield strong influence in health policy discussions and through the ability to set training standards, thereby regulating entry to the field through medical education. The emphasis on high-quality clinical care often translates into a reliance upon high-technology interventions in a complex and highly differentiated health care division of labor, as opposed to a focus on primary care and prevention (see also Chapter 10). As a result, costs are high in the professional model, largely because third-party payers historically reimbursed charges from providers almost without question, in deference to the expertise of their clinical judgment. This reflects the central role of health professionals (typically physicians), buttressed by the autonomy, power, and prestige given to those professionals. While payers have more recently embraced greater cost containment measures, systems reflecting this model remain expensive, in large part due to the focus on diagnostic and treatment procedures and resistance to cost control measures that might interfere with the clinical autonomy of providers.

Throughout its historical development, the American health care system most closely adheres to the principles of this model. This is a system that largely reflects the pursuits and priorities of elite business and political interests, along with minimal government regulation. It leaves room for relatively unimpeded choice for both patients and providers, thereby opening the door for various phenomena described below like moral hazard, provider-induced demand, overdiagnosis, and over-treatment (Light 2000). As a result, this system promotes a more liberal approach to tests and procedures that might offer disproportionately small benefits to the individual patient relative to his or her costs to the system, because the commitment of the professional to the patient does not require an accounting of costs at the system level. These features help explain some of the paradoxes in U.S. system, underscoring why a top health care system shows tepid returns (health outcomes) on its investments (cost) and has such dramatic inequities in terms of access.

The rise of the professional model in the United States continued largely unabated throughout much of the twentieth century. But more recently, there has been a decline in private physicians' practices in American health care delivery, along with the deprofessionalization of medicine, coinciding with the rise of corporate health care, where large health care and insurance corporations employ more and more practitioners and own more and more facilities. Nonetheless, while their power and autonomy have declined, physicians still play a major role in American health care, although other professional groups like nurse practitioners and physician assistants continue to encroach upon the terrain historically claimed by professional medicine (see Chapter 10). Even before recent health care reforms, Wendt et al. (2009:85) notes, "The U.S. healthcare system has often been taken as an ideal-type private model. However, today, it is mainly financed out of public funds since it is heavily tax-subsidized ... today [it] can be described as a private-based mixed type." So while American health care delivery still closely adheres to the professional model, it is now very much in a period of contested transition, particularly on the heels of the Patient Protection and Affordable Care Act of 2010.

The Corporatist Model

Quite distinct from the notion of corporate health care that now exists in the United States, the fourth model is a corporatist model. This is a hybrid model that draws upon attributes of the other three types described above, "a structured counterbalancing of the conflicting priorities and values of citizen/consumers (mutual-aid), providers (profession), and payers (the state and employers)" (Light 2013:552). The key values involve (1) joining together buyers and sellers, and providers and patients, to decide the range and costs of services and an acceptable budget to deliver those services; (2) minimizing conflict through negotiation and consensus; and (3) balancing costs against provider interests (Light 2013:552). Many European systems have moved toward corporatist models where they have tried to capitalize on the efficiency of private markets, without undermining access and the ability to control costs. The result is that governments retain oversight and regulate the roles of different players, often mandating that they arrive at agreements that achieve particular benchmarks in terms of cost, quality, and access. In the Netherlands, for example:

> Officially recognized representative associations of providers, health insurers, employers, and employees are given substantial authority to negotiate health care prices and other contractual conditions, to determine the supply of medical manpower, and to establish premiums and benefits for social health insurance programs. They are granted a majority of seats in the national advisory and superintendent bodies, which play a determining role in the decision-making process. Examples include the COTG, which monitors health care prices; the Sickness Fund Council, which supervises the administration of the social health insurance programs; and the National Council for Public Health, which is the main advisory body on general health policy matters. The associations are given a representative monopoly in exchange for their compliance with public interest by disciplining members according to public goals. Generally, the associations are encouraged to comply with the public interest under threat of direct state intervention. (Schut 1995:622–23)

Other national health insurance systems have adopted similar corporatist strategies in an attempt to capitalize on the respective strengths of private and public systems, including Canada, Taiwan, and South Korea (Frogner et al. 2011).

As described above, the German system originated in the mutual aid model, but German physicians eventually professionalized and institutionalized the goals of the professional model (including greater autonomy, fee-for-service, and an emphasis on acute intervention) (Light 2013). But the rising costs that emerged as an effect of the professional model compelled restructuring more akin to corporatism. This is good illustration of how, in the real world, most systems blend elements of these four ideal type models, in response to the relentless pressures of delivering quality care to large populations at a price that is both affordable and acceptable to all players involved. During the period when the mutual aid model emerged, there were limited technologies available to medicine, and acute injury and infection were the most significant mortality risks. That was a landscape where health care was, relatively speaking, inherently low-cost and relationships between patients and providers were relatively straightforward. Today, chronic illness management is organized around clinical expertise and practice that utilizes a variety of high-tech and constantly emerging treatment options, along with a highly specialized division of labor necessitating the coordination of multiple practitioners to address complex disorders. This requires a health care model matched to that complexity. In short, health care systems of all types emerge to solve the problems emerging from epidemiology, but as they evolve they are molded by the social and political interests of various constituencies (patients, providers, and states) participating in the institution and administration of health care.

Health Care in the United States

Complex, intersecting, and sometimes competing social and political values underlie American health care delivery. These values change over time in response to the needs and interests of various stakeholders, as well as disease patterns; so, what we have today is largely the end result of the building block metaphor described previously. That is, over time those responsible for maintaining health care added or subtracted various aspects in response to various challenges. But insofar as our primary objective in this book involves cultivating a sociological imagination, it is important for providers to be able to see *themselves* within the health *system*. That is, unpacking the real significance of health system insights, and the relative strengths and weaknesses of different approaches, requires examining how what is unfolding at the systems levels of health care delivery affects the behavior, expectations, and experiences of providers, patients, family members, colleagues, and others.

Provider-Induced Demand and Overtreatment

An affinity for health care is firmly rooted in American culture. In the United States, we possess a widespread tendency to look to medical care to solve many of our problems (see Chapter 7 on medicalization; Conrad 2005). When the practitioner autonomy of the professional model is combined with the value of providing the most sophisticated care possible to individual patients, along with payments to providers based on treatments and services (e.g., prescribing medications, treatments, and surgeries), and where concerns about cost are far removed from the provider–patient interaction,[9] social forces align in ways that promote overdiagnosis and overtreatment. Our first example shows how providers can drive these dynamics, leading to overtreatment and high system costs (later we examine patients' roles as well):

> Jake Waterman routinely had sinus problems since puberty, but they typically were well-managed with over-the-counter medications. However, one day he developed a particularly bad sinus infection with accompanying headache that persisted into the night, and multiple over-the-counter sinus and analgesic medications did little to alleviate the pain. At 2am, only an hour or so after having taken a dose of a phenylephrine-based sinus medication, he took a stronger, pseudoephedrine-based medicine. Still nothing worked, so he went to an urgent care clinic hoping to get a prescription for a cortico-steroid inhalant that might reduce the inflammation.

> The nurse and physician at the urgent care noted Jake's elevated blood pressure (146 over 118). Despite the fact that he had no history of high blood pressure and the sinus medications he took were the most obvious explanation for his elevated blood pressure, they sent him straight to the emergency room, with no treatment for his sinus headache. At the emergency room his blood pressure was recorded as 138/97 and an electrocardiogram test showed that everything was normal.

> Still, Jake was taken back to a room, where he was seen by two nurses, one resident, and the attending physician over the next two hours. Each asked him a series of largely routine questions, took his blood pressure, which remained slightly elevated, and examined his vitals. Jake explained to each that he had taken a higher-than-recommended amount of sinus medication, including 12-hour release dose of pseudoephedrine at 2am. Nonetheless, the attending physician referred him for a CT scan of the head and sinuses to rule out a stroke and conducted a basic metabolic panel, complete blood count, and urinalysis. Jake considered leaving against medical advice, feeling rather certain that his blood pressure would return to normal after the sinus medication wore off, but worried that if he did so, his insurance company would not pay for the services he had already received.

> When the results of the CT scans and the lab tests were normal, the physicians decided to simply observe Jake and see if his blood pressure returned to normal

---

[9] Health care markets are fundamentally different than other markets because, in short, the *payer* is typically removed from the transaction between who we *think* are the *buyer* and/or *seller*. If a buyer purchases a computer, for example, (s)he ideally possesses knowledge of the upsides and downsides of that particular computer compared with others like it, and is responsible for paying a seller for that computer. In health care, the patient has limited knowledge of the goods or services being purchased; knows of few, if any, feasible alternatives that might offer greater value; and rarely pays on his or her own behalf. The buyer is typically a third party insurer, while the seller is often the hospital or system that employs the provider (or in increasingly rare instances of private practice, a billing office or specialist is responsible for such financial matters). As a result, both providers and patients are insulated from the effects of cost, supply, and demand that typify "normal" markets of goods and services.

around 2pm, 12-hours after taking the pseudoephedrine. When it did, he was discharged, but not before a bill for well over $2500 had been amassed. His insurance
paid all but Jake's co-pay of $150.

In this passage we can make many connections between the structure of the health
care system and the clinical experience. Reflecting the professional model, the
physician lies at the center of the interaction and the delivery of health services.
As a result, the patient experiences pressure to conform to the doctor's recommendations. In this scenario, the patient even wanted to go against the recommendations of the provider to have a CT scan, but like the majority of patients went
along with the expert advice of his providers, partially out of deference to their
expertise and partially for fear that there would be ramifications for his insurance
coverage.[10] Of course, the physicians in this case also experience pressure, most
notably the fear of litigation. That is, while the most prudent course of action in
this case would have been to wait to see if Jake's blood pressure returned to normal
before doing CT scans, if something serious had gone undetected, the physicians
could face a lawsuit, even if they would likely be held harmless in the end. In other
contexts, providers face the pressure of professional norms and financial incentives, because in American health care delivery, payments are closely tied to diagnoses and treatment procedures. In short, if there is a financial incentive tied to
doing things to patients, then there is pressure to be active rather than passive
in the diagnostic and treatment process, even if a wait-and-see approach is more
sensible. Also, providers have expenses associated with facilities, personnel, and
technology, and they too need to earn a living, often made more difficult by sizable
debt amassed in pursuit of a costly education. Finally, overtreatment emerges from
the norms of medical training and practice, where providers are trained to locate
abnormalities within very specialized human systems, and to fix those abnormalities, even when "the distinction between abnormal and normal can be quite arbi-
trary" (Welch et al. 2011:32).

The abundance of technology also serves to encourage its use, in part
because the costs of purchasing that technology must somehow be recovered.
This equipment is also frequently updated, because both patients and providers
want the newest version of any diagnostic instrument available (Budrys 2015).
This is attributable to the idea that "more and newer technology is *better*," a
general overreliance on technology in the diagnostic process, and the ubiquitous
risk among providers of facing malpractice litigation should they fail to use all
resources available to them. Even the massive size of American health care, along
with its available personnel and technological resources, may orient many toward
a decidedly medical approach to their problems. Highly specialized providers, for
example, are compelled by their own training and incentives to oblige. As cardiologist Andrey Espinoza explains in the documentary *Money-Driven Medicine*
(2009) (documentary film by California Newsreel: http://moneydrivenmedicine.
org/about-mdm, "[I]f you're a hammer, everything looks like a nail ... I'm an

---

[10] This is a commonly held myth among both patients and providers, but is not true in the majority of
cases where patients leave against medical advice. One study even found that some providers counsel
patients that this might happen (Schaefer et al. 2012), presumably in an effort to persuade them to
follow medical advice, though they likely, at the same time, also believe genuinely that to be the case.

interventional cardiologist and that's what I do for a living is I fix blockages." This approach also sets the stage for *cascading medical events*, which like falling dominoes, once begun, are difficult to interrupt. Welch and colleagues (2011), for example, describe a woman whose osteoporosis screening yielded a marginal result. Despite having no additional risk factors she attempted a series of treatments, each of which produced significant and unpleasant side effects. Throughout this course of events, multiple specialists each focused on treating various ailments and complications arising from those same treatments:

> Ideally the specialist would rethink the most fundamental question: is this a condition that warrants treatment? Based on [her] T score[11] and the absence of other fracture risk factors, her chances of having a fracture were low; consequently, the benefit of treatment would be small at best ... But the endocrinologist didn't raise this point; he was dealing with a medical challenge.

In fact, for a while none of the many specialists she saw raised this question. She was sent to each of them for treatment of a particular ailment and that is where they focused their efforts. No one stepped back from the situation to examine it as a whole; each acted as a hammer, finding and driving the nails of their own specialties, until a surgeon finally stopped the cascade of interventions.

We stress here that this is best understood not as a failure of any given practitioner, but rather a system that is set up to encourage particular ways of thinking about and treating illness. The experiences recounted above highlight the roles played by financial incentives, the available technology in overtreatment, the tepid accountability for system-level health care costs at the clinical level, and the practice of defensive medicine. All of these drive up system-level health care costs. But such practices do not only emerge from the professional norms and tendencies of providers. Patients play a significant role as well.

Patient-Induced Demand and Overtreatment

A second case presents another perspective where patients push for care that is not clinically indicated in an effort to achieve diagnostic certainty and because they are often not individually responsible for the costs:

> George Palmer was a 10-year-old patient whose mother brought him to a developmental-behavioral pediatrician because he had a hard time concentrating and following directions, and his grades in school were marginal (C's), whereas his older sister had always excelled scholastically. After a thorough evaluation, his physician, Dr. Sarah Hemming, diagnosed him with ADHD and prescribed Ritalin. The boy responded reasonably well to the medication, and his grades improved.

> At a follow-up visit 3 months later, however, the boy's mother told Dr. Hemming that she had read on the Internet that impulsive behavior could be caused by tumors or cysts in the brain and insisted that she order an EEG and CT brain scan.

[11] A measure of bone density that quantifies the patient's bone density compared to "normal," which is the average bone density of white women aged 20–29. In this case, the 65-year-old patient exhibited slightly lower bone density compared to someone 40 years her junior, thereby triggering medical intervention in the absence of other risk factors (Welch et al. 2011).

Dr. Hemming assured her that there was no clinical indication of a cyst or tumor and that those kinds of imaging studies normally should only be used to confirm findings for which there was something observed clinically that needed to be explained.

At the next visit, George, who had now turned 11, told Dr. Hemming that he didn't like being on the medication. He told her that while he was able to concentrate in school, he didn't feel like himself. He said he didn't make jokes like he used to and missed being the person all his friends thought was the "funny one." Dr. Hemming discussed this with Mrs. Palmer, noting that George's academic performance hadn't been so bad before taking the medication and that behavioral techniques might be sufficient to manage his relatively mild dysfunction. Mrs. Palmer insisted he stay on the medicine, noting that if he didn't excel in school now, he would get "put in the slow classes" and would never catch up.

Two months later Dr. Hemming was notified by the hospital attorney that she was named in a lawsuit against the health system that employed her. Apparently, after an episode where George had thrown dishes at a babysitter during dinner, his mother took him to a pediatric neurologist, who performed an EEG and CT brain scan and discovered a very small arachnoid cyst bordering the left temporal lobe. Mrs. Palmer claimed that Dr. Hemming had failed to properly diagnose George, and cited the fact that she had refused to order an EEG and CT scan, and had even suggested stopping the medication. While it is highly unlikely that the small cyst explained the child's outburst, let alone his impulsivity and short attention span, the hospital settled the suit for an undisclosed amount of money. For her part, Dr. Hemming reported feeling compelled to start ordering more diagnostic screening tests for her patients, even when, in her best clinical judgment, they were not warranted.

Here the provider is in a tough position. The pediatrician clearly is using her best clinical judgment to treat the patient while at the same time being mindful about what sorts of tests are really necessary. But the patient's mother sees what constitutes a reasonable course of action very differently.

It is not difficult to see how a provider (as the pediatric neurologist appears to have done in this situation) might order the imaging tests despite clinical indications that are marginal at best, noting the family's insurance status or by appealing to the idea of *patient-centered care*, which is by definition attentive to patient preferences, needs, and values. Providers might also be motivated to maintain high patient ratings in a very competitive professional marketplace, ratings that are used as a proxy for quality care and are becoming more significant in the evaluation of providers within many institutions. Additionally, the threat of legal action exerts significant pressure to utilize excessive and expensive diagnostic tests and treatments for fear of overlooking something. Indeed, Dr. Hemming's clinical behavior may have been significantly altered after this situation in ways that draw her away from her best clinical judgment and toward a more defensive practice. This aspect of the case also highlights how patient- and provider-induced overtreatment are related and can feed each other.

In this situation we can also discern a different phenomenon called *moral hazard*, which refers to situations where patients are so far removed from the financial risk of a choice, behavior, or activity that they will alter their behavior to take on more of that risk (White 2011). In other words, unlike other markets, in the health care system patients are insulated from the costs of their choices (to ask for additional services or procedures, which are typically paid by a third-party insurer), and so they are more likely to opt for additional tests and treatments. In the situation above, the choices involved increased the health care costs to the system, and ultimately to other patients within and across insurance groups. Had the patient's mother been individually responsible for the costs of the imaging studies, she may have not pushed for them, particularly in light of the lack of clinical indication for them.

Patient-induced demand is also driven by a quest for medical certainty. Here patients and families (but other times providers) make decisions to utilize health care services in an attempt to approach 100% certainty in medical diagnosis and treatment. Unfortunately, in the contemporary chronic disease era, as we have previously discussed, the notion of medical certainty is elusive. Still, well-meaning attempts to get certain answers about their own conditions or those of loved ones can represent a virtually endless series of tests and treatments that predictably offer little benefit and tremendously increase the costs to the larger system. In both cases summarized here, underlying personal and system values, as well as self-interest, motivate both patient and provider behavior in American health care delivery. As Bradley and Taylor (2013:168–69) explain:

> Health care providers are trying to make the best living possible by structuring days to see a maximum number of patients, in light of the demands that administra[tion] and paperwork place on their time. Patients and their families are trying to extract as much certainty as they can from the medical complex and, in the case of well-insured families, are insulated from the costs of this effort. None of the actors in the American health care landscape deserves full blame … All are merely acting in accordance with what the system allows and rewards.

Bureaucratic Complexity

The final scenario takes us back to where we began in this chapter: the complexity of American health care delivery. Undoubtedly, many patients and their families struggle to navigate the system, and even many providers might at times find themselves lost in a complex sea of paperwork and administrative bloat. This comes into sharp relief in accounts of physicians who become patients. Theoretically, a physician is the best positioned of any patient to understand what is happening in the course of his or her care. Indiana University School of Medicine Professor of Pediatrics Aaron Carroll (2015) provides a personal narrative that illustrates how difficult that system can be to navigate. For Carroll, the discovery that a cheap generic drug was effective for treating his ulcerative colitis was welcomed news. But he describes how getting the drug, even as a physician at a major academic medical center with excellent insurance coverage, is anything but simple:

> Every three months, I run out of my medication. In order to get more, I need a new prescription. In order to get the prescription, I need to have lab testing to prove to my doctor that I don't have anemia. This all sounds simple, and it's the same process every three months. But it's never the same, and it's never easy.

Let's start with the lab testing. At various times, my insurance plan (which is excellent, by the way) changes which laboratory facilities it will cover fully. Often, these are not labs that are housed in the huge health care system for which I work. I often have to get a new prescription for the labs, since they can't share with one another.

Further, even though my lab orders are good for a year—and I need to have them drawn basically forever—the labs recognize them for only six months. So sometimes I have to get in touch with my doctor and get a new lab order. Often, they send over the old order, because they think it's good for a year, in which case I have to go back to them and ask for a newly written one, because the lab won't recognize the really-still-valid old one. Worse, they often just fax the order to the lab itself, thinking they're helping me, so that I don't realize they sent over an old one until I'm already there, and it's too late.

After I get that sorted out, I have my blood drawn and analyzed. But because the laboratory and my doctor are in completely different health care systems, the lab results won't show up in my doctor's electronic database. I have to beg the lab to remember to fax over the results—using paper—which it often fails to do.

My next step is to check if the pharmacy I use is still under contract with my insurance plan. The medication I use needs to be ordered at a mail-order pharmacy, because my insurance won't cover it at a local facility. My insurance plan has changed its mail-order pharmacy of choice more than once in the last few years, which necessitates that I inform my physician about the change.

I also have to open a new account with the new pharmacy and give it my payment information so that it can process everything once it has the order from the doctor. I do this before getting the prescription called in because I don't want anything to get slowed down.

It's at this point that I try to get in touch with my doctor, previously through a phone message, and more recently through an online site. If I'm lucky, which usually isn't the case, the doctor will already have the lab results. If not, I have to go back to the lab and beg it again to fax over the results. If they doctor has the lab results, and they're normal (they always are), a nurse will then call in the prescription. This usually takes a few days.

Then the pharmacy will finally start to move. Even that is painful. Once my drug was on "back order," and since it was the only pharmacy I was permitted to go to, I just had to wait. It always takes at least a few days for me to get the drug, though, because processing takes time. I always, no matter how hard I try, run out of medication before I get the new bottle, during which I hold my breath and hope nothing goes wrong.

I do this four times a year. It's always a stressful time for me, and stress isn't a good thing for a person with my disease.

As a professional, Dr. Carroll likely possesses a level of familiarity and training, as well as a set of social characteristics, that permits him to make the best of a complex system that regularly creates a sense of alienation among many patients and families. Many other people, however, simply become lost in that system, often to the detriment of their health.

Conclusion: The End of Modern Health Care

Earlier in this book and elsewhere, we explain how the structure of American health care delivery is now poorly matched to the types of diseases and experiences that patients most commonly experience today (see also Wasserman & Hinote 2012). The same is true of etiological profiles and how they extend well past a purely *disease* state and into the realm of the social and psychological. We characterize these mismatches, and the problems emanating from them, as the *end of modern health care*. Now this does not mean that health care will soon disappear, leaving a nearly $3 trillion dollar hole in our economy; tens of thousands unemployed; and millions of patients sick, suffering, and in need of care. Instead, it means that clinicians and health professionals should consider shifting the focus and character of the health care system as a whole, and their individual practices within it, toward a more humanistic and patient-centered practice that is able to incorporate many of the social and psychological insights that we described in the previous chapters. In other words, this means the *birth* of a new type of health care that emerges as we leave the vestiges of outdated modernist modes of care behind (see Chapter 2).

In this chapter we directly link the values underlying health care to the structures of various delivery systems around the world and emphasize how they influence, or even channel, the experiences and behavior of clinicians in the United States. With the rise of social determinants of health and shifts toward increasingly complex epidemiology, the elements of health and disease that professionals will inevitably confront in their work today defy many elements of a system built around acute intervention and relatively simpler disease models. This insight possesses particularly important consequences for health care system as a whole (and within it the role of the clinic, diagnostic and treatment processes, divisions of labor, medical education, reimbursement structures, etc.). For example, many of the paradoxes of American health care arise because the health challenges today have to be confronted with preventative measures, and with interventions that are nested within or at least take serious account of community and environmental factors. A health care system designed around the clinical treatment of infectious and acute ailments will likely struggle to promote quality outcomes and cost containment in an era of increased epidemiological complexity. But perhaps even more importantly, there are consequences for the professionals who work within that system, because:

> [B]eing obliged to practice in a way that is not responsive to the diseases patients increasingly face likely contributes significantly to professional dissatisfaction. The strictures and rigidity of bureaucracy often can be annoying, but the way in which the rules and procedures of modern medical bureaucracies contribute to the fissure between contemporary illness and medical practice may signal a deeper existential crisis within the practice of medicine—one that we believe is only beginning to materialize. (Wasserman & Hinote 2012:151)

One of the overarching goals of this book and the approaches outlined within it involves integrating new and relevant insights into one's clinical work, which we believe is key to professional satisfaction. Approaching patient care critically, creatively, and reflexively can engender better communication, more effective diagnosis, improved treatment plans, and hopefully a provider–patient relationship built on trust and rapport, with overall better care and improved patient outcomes as a result. And those same individual-level, clinical insights can also show us how to reshape a health care system that empowers providers to practice in those ways.

Getting a sense of the various systems that comprise U.S. health care, along with the often-hidden connections between the actors within those structures, is an essential element of the sociological imagination, of seeing the bigger picture and your place within it, and of your capacity to creatively carry out your work. Indeed, this approach also brings us back to the originally stated goal of this book—the direct *application* of social and behavioral science insights most relevant to health professionals and delivering health care in the United States. As we also described very early on, this is a very important part of how professionals go about their work; set goals for themselves and their broader professions; respond to new and not-so-new health threats as individual practitioners, teams, and institutions; collaborate and communicate successfully with both colleagues and patients in increasingly complex situations and organizations; and do all of these while continuously honing their skills in ways that enable them to do their work most effectively.

The variety of insights explored above must not only inform providers at the clinical level, but should also be carried forward into the design of health care systems. As in most contemporary models of health care delivery, providers will play a critical role in how those systems are shaped in the future. Just as we began our discussion in Chapter 1 with a reflexive model of the world, so too can we apply it here. Health care delivery influences professional behavior in observable ways, but recognizing the responsible social and psychological influences inspires the possibility of charting a new course—for professional behavior and engagement, but also for American health care. After all, systems change because the actors, behaviors, and values that sustain them change. Grasping this insight, and understanding ways to navigate the challenges associated with today's health landscape, is vital to the success of health care in the twenty-first century.

CHAPTER 12 ACTIVITY

Matching Health System Design to the Health and Illness Landscape

Helpful Hint: In addition to the directly applicable material from Chapter 12, you may want to review material from Chapter 2 regarding the shifting landscape of health and illness from the premodern era to the present.

Part 1

Imagine that it is the year 1831 and you're elected as the first Minister of Health Systems in the (fictitious) country of Florin. In terms of medical science, Florin is quite advanced for the time, but curing infectious diseases still eludes the practitioners of the day. While most diseases are self-limiting, average life expectancy in Florin is only 45 years for men and 50 years for women.

The vast majority of citizens work on farms or factories doing difficult manual labor. In fact, most of the towns and villages in Florin are organized around particular labor opportunities. Some towns cropped up around steel mills, others around cotton farming and ginning, and likewise. Medical treatments typically consist of basic injury repair or amputation and the prescription of medicinals and tinctures that are compounded locally from plant or mineral sources, and which have modest effects on symptoms.

Discussion Questions

1. What sorts of challenges do you face in designing a health care system in terms of cost, quality, and access? Would any of these be more challenging than the others? Why or why not?

2. How would you organize health care delivery (i.e., what classes of professionals would perform what kinds of tasks and where)? In other words, what does health care look like (use your sociological imagination to describe that social sphere)?

3. Describe which of the four models of health care delivery would be best suited for this health landscape and why? You also may pick more than one and describe the relative strengths of each. Describe the various ways in which the other models of health care delivery would be ill suited.

Part 2

It's 1955 and you've been elected to serve as the fourteenth Minister of Health Systems in the (fictitious) country of Florin. Medical science has advanced tremendously over the last seventy years, particularly in the areas of antiseptic practices, vaccines for preventing disease, antibiotics for fighting infection, and many surgical interventions. Polio and small pox, which had been prevalent, are now on the verge of eradication. Average life expectancy has risen to about 66 years for men and 72 years for women.

Much has changed socially in Florin over the last seventy years as well. Urbanization and ongoing industrialization have brought most people to live in cities or suburbs. While labor opportunities remain mostly in factory production, there are an increasing number of people who are becoming college educated and working in skilled technical and service positions (engineers, lawyers, accountants, etc.).

Medical practitioners can now do a great deal for people with acute injuries or illnesses and, in terms of public health, great strides have been made at controlling the spread of infection. Medical technology used in clinical practice is now relatively advanced, particularly in terms of laboratory testing and imaging, which are now routinely utilized in the diagnostic process.

Discussion Questions

1. What sorts of challenges do you face in designing a health care system in terms of cost, quality, and access? Would any of these be more challenging than the others? Why or why not?

2. How would you organize health care delivery (i.e., what class of professionals would perform what kinds of tasks and where)? In other words, what does health care look like (use your sociological imagination to describe that social sphere)?

3. Describe which of the four models of health care delivery would be best suited for this health landscape and why? You also may pick more than one and describe the relative strengths of each. Describe the various ways in which the other models of health care delivery would be ill suited.

Part 3

It is the year 2020 and you've just been elected as the twenty-fourth Minister of Health Systems for the (fictitious) country of Florin. Medical science has continued to advance at an increasingly rapid pace since the 1950s. Many infectious diseases have been nearly totally eradicated, while others that used to be fatal are now curable or have been rendered significantly less serious. Life expectancy has risen to about 79 years for men and 84 years for women, but gains in life expectancy have tapered off in recent years. Among some groups in Florin, life expectancy has actually begun to decline. According to many experts, the reason has to do with the growing prevalence of chronic diseases that emerge from, and are largely managed by, health behaviors and lifestyles.

Social life in Florin has also continued to change. Urbanization has continued to a degree that most rural areas have seen dramatic population and economic declines. Cities have become more populated, but also more stratified. Class-based disparities persist on nearly every measure of achievement and status. Declines in both the farming and manufacturing industries mean that most people work in service occupations of some kind. Wages have been declining against inflation. Full-time positions with benefits, including health insurance, are increasingly difficult to find, while part-time, contractual, and temporary job opportunities are increasing in number.

Medical technology has increased in sophistication exponentially, especially with respect to robotic and laparoscopic surgeries. While new drugs continue to render infectious diseases less significant, the pharmacological management of chronic illnesses has demonstrated comparatively modest effects, depending heavily on other factors related to the patient's life and behavior. In managing their chronic conditions or factors leading to them (i.e., body mass index), many citizens of Florin engage in a range of lifestyle modifications, exercise programs, dietary plans, and so on. However, many of them undertake no intentional lifestyle plans at all.

Discussion Questions

1. What sorts of challenges do you face in designing a health care system in terms of cost, quality, and access? Would any of these be more challenging than the others? Why or why not?

2. How would you organize health care delivery (i.e., what class of professionals would perform what kinds of tasks and where)? In other words, what does health care look like (use your sociological imagination to describe that social sphere)?

3. Describe which of the four models of health care delivery would be best suited for this health landscape and why? You also may pick more than one and describe the relative strengths of each. Describe the various ways in which the other models of health care delivery would be ill suited.

CHAPTER 13

Conclusion

Throughout this book we have highlighted various ways that social and psychological features of human life affect health and health care. While there are many texts that catalogue insights from medical sociology or health psychology, we have tried to bring a number of ideas together to directly inform clinical practice and the work of health professionals. These span multiple disciplines from sociology, psychology, history, counseling, ethics, and others, but all coalesce into a robust picture depicting the most important social and behavioral components of health and health care. In the brief closing remarks presented here, we bring together various insights from the different sections and chapters of this book to underscore once again the broader picture of health care delivery and practice, informed by social and behavioral science, that we have hoped to portray.

In Part I of the book (Chapters 1–3), we presented core concepts and insights for thinking about health and illness. From there, the second part of the book (Chapters 4–6) incrementally works insights across multiple levels of scale, and deals with epidemiological issues and the ways that population health is shaped through social forces like socioeconomic status (SES), race, gender, age, culture, and related factors. Additionally, in Chapter 6, we explored how various demographic and social contexts affect health behaviors and practices through different behavioral and lifestyle models. This chapter in particular illustrates the connections between macro-level social structures like SES and lifestyles, which are closely tied to particular health and disease outcomes.

Part III of the book (Chapters 7–11) explores more micro-level phenomena. This is not to say that these issues are not affected by powerful social forces rooted in large-scale social constructs like race and SES. Nonetheless, they manifest most clearly in our interactions and communication with each other, as well as the ways that we think about particular phenomena. This includes how we define and classify experiences as disease; the significant ways that the physical experience of disease extends into the social experience of illness; and the social structure of interpersonal communication, including that between providers and patients; as well as the ways that individuals socialized into different professional roles interact with each other. This part concludes with an exploration of moral frameworks used in making critical health care decisions, as well as the social psychological forces that influence those decisions, often in unrecognized ways.

The final part of the book, Part IV (Chapter 12), instead of explicating American health care delivery from top to bottom (which would require much more than a single chapter), explores the ways that cultural values underpin the structures of health care systems around the world. Despite the tentative and ever-changing nature of health care systems, we focus on core sociological considerations that help characterize various *kinds* of systems and what those structures mean for clinical practice, health care divisions of labor, provider–patient interaction, interprofessional communication, and so on, along with the ubiquitous concerns of costs, access, and quality. In doing so, we raise important questions that can be asked of any system or set of health policies, and provide a useful application of the sociological imagination that can directly inform the work of health professionals.

Throughout the entire book we account for a broad range of important phenomena. Consider, for example, the popular diagram of conveying the *social determinants of health* by Dahlgren and Whitehead ([1991] 2007; see Figure 13.1). You will undoubtedly recognize how our coverage of class, neighborhood, race/ethnicity, social support systems, and the like captures concepts in the outer rings of this illustration, while lifestyle and health behavior begin to connect those macro-level social features to individual health outcomes. Additionally, as we have explained, health systems are socially and historically structured collections of policies, institutions, and actors, which emerge from unique political, economic, and cultural conditions, and ultimately affect the character of health care services as well as the behavior and perspectives of frontline providers. As such, these insights also can be mapped onto this now classic depiction of how social and psychological

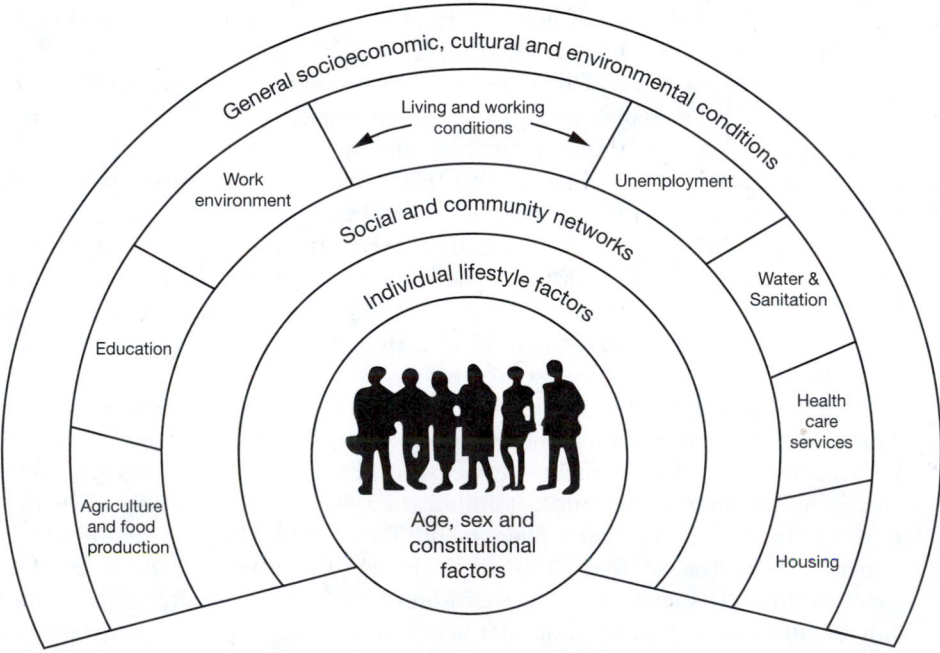

FIG. 13.1 Social determinants of health.

Source: Dahlgren, Göran & Margaret Whitehead. ([1991] 2007). *Policies and Strategies to Promote Social Equity in Health.* Stockholm, Sweden: Institute for Futures Studies.

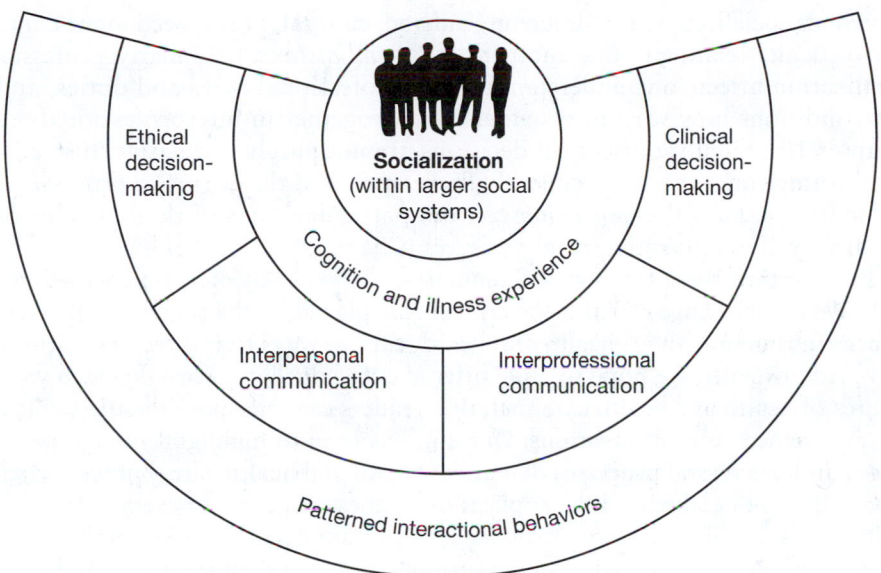

FIG. 13.2 Micro/interactional features of health and health care.

factors impact health. Yet, this only depicts half of what we have presented. While the ways that larger social and cultural forces influence health through multiple pathways are undoubtedly important, the interactions between individuals within various social and professional settings (e.g., the clinic, the workplace, the landscape of health, and medicine itself) are also important. To that end, we might diagram that portion of this book as depicted in Figure 13.2.

Clearly the large-scale social, demographic, and contextual features articulated in Figure 13.1 not only function to establish aggregate patterns, but also serve as contexts within which individuals are socialized. That is, as people experience the various social contexts in which they live, study, and work, they learn to think about the world in particular ways. This includes ways of thinking about health and the body; how someone experiences disease and illness is significantly affected by the expectations and understandings that they have developed over time. This also includes professional socialization, which confers particular ways of looking at patients, disease, and illness. Socialization also powerfully shapes how we interact with others and evaluate treatment plans and courses of action, which include ethical and clinical decisions. Medicalization, for example, emerges from socialization processes that confer expectations about the ability of medicine to define and treat an illness, as well as social norms for acceptable and unacceptable behaviors and conditions. These, in turn, affect clinical decision-making in the diagnostic process, eventually culminating in patterned overdiagnosis and overtreatment for certain conditions and in particular subpopulations (see Chapter 7). Similarly, individuals and families experience illness in ways that are inextricably linked to how they think about health and the body, as well as the various social roles and functions that they inhabit and perform (Chapter 8). Chapter 9 deals with patient–provider communication. As we discuss, communication problems often arise where individuals socialized within different gendered, cultural, or socioeconomic contexts have difficulty relating to one another (i.e., *social distance*). Similarly, professional socialization affects our understandings of professional roles and duties, and in turn conditions how various providers work together in interprofessional teams (Chapter 10). Finally, our ethical decisions are not purely normative. Instead, the moral frameworks that we frequently draw upon and the cognitive processes that culminate in ethical decisions emerge from particular ways of thinking about the world, as well as influential social pressures (Chapter 11).

Put together, these two figures summarize the expansive terrain covered in this book. We hope to have clarified the critical role played by the social and behavioral sciences in thinking about health and health care in ways that directly inform your work. Additionally, we hope to have offered core conceptual insights into various features of health and health care such that readers can transpose these insights into new experiences and observations. Our aim has been to highlight influential social factors and behavioral processes that affect health and health care, but we recognize that we have not elaborated the application of these concepts in every corner of the health landscape. Instead, we introduce and explain concepts in ways that readers can use to think through and examine various aspects of their own lives and careers, drawing on and adapting them to better understand situations that they encounter.

Finally, we hope to elucidate the need for clinical practitioners to think more deeply, critically, and reflexively across various domains of health and health care. It is not always obvious how social science insights, particularly those that speak primarily to aggregate patterns observed in large groups, are informative for practitioners working to improve the health of individual patients. Throughout this work, however, we articulate how the various concepts under discussion can directly inform your practice in medicine, nursing, or any number of allied health fields. When it comes to issues like ethical decision-making, provider–patient interaction, and the like, this comes more naturally. However, even macro-level concerns like the relationship between SES and health are informative for practice because such concepts sensitize providers to the particular trends and tendencies of the subpopulations in which they work and from which their individual patients come. Herbert Blumer (1954:7) defined *sensitizing concepts* and elaborated their utility for social science research, but clinical practitioners face the same problems that are addressed by the notion:

> A definitive concept refers precisely to what is common to a class of objects, by the aid of a clear definition in terms of attributes or fixed bench marks. This definition, or the bench marks, serve as a means of clearly identifying the individual instance of the class and the make-up of that instance that is covered by the concept. A sensitizing concept lacks such specification of attributes or bench marks and consequently it does not enable the user to move directly to the instance and its relevant content. Instead, it gives the user a general sense of reference and guidance in approaching empirical instances. Whereas definitive concepts provide prescriptions of what to see, sensitizing concepts merely suggest directions along which to look.

Certainly, clinical practitioners should avoid reductionist assumptions about, for example, the health of any particular poor person and the challenges they may or may not face. That is, SES is not a *definitive concept* for health. But SES can serve as a *sensitizing concept*, insofar as its relationship to health can inform practitioners about what sorts of questions they might need to ask in order to best treat individuals that experience and manage their illnesses in particular social contexts.

Our book is saturated with these sorts of sensitizing concepts. We hope that in learning about various social and behavioral science insights, your awareness of phenomena surrounding health and health care has expanded, along with your curiosity. That is, we hope that the core concepts presented in each chapter have changed how readers understand health, illness, and clinical practice, as you experience it. Over the course of one's professional life, we hope these will evolve from the academic concepts described in this text into an inherent part of your practice experience, that they will crystallize and expand as you see them manifest in your real-world health care endeavors.

References

Abel-Smith, Brian. (1976). *Value for Money in Health Services: A Comparative Study*. London: Heinemann.

Abrums, Mary E. (2000). "'Jesus Will Fix It after a While': Meanings and Health." *Social Science & Medicine* 50, 89–105.

Adams, Brad, Maria P. Aranda, Bryan Kemp, & Kellie Takagi. (2002). "Ethnic and Gender Differences in Distress among Anglo American, African American, Japanese American and Mexican American Spousal Caregivers of Persons with Dementia." *Journal of Clinical Geropsychology* 8, 279–301.

Adelman, Larry. (2008). *Unnatural Causes: Is Inequality Making Us Sick?* San Francisco, CA: California Newsreel.

Adelman, Ronald D., Lyubov L. Tmanova, Diana Delgado, Sarah Dion, & Mark S. Lachs. (2014). "Caregiver Burden: A Clinical Review." *Journal of the American Medical Association* 311, 1052–59.

Agency for Healthcare Research and Quality. (2003). *Patient Safety Initiative: Building Foundations, Reducing Risk*. Rockville, MD: Agency for Healthcare Research and Quality. http://archive.ahrq.gov.

Ahgren, Bengt. (2014). "Health Care Delivery System: Sweden." Pp. 866–72 in *The Wiley-Blackwell Encyclopedia of Health, Illness, Behavior & Society*. William C. Cockerham, Robert Dingwall, & Stella Quah, eds. Malden, MA: John Wiley & Sons.

Ajzen, Icek. (1991). "The Theory of Planned Behavior." *Organizational Behavior & Human Decision Processes* 50, 179–211.

Ajzen, Icek & B. L. Driver. (1991). "Prediction of Leisure Participation from Behavioral, Normative, and Control Beliefs: An Application of the Theory of Planned Behavior." *Leisure Sciences* 13, 185–204.

American Psychiatric Association. (2013). *Diagnostic and Statistical Manual of Mental Disorders*, 5th edition. Washington, DC: American Psychiatric Publishing.

Anspach, Renee R. (1988). "Notes on the Sociology of Medical Discourse: The Language of Case Presentation." *Journal of Health and Social Behavior* 29, 357–75.

Arora, Vineet, Sandeep Gangireddy, Amit Mehrotra, Ranjan Ginde, Megan Tormey, & David Meltzer. (2009). "Ability of Hospitalized Patients to Identify Their In-Hospital Physicians." *Archives of Internal Medicine* 169, 199–201.

Aruguete, Mara S. & Carlos A. Roberts. (2002). "Participants' Ratings of Male Physicians Who Vary in Race and Communication Style." *Psychological Reports* 91, 793–806.

Asch, Solomon E. (1955). "Opinions and Social Pressure." *Scientific American* 193, 31–35.

Aspinall, Peter J. (2001). "Operationalizing the Collection of Ethnicity Data in Studies of the Sociology of Heath and Illness." *Sociology of Health & Illness* 23, 829–62.

Avdi, Elma, Petrina Barson, & Ilana Rischin. (2008). "Empathic Communication Skills in CALD Medical Student Interviews." *Prospect* 23, 4–11.

Azjen, Icek & Martin Fishbein. (1980). *Understanding Attitudes and Predicting Health Behavior*. Englewood Cliffs, NJ: Prentice-Hall.

Babcock, Linda & Sara Laschever. (2003). *Women Don't Ask: Negotiation and the Gender Divide*. Princeton, NJ: Princeton University Press.

Badiou, Alain. (2003). *Saint Paul: The Foundation of Universalism*. Stanford, CA: Stanford University Press.

Baker, David P., Sigrid Gustafson, Jeff Beaubien, Eduardo Salas, & Paul Barach. (2005). *Medical Teamwork and Patient Safety: The Evidence-based Relation*. Final Report. Rockville, MD: Agency for Healthcare Research and Quality.

Baldwin, DeWitt C. (1996). "Some Historical Notes on Interdisciplinary and Interprofessional Education and Practice in Healthcare in the U.S.A." *Journal of Interprofessional Care* 10, 173–87.

Bandura, Albert. (1997). *Self-Efficacy: The Exercise of Control*. New York: W.H. Freeman.

Bardon, Adrian. (2003). "Ethics Education and Value Prioritization among Members of US Hospital Ethics Committees." *Kennedy Institute of Ethics Journal* 14, 395–406.

Barnes, Patricia M., Eve Powell-Griner, Kim McFann, & Richard L. Nahin. (2004). "Complementary and Alternative Medicine Use among Adults: United States, 2002." *Seminars in Integrative Medicine* 2, 54–71.

Bärninghausen, Till & Rainer Sauerborn. (2002). "One Hundred and Eighteen Years of the German Health Insurance System: Are There Any Lessons for Middle- and Low-Income Countries?" *Social Science & Medicine* 54, 1559–87.

Barr, Hugh & Julia Coyle. (2013). "Introducing Interprofessional Education." Pp. 185–96 in *Educating Health Professionals: Becoming a University Teacher*. S. Loftus et al., eds. Rotterdam, The Netherlands: Sense Publishers.

Bastra, Laura & Allen Frances. (2012). "DSM-5 Further Inflates Attention Deficit Hyperactivity Disorder." *Journal of Nervous and Mental Disease* 200, 486–88.

Bauer, Ursula E., Peter A. Briss, Richard A. Goodman, & Barbara A. Bowman. (2014). "Prevention of Chronic Disease in the 21st Century: Elimination of the Leading Preventable Causes of Premature Death and Disability in the USA." *The Lancet* 384, 45–52.

Bauman, Zygmunt. (1999). *In Search of Politics*. Stanford, CA: Stanford University Press.

Beauchamp, Tom L. & James F. Childress. (2001) *The Principles of Biomedical Ethics*, 5th edition. New York: Oxford University Press.

Beck, Ulrich. (1992). *Risk Society*. London: Sage.
———. (1999). *World Risk Society*. Cambridge: Polity.

Becker, E. (1973). *The Denial of Death*. New York: Free Press.

Beecher, Henry K. (1966). "Ethics and Clinical Research." *The New England Journal of Medicine* 274, 1354–60.

Bell, Ann V. (2014). "'I think about Oprah': Social Class Differences in Sources of Health Information." *Qualitative Health Research* 24, 506–16.

Benestad, Haakon Breien & Petter Laake. (2007). "Research Methodology: Strategies, Planning and Analysis." Pp. 93–124 in *Research Methodology in the Medical and Biological Sciences*. Petter Laake, Haakon Breien Benestad, & Bjørn Reino Olsen, eds. London: Academic Press.

Bernard, Jessie. (1972). *The Future of Marriage*. New Haven, CT: Yale University Press.

Bertakis, Klea D. & Rahman Azari. (2012). "Patient-Centered Care: The Influences of Patient and Resident Physician Gender and Gender Concordance in Primary Care." *Journal of Women's Health* 21, 326–33.

Bertrand, Marrianne & Sendhil Mullainathan. (2004). "Are Emily and Greg More Employable Than Lakisha and Jamal? A Field Experiment on Labor Market Discrimination." *The American Economic Review* 94, 991–1013.

Berwick, Donald M., Thomas W. Nolan, & John Whittington. (2008). "The Triple Aim: Care, Health, and Cost." *Health Affairs* 27, 759–69.

Bes-Rastrollo, Maira, Matthias B. Schulze, Miguel Ruiz-Canela, & Miguel A. Martinez-Gonzalez. (2013). "Financial Conflict of Interest and Reporting Bias Regarding the Association between Sugar-Sweetened Beverages and Weight Gain: A Systematic Review of Systematic Reviews." *PLOS Medicine* 10(12), e1001578. doi:10.1371/journal.pmed.1001578.

Bevans, Margaret & Esther M. Sternberg. (2012). "Caregiving Burden, Stress, and Health Effects among Family Caregivers of Adult Cancer Patients." *Journal of the American Medical Association* 307, 398–403.

Billings, John, Joel C. Cantor, & Chelsea Clinton. (2011). "Access to Care." Pp. 151–80 in *Jonas & Kovner's Health Care Delivery in the United States*. Anthony R. Kovner & James R. Knickman, eds. New York: Springer.

Bird, Chloe E. & Martha E. Lang. (2014). "Gender, Health, and Constrained Choice." Pp. 602–11 in *The Wiley-Blackwell Encyclopedia of Health, Illness, Behavior and Society*. William C. Cockerham, Robert Dingwall, & Stella Quah, eds. Malden, MA: John Wiley & Sons.

Bird, Chloe E. & Patricia P. Rieker. (2008). *Gender and Health: The Effects of Constrained Choices and Social Policies*. New York: Cambridge University Press.

Bishop, Jeffrey P., Joseph B. Fanning, & Mark J. Bilton. (2009). "Of Goals and Goods and Floundering About: A Dissensus Report on Clinical Ethics Consultation," *Healthcare Ethics Forum* 21, 275–91.

Black, Lewis. (2000). *The White Album*. Audio recording. Minneapolis, MN: Stand Up Records, #001.

Blinder, Alan. (2016). "Outbreak is Fueled by Mistrust in Rural Alabama." *New York Times*, January 18, A9.

Bloom, Samuel W. (1965). *The Doctor and His Patient: A Sociological Interpretation*. New York: Free Press.

Bloom, Samuel W. (2002). *The Word as Scalpel: A History of Medical Sociology*. New York: Oxford University Press.

Bloomgarden, Z. T. (2009). A1C: Recommendations, debates, and questions. *Diabetes Care* 32 (12), e141–e147.

Blumer, Herbert. (1954). "What Is Wrong with Social Theory?" *American Sociological Review* 18, 3–10.

Bonanno, George A. (2004). "Loss, Trauma, and Human Resilience: Have We Underestimated the Human Capacity to Thrive after Extremely Aversive Events?" *The American Psychologist* 59, 20–28.

Bosk, Charles L. (2010). "Bioethics, Raw and Cooked: Extraordinary Conflict and Everyday Practice." *Journal of Health and Social Behavior* 51(Suppl.), S133–46.

Bourdieu, Pierre. ([1972] 1977). *Outline of a Theory of Practice*. Cambridge, MA: Cambridge University Press.

———. (1984). *Distinction: A Social Critique of the Judgement of Taste*. Cambridge, MA: Harvard University Press.

———. (1990). *The Logic of Practice*. Stanford, CA: Stanford University Press.

Boysen, Philip G. (2013). "Just Culture: A Foundation for Balanced Accountability and Patient Safety." *The Ochsner Journal* 13, 400–06.

Bradley, Elizabeth H. & Lauren A. Taylor. (2013). *The American Health Care Paradox: Why Spending More Is Getting Us Less*. New York: PublicAffairs.

Braveman, Paula A., Catherine Cubbin, Susan Egerter, David R. Williams, & Elsie Pamuk. (2010). "Socioeconomic Disparities in Health in the United States: What the Patterns Tell Us." *American Journal of Public Health* 100, S186–96.

Brenton, Joslyn. (2014). "Gendered Health Discourse." In *The Wiley Blackwell Encyclopedia of Health, Illness, Behavior, and Society*. W. C. Cockerham, R. Dingwall, & S. R. Quah, eds. West Sussex: Wiley-Blackwell.

Brockmann, Hilke & Maike Schulz. (2014). "Health Care Delivery System: Germany." Pp. 809–16 in *The Wiley-Blackwell Encyclopedia of Health, Illness, Behavior & Society*. William C. Cockerham, Robert Dingwall, & Stella Quah, eds. Malden, MA: John Wiley & Sons.

Brown, Carolyn & Richard Segal. (1996). "Ethnic Differences in Temporal Orientation and Its Implications for Hypertension Management." *Journal of Health and Social Behavior* 37(4), 350–61.

Brown, Phil R., Rachel Morello-Frosch, Stephen Zavestoski, Sabrina McCormick, Brian Mayer, Rebecca Gasior Altman, et al. (2012). "Embodied Health Movements." Pp. 15–32 in *Contested Illnesses: Citizens, Science, and Health Social Movements*. Phil R. Brown, Rachel Morello-Frosch, & Stephen Zavestoski, eds. Berkeley, CA: University of California Press.

Brueggemann, John. (2010). *Rich, Free, and Miserable: The Failure of Success in America*. Lanham, MD: Rowman & Littlefield.

Bruhn, J. G. & H. M. Rebach. (2014). *The Sociology of Caregiving*. New York: Springer.

Bruhn, John G. & Stewart Wolf. (1979). *The Roseto Story: An Anatomy of Health*. Norman, OK: University of Oklahoma Press.

Budrys, Grace. (2005). *Our Unsystematic Health Care System*. Lanham, MD: Rowman & Littlefield.

———. (2014). "Health Care Delivery System: United States." Pp. 895–901 in *The Wiley-Blackwell Encyclopedia of Health, Illness, Behavior & Society*. William C. Cockerham, Robert Dingwall, & Stella Quah, eds. Malden, MA: John Wiley & Sons.

———. (2015). *Our Unsystematic Health Care System*, 4th edition. Lanham, MD: Rowman & Littlefield.

Burke, Peter J. & Donald C. Reitzes. (1981). "The Link between Identity and Role Performance." *Social Psychology Quarterly* 44, 83–92.

Butler, Robert N. (1969). "Age-Ism: Another Form of Bigotry." *Gerontologist* 9, 243–46.

Bylund, Carma L. & Gregory Makoul. (2002). "Empathic Communication and Gender in the Physician-Patient Encounter." *Patient Education and Counseling* 48, 207–16.

Caronna, Carol A. & Michael K. Ong. (2011). "Organization of Medical Care." Pp. 181–204 in *Jonas & Kovner's Health Care Delivery in the United States*. Anthony

R. Kovner & James R. Knickman, eds. New York: Springer.

Carroll, Aaron E. (2014). "Calling an Ordinary Health Problem a Disease Leads to Bigger Problems." *New York Times.* June 2, 2014.

———. (2015). "Trapped in the System: A Sick Doctor's Story." *New York Times.* September 21.

Case, Anne & Angus Deaton. (2015). "Rising Morbidity and Mortality in Midlife among White Non-Hispanic Americans in the 21st Century." *Proceedings of the National Academy of Sciences of the United States* 112, 15078–83.

Cass Alan, Anne Lowell, Michael Christie, Paul L. Snelling, Melinda Flack, Betty Marrnganyin, & Isaac Brown. (2002). "Sharing the True Stories: Improving Communication between Aboriginal Patients and Healthcare Workers." *Medical Journal of Australia* 176, 466–70.

Cassell, Eric J. (1991). *The Nature of Suffering and the Goals of Medicine.* New York: Oxford University Press.

Cauce, Ana Mari, Matthew Paradise, Joshua A. Ginzler, Lara Embry, Charles J. Morgan, Yvette Lohr, et al. (2000). "The Characteristics and Mental Health of Homeless Adolescents: Age and Gender Differences." *Journal of Emotional and Behavioral Disorders* 8, 230–39.

Chadwick, Edwin. (1842). *Report on the Sanitary Condition of the Labouring Population and on the Means of Its Improvement.* London: W. Clowes & Sons.

Chae, David H., Amani M. Nuru-Jeter, Nancy E. Adler, Gene H. Brody, Jue Lin, Elizabeth H. Blackburn, et al. (2014). "Discrimination, Racial Bias, and Telomere Length in African-American Men." *American Journal of Preventive Medicine* 46, 103–11.

Champion, Victoria L. & Celette S. Skinner. (2008). "The Health Belief Model." Pp. 45–65 in *Health Behavior: Theory, Research and Practice,* 4th edition. Karen Glanz, Barbara K. Rimer, & K. Viswanath, eds. San Francisco, CA: John Wiley & Sons.

Charmaz, Kathy. (1991). *Good Days, Bad Days: The Self in Chronic Illness and Time.* New Brunswick, NJ: Rutgers University Press.

———. (1995). "The Body, Identity, and Self: Adapting to Impairment." *The Sociological Quarterly* 36, 657–80.

Charon, Rita. (2006). *Narrative Medicine: Honoring the Stories of Illness.* New York: Oxford University Press.

Chen, Edith, Margaret D. Hanson, Laurel Q. Paterson, Melissa J. Griffin, Hope A. Walker, & Gregory E. Miller. (2006). "Socioeconomic Status and Inflammatory Processes in Childhood Asthma: The Role of Psychological Distress." *The Journal of Allergy & Clinical Immunology* 117, 1014–20.

Christiansen, Clayton M. (2011). *The Innovator's Dilemma: The Revolutionary Book That Will Change the Way You Do Business.* New York: Harper.

Clair, Jeffrey Michael. (1990). "Regressive Intervention: The Discourse of Medicine during Terminal Encounters." *Advances in Medical Sociology* 1, 57–97.

Clair, Jeffrey Michael, Cullen Clark, Brian P. Hinote, Caroline O. Robinson, & Jason Adam Wasserman. (2007). "Developing, Integrating, and Perpetuating New Ways of Applying Sociology to Health, Medicine, Policy, and Everyday Life." *Social Science and Medicine* 64, 248–58.

Clark, Jack A., Deborah A. Potter, & John B. McKinlay. (1991). "Bringing Social Structure back into Clinical Decision Making." *Social Science & Medicine* 32, 853–66.

Coburn, David. (1994). "Professionalization and Proletarianization: Medicine, Nursing, and Chiropractic in Historical Perspective." *Labour/LeTravail* 34, 139–62.

Cockerham, William C. (1999). *Health and Social Change in Russia and Eastern Europe.* New York: Routledge.

———. (2005). "Health Lifestyle Theory and the Convergence of Agency and Structure." *Journal of Health and Social Behavior* 46, 51–67.

———. (2012). *Medical Sociology.* Upper Saddle River, NJ: Prentice-Hall.

———. (2013). *Social Causes of Health and Disease.* Cambridge: Polity.

———. (2016). *Medical Sociology.* 13th edition. New York: Routledge.

Cockerham, William C. & Brian P. Hinote. (2015). "PAs in a Changing Society: A Sociologic Perspective." *Journal of the American Academy of Physician Assistants* 28, 18–20.

Cockerham, William C., Hiroyuki Hatton, & Yukio Yamori. (2000). "The Social Gradient in Life

Expectancy: The Contrary Case of Okinawa in Japan." *Social Science & Medicine* 51, 115–22.

Cockerham, William C., Brian P. Hinote, Geoffrey B. Cockerham, & Pamela Abbott. (2006a). "Health Lifestyles and Political Ideology in Belarus, Russia, and Ukraine." *Social Science & Medicine* 62, 1799–1809.

Cockerham, William C., Brian P. Hinote, & Pamela Abbott. (2006b). "Psychological Distress, Gender, and Health Lifestyles in Belarus, Kazakhstan, Russia, and Ukraine." *Social Science & Medicine* 63, 2381–94.

Cohen, Marie Seren. (1999). "Families Coping with Childhood Chronic Illness: A Research Review." *Family Systems and Health* 17, 149–64.

Cohen, Sheldon, Lynn G. Underwood, & Benjamin H. Gottlieb, eds. (2000). *Social Support Measurement and Intervention: A Guide for Health and Social Scientists*. New York: Oxford University Press.

Cole, Steven A. & Julian Bird. (2014). *The Medical Interview: The Three-Function Approach*. Philadelphia: Elsevier.

Collins, Patricia Hill. (1990). *Black Feminist Thought: Knowledge, Consciousness, and the Politics of Empowerment*. New York: Routledge.

Colpo, Anthony. (2012). "The Full Story: Why Eggs Do Not Cause Cardiovascular Disease." http://anthonycolpo.com/the-full-story-why-eggs-do-not-cause-cardiovascular-disease/. Accessed March 2015.

Commission on Social Determinants of Health (CSDH). (2008). *Closing the Gap in a Generation: Health Equity Through Action on Social Determinants of Health*. Geneva: World Health Organization.

Conrad, Peter. (1975). "The Discovery of Hyperkinesis: Notes on the Medicalization of Deviant Behavior." *Social Problems* 23, 12–21.

———. (1992). "Medicalization as Social Control." *Annual Review of Sociology* 18, 209–32.

———. (2005). "The Shifting Engines of Medicalization." *Journal of Health and Social Behavior* 46, 3–14.

Conrad, Peter & Valerie Leiter. (2004). "Medicalization, Markets, and Consumers." *Journal of Health and Social Behavior* 45, 158–76.

Coombs, Robert H., Sangeeta Chopra, Debra R. Schenk, & Elaine Yutan. (1993). "Medical Slang and Its Functions." *Social Science & Medicine* 36, 987–98.

Cooper, Lisa A., Debra L. Roter, Kathryn A. Carson, Mary Catherine Beach, Janice A. Sabin, Anthony Greenwald, et al. (2012). "The Associations of Clinicians' Implicit Attitudes about Race with Medical Visit Communication and Patient Ratings of Interpersonal Care." *American Journal of Public Health* 102, 979–87.

Courtenay, Will H. (2000). "Constructions of Masculinity and Their Influence on Men's Well-Being: A Theory of Gender and Health." *Social Science & Medicine* 50, 1385–401.

Cousins, Glynis. (2006). "An Introduction to Threshold Concepts." *Planet* 17, 4–5.

Cox, Carole & Abraham Monk. (1996). "Strain Among Caregivers: Comparing the Experiences of African American and Hispanic Caregivers of Alzheimer's Relatives." *The International Journal of Aging and Human Development* 43, 93–105.

Cruess, Sylvia R. (2006). "Professionalism and Medicine's Social Contract with Society." *Clinical Orthopaedics and Related Research* 449, 170–76.

CSDH (2008). *Closing the Gap in a Generation: Health Equity through Action on the Social Determinants of Health. Final Report of the Commission on Social Determinants of Health*. Geneva, World Health Organization.

Curran, Vernon R., Dennis Sharpe, & Jennifer Forristall. (2007). "Attitudes of Health Sciences Faculty Members towards Interprofessional Teamwork and Education." *Medical Education* 41, 892–96.

Dahlgren, Göran & Margaret Whitehead. ([1991] 2007). *Policies and Strategies to Promote Social Equity in Health*. Stockholm, Sweden: Institute for Futures Studies.

Dahrendorf, Ralf. (1979) *Life Chances: Approaches to Social and Political Theory*. Cambridge: Polity.

De Vries, Nanne. (2014). "Health Psychology and Behavior Change." Pp. 1085–87 in *The Wiley-Blackwell Encyclopedia of Health, Illness, Behavior and Society*. William C. Cockerham, Robert Dingwall, & Stella Quah, eds. Malden, MA: John Wiley & Sons.

De Vries, Raymond, Leigh Turner, Kristina Orfali, & Charles L. Bosk. (2007). *The View from Here: Bioethics and the Social Sciences*. Malden, MA: Blackwell Publishing.

Department of Health and Human Services. (2003). "Summary of the HIPAA Privacy Rule." http://www.hhs.gov/sites/default/files/privacysummary.pdf. Accessed April 9, 2016.

Deutsch, Morton & Harold B. Gerard. (1955). "A Study of Normative and Informational Social Influences upon Individual Judgment." *Journal of Abnormal and Social Psychology* 51, 629–36.

Di Cimbrini, Tiziana. (2015). "Welfare or Politics?: The Identity of Mutual Aid Societies as Revealed by a Latent Class Cluster Analysis of Their Annual Reports." *Accounting History* 20, 310–41.

DiMaggio, Paul. (2012). "Sociological Perspectives on the Face-to-Face Enactment of Class Distinction." Pp. 15–38 in *Facing Social Class: How Societal Rank Influences Interaction.* Susan T. Fiske & Hazel Rose Markus, eds. New York: Russell Sage Foundation.

Dohrenwend, Bruce P. & Barbara S. Dohrenwend (1976). "Sex Differences and Psychiatric Disorders." *American Journal of Sociology* 81, 1447–54.

Dolnick, Edward. (1993). "Deafness as Culture." *The Atlantic Monthly* 272, 37–53.

Donelan, Karen, Craig A. Hill, Catherine Hoffman, Kimberly Scoles, Penny Hollander Feldman, Carol Levine, & David Gould. (2002). "Challenged to Care: Informal Caregivers in a Changing Health System." *Health Affairs* 21, 222–31.

Dorsey, E. Ray, Jason de Roulet, Joel P. Thompson, Jason I. Reminick, Ashley Thai, Zachary White-Stellato, et al. (2010). "Funding of US Biomedical Research, 2003–2008." *Journal of the American Medical Association* 303(2), 137–43.

Dovidio, John F. & Samuel L. Gaertner. (2000). "Aversive Racism and Selection Decisions: 1989 and 1999." *Psychological Science* 11, 315–19.

Drentea, Patricia. (2014). "Caregiving and Gender Roles." In *The Wiley Blackwell Encyclopedia of Health, Illness, Behavior, and Society.* W. C. Cockerham, R. Dingwall, & S. R. Quah, eds. West Sussex: Wiley-Blackwell.

Drife, J. (2002). "The Start of Life: A History of Obstetrics." *Postgraduate Medical Journal* 78, 311–15.

Dubois, W. E. B. (1899). *The Philadelphia Negro.* Philadelphia, PA: University of Pennsylvania Press.

Dubos, Rene. (1959). *Mirage of Health.* New York: Harper & Row.

Duffy, John. (1993). *From Humors to Medical Science: A History of American Medicine.* Champaign, IL: University of Illinois Press.

Durkheim, Emile. (1897 [1951]). *Suicide: A Study in Sociology.* J.A. Spaulding & G. Simpson, trans. Glencoe, IL: Free Press.

———. (1933 [1997]). *The Division of Labor in Society.* New York: The Free Press.

Eisenberg, John M. (1979). "Sociologic Influences on Decision-Making by Clinicians." *Annals of Internal Medicine* 90, 957–64.

Eisenkroft, James B. (2008). "Anaesthesia Delivery System." Pp. 767–820 in *Anaesthesiology.* Longnecker David, David L. Brown, Mark F. Newman, & Warren M. Zapol, eds. New York: McGraw Hill Medical.

Ekdahl, Anne W., Ingrid Hellström, Lars Andersson, & Maria Friedrichsen. (2012). "Too Complex and Time-consuming to Fit In! Physicians' Experiences of Elderly Patients and Their Participation in Medical Decision Making: A Grounded Theory Study." *BMJ Open* 2:e001063. doi:10.1136/bmjopen-2012-001063.

Elliott, Andrea M., Stewart C. Alexander, Craig A. Mescher, Deepika Mohan, & Amber E. Barnato. (2016). "Differences in Physicians' Verbal and Nonverbal Communication with Black and White Patients at the End of Life." *Journal of Pain and Symptom Management* 51, 1–8.

Emslie, Carol & Kate Hunt. (2008). "The Weaker Sex? Exploring Lay Understandings of Differences in Life Expectancy: A Qualitative Study." *Social Science & Medicine* 67, 808–16.

Engel, George L. (1977). "The Need for a New Medical Model: A Challenge for Biomedicine." *Science* 196, 129–36.

Engels, Friedrich. (1845 [2009]). *The Condition of the Working Class in England.* London: Oxford University Press.

Erchak, Gerald M. (1992). *The Anthropology of Self and Behavior.* New Brunswick, NJ: Rutgers University Press.

Eymard, Amanda S. & Dianna H. Douglas. (2012). "Ageism among Health Care Providers and Interventions to Improve Their Attitudes toward Older Adults: An Integrative Review." *Journal of Gerontological Nursing* 38, 26–35.

Fein, Stephanie, Lee Hilborne, Margie Kagawa-Singer, Eugene Spiritus, Craig Keenan, Gregory Seymann, et al. (2014). "A Conceptual Model for Disclosure of Medical Errors." In *Advances in Patient Safety*. Rockville, MD: Agency for Healthcare Research and Quality.

Fiske, Susan T. & Hazel Rose Markus, eds. (2012). *Facing Social Class: How Societal Rank Influences Interaction*. New York: Russell Sage Foundation.

Fitzpatrick, Kevin & Mark LaGory. (2011). *Unhealthy Cities: Poverty, Race, and Place in America*. New York: Routledge.

Flannery, Michael A. (2002). "The Early Botanical Medical Movement as a Reflection of Life, Liberty, and Literacy in Jacksonian America." *Journal of the Medical Library Association* 90, 442–54.

Flexner, Abraham. (1910). *Medical Education in the United States: A Report to the Carnegie Foundation for the Advancement of Teaching*. New York: Carnegie Foundation for the Advancement of Teaching.

Folkman, Susan. (1984). "Personal Control and Stress and Coping Processes: A Theoretical Analysis." *Journal of Personality and Social Psychology* 46, 839–52.

———. (1963 [1994]). *The Birth of the Clinic: An Archaeology of Medical Perception*. New York: Vintage Books.

Foucault, Michel. (1963 [2003]). *The Birth of the Clinic: An Archaeology of Medical Perception*. New York: Taylor & Francis.

———. (1975 [1995]). *Discipline and Punish: The Birth of the Prison*. New York: Vintage Books.

Frakt, Austin. (2015). "How to Know Whether to Believe a Health Study." *New York Times*. August 17.

Frank, Arthur W. (1991[2000]). *At the Will of the Body: Reflections on Illness*. Boston, MA: Houghton &Mifflin.

Frankel, Richard M. & Howard B. Beckman. (1989). "Evaluating the Patient's Primary Problem(s)." Pp. 86–98 in *Communicating with Medical Patients*. Moira Stewart & Debra Roter, eds. Newbury Park, CA: Sage Publications.

Frankfort-Nachmias, Chava & David Nachmias. (2000). *Research Methods in the Social Sciences*. New York: Worth.

Franzini, Luisa, John C. Ribble, & Arlene M. Keddie. (2002). "Understanding the Hispanic Paradox." Pp. 280–310 in *Race, Ethnicity, and Health: A Public Health Reader*. Thomas A. LaVeist, ed. San Francisco, CA: Jossey-Bass.

Freidson, Eliot. (1970). *The Profession of Medicine: A Study of the Sociology of Applied Knowledge*. New York: Harper & Row Publishers.

Freud, Sigmund. (1926 [1959]). "The Question of Lay Analysis." Pp. 177–258 in *The Standard Edition of the Complete Psychological Works of Sigmund Freud. Volume 20*. J. Strachey, ed. London: Hogarth Press.

Frogner, Bianca K., Hugh R. Waters, & Gerard F. Anderson. (2011). "Comparative Health Systems." Pp. 67–84 in *Jonas & Kovner's Health Care Delivery in the United States*. Anthony R. Kovner & James R. Knickman, eds. New York: Springer.

Frohlich, Katherine L., Ellen Corin, & Louise Potvin. (2001). "A Theoretical Proposal for the Relationship between Context and Disease." *Sociology of Health and Illness* 23, 776–97.

Furman, David, Boris P. Hejblum, Noah Simon, Vladimir Jojic, Cornelia L. Dekker, Rodolphe Thiébaut, et al. (2014). "Systems Analysis of Sex Differences Reveals and Immunosuppressive Role for Testosterone in the Response to Influenza Vaccination." *Proceedings of the National Academy of Sciences of the United States of America* 111, 869–74.

Gadbois, Emily A., Edward Alan Miller, Denise Tyler, & Orna Intrator. (2014). "Trends in State Regulation of Nurse Practitioners and Physician Assistants, 2001 to 2010." *Medical Care Research and Review* 72, 200–19.

Gallagher, Thomas H., Amy D. Waterman, Alison G. Ebers, Victoria J. Fraser, & Wendy Levinson. (2003). "Patients' and Physicians' Attitudes Regarding the Disclosure of Medical Errors." *Journal of the American Medical Association* 289, 1001–07.

Gamble, Vanessa Northington. (1997). "Under the Shadow of Tuskegee: African Americans and Health Care." *American Journal of Public Health* 87, 1773–78.

Garrioch, David. (2011). "Mutual Aid Societies in Eighteenth Century Paris." *French History and Civilization* 4, 22–33.

Gawande, Atul. (2011). "Cowboys and Pit Crews." *New Yorker*, May 26. http://www.newyorker.com/news/news-desk/cowboys-and-pit-crews.

Giddens, Anthony. (1987). *Social Theory and Modern Sociology*. Stanford, CA: Stanford University Press.

———. (1991). *Modernity and Self-Identity: Self and Society in the Late Modern Age*. Stanford, CA: Stanford University Press.

Gittell, Ross & Avis Vidal. (1998). *Community Organizing: Building Social Capital as a Development Strategy*. Newbury Park, CA: Sage.

Gladwell, Malcolm. (2008). *Outliers: The Story of Success*. New York: Little, Brown & Company.

Glanz, Karen, Barbara K. Rimer, & K. Viswanath, eds. (2015). *Health Behavior: Theory, Research and Practice*, 5th edition. San Francisco, CA: John Wiley & Sons.

Glaser, Barney G. & Anselm L. Strauss. (1965). *Awareness of Dying*. New York: Aldine.

Glymour, M. Maria, Mauricio Avendano, & Ichiro Kawachi. (2014). "Socioeconomic Status and Health." Pp. 17–62 in *Social Epidemiology*. Lisa F. Berkman, Ichiro Kawachi, & M. Maria Glymour, eds. New York: Oxford.

Gochman, David S. (1982). "Labels, Systems & Motives: Some Perspectives for Future Research." *Health Education Quarterly* 9, 167–74.

———, ed. (1988). *Health Behavior: Emerging Research Perspectives*. New York: Springer.

Goetz Goldberg, Debra, Trisha Beeson, Anton J. Kuzel, Linda E. Love, Mary C. Carver. (2013). "Team-based Care: A Critical Element of Primary Care Practice Transformation." *Population Health Management* 16, 150–56.

Goffman, Erving. (1959). "The Moral Career of the Mental Patient." *Psychiatry: Journal for the Study of Interpersonal Processes* 22, 123–42.

Goldacre, Ben. (2012). *Bad Pharma: How Drug Companies Mislead Doctors and Harm Patients*. New York: Faber & Faber.

———. (2013). "Health Care's Trick Coin." *New York Times*. February 2, 2014, A23.

Gönül, Füsun F., Franklin Carter, Elina Petrova, & Kannan Srinivasan. (2001). "Promotion of Prescription Drugs and Its Impact on Physicians' Choice Behavior." *Journal of Marketing* 65, 79–90.

Goode, William J. 1957. "Community within a Community." *American Sociological Review* 22, 194–200.

Gordon, Howard S., Richard L. Street Jr., Barbara F. Sharf, P. Adam Kelly, & Julianne Souchek. (2006). "Racial Differences in Trust and Lung Cancer Patients' Perceptions of Physician Communication." *Journal of Clinical Oncology* 24, 904–09.

Gove, Walter R. & Jeannette F. Tudor. (1973). "Adult Sex Roles and Mental Illness." *American Journal of Sociology* 78, 812–35.

Graber, Mark, Ruthanna Gordon, & Nancy Franklin. (2002). "Reducing Diagnostic Errors in Medicine: What's the Goal? *Academic Medicine* 77, 981–92.

Graham, Judith. (2014). "Older People Often Overtreated for Diabetes, Study Suggests." *New York Times*. June 30, 2014.

Greene, Michelle G., Ronald Adelman, Rita Charon, & Susie Hoffman. (1986). "Ageism in the Medical Encounter: An Exploratory Study of the Doctor-Elderly Patient Relationship." *Language and Communication* 6, 113–24.

Greenhalgh, Trisha. (1997a). "Getting Your Bearings (Deciding What the Paper Is About)." (Part 2). *British Medical Journal* 315 (7102), 243–46.

———. (1997b). "Assessing the Methodological Quality of Published Papers." (Part 3). *British Medical Journal* 315(7103), 305–08.

———. (1997c). "Different Types of Data Need Different Statistical Tests (Statistics for the Non-Statistician I)." (Part 4). *British Medical Journal* 315(7104), 363–66.

———. (1997d). "Significant Relations and Their Pitfalls (Statistics for the Non-Statistician II)." (Part 5). *British Medical Journal* 315(7105), 422–25.

———. (1997e). "Papers That Report Drug Trials." (Part 6). *British Medical Journal* 315(7106), 480–83.

———. (1997f). "Papers That Report Diagnostic or Screening Tests." (Part 7). *British Medical Journal* 315(7107), 540–43.

———. (1997g). "Papers That Tell You What Things Cost (Economic Analyses)." (Part 8). *British Medical Journal* 315(7108), 596–99.

———. (1997h). "Papers That Summarise Other Papers (Systematic Reviews and

Meta-Analyses).” (Part 9). *British Medical Journal* 315(7109), 672–75.

———. (1997i). “Papers That Go beyond Numbers (Qualitative Research).” (Part 10). *British Medical Journal* 315(7110), 740–43.

———. (2014). *How to Read a Paper: The Basics of Evidence-Based Medicine*. Oxford: John Wiley & Sons.

Gregory, Stanford W. & Richard O’Toole. (1987). “Teaching Sociological Research Methods to Medical Students.” *Teaching Sociology* 15(2), 128–35.

Grell, Ole Peter. (1998). *Paracelsus: The Man and His Reputation, His Ideas, and Their Transformation*. Boston, MA: Brill.

Grimen, Harald & Benedicte Ingstad. (2007). “Qualitative Research.” Pp. 281–309 in *Research Methodology in the Medical and Biological Sciences*. Petter Laake, Haakon Breien Benestad, & Bjørn Reino Olsen, eds. London: Academic Press.

Guttman, Matthew C. (1999). “Ethnicity, Alcohol, and Acculturation.” *Social Science & Medicine* 48, 173–84.

Hafferty, Frederick W. & Ronald Franks. (1994). “The Hidden Curriculum, Ethics Teaching, and the Structure of Medical Education.” *Academic Medicine* 69, 861–71.

Haider, Adil H., Janel Sexton, N. Sriram, Lisa A. Cooper, David T. Efron, Sandra Swoboda, et al. (2011). “Association of Unconscious Race and Social Class Bias with Vignette-Based Clinical Assessments by Medical Students.” *Journal of the American Medical Association* 306, 942–51.

Haider, Adil H., Eric B. Schneider, N. Sriram, Deborah S. Dossick, Valerie K. Scott, Sandra M. Swoboda, et al. (2014). “Unconscious Race and Class Bias: Its Association with Decision Making by Trauma and Acute Care Surgeons.” *Journal of Trauma and Acute Care Surgery* 77, 409–16.

Haider, Adil H., Eric B. Schneider, N. Sriram, Valerie K. Scott, Sandra Swoboda, Cheryl K. Zogg, et al. (2015). “Unconscious Race and Class Biases among Registered Nurses: Vignette-Based Study Using Implicit Association Testing.” *Journal of the American College of Surgeons* 6, 1077–86.

Hall, Judith A. & Debra L. Roter. (2002). “Do Patients Talk Differently to Male and Female Physicians? A Meta-analytic Review.” *Patient Education and Counseling* 48, 217–24.

Hall, Judith A., Julie T. Irish, Debra L. Roter, Carol M. Ehrlich, & Lucy H. Miller. (1994). “Gender in Medical Encounters: An Analysis of Physician and Patient Communication in a Primary Care Setting.” *Health Psychology* 5, 384–92.

Hall, Pippa. (2005). “Interprofessional Teamwork: Professional Cultures as Barriers.” *Journal of Interprofessional Care* Supplement 1, 188–96.

Hankivsky, Olena. (2012). “Women’s Health, Men’s Health, and Gender and Health: Implications of Intersectionality.” *Social Science & Medicine* 74, 1712–20.

Hankivsky, Olena & Cormier, Renée. (2009). *Intersectionality: Moving Women’s Health Research and Policy Forward*. Vancouver, BC: Women’s Health Research Network.

Harris, Margaret & Emmanouela Terleksti. (2011). “Reading and Spelling Abilities of Deaf Adolescents with Cochlear Implants and Hearing Aids.” *Journal of Deaf Studies and Deaf Education* 16, 24–34.

Harvard T. H. Chan School of Public Health. “Eggs and Nutrition.” http://www.hsph.harvard.edu/nutritionsource/eggs/. Accessed April 3, 2016

Havey, J. Michael, Julie M. Olson, Christine McCormick, & Gary L. Cates. (2010). “Teachers’ Perceptions of the Incidence and Management of Attention-Deficit Hyperactivity Disorder.” *Applied Neuropsychology* 12, 120–27.

Havranek, Edward P., Mahasin S. Mujahid, Donald A. Barr, Irene V. Blair, Meryl S. Cohen, Salvador Cruz-Flores, et al. (2015). “Social Determinants of Risk and Outcomes for Cardiovascular Disease: A Scientific Statement from the American Heart Association.” *Circulation* 132, 873–98.

Hayden, Joanna. (2014). *Introduction to Health Behavior Theory*. Burlington, MA: Jones & Bartlett.

Higgs, Joy, Rola Ajjawi, Lindy McAllister, Franziska Trede, & Stephen Loftus. 2012. *Communicating in the Health Sciences*, 3rd edition. Sydney, Australia: Oxford University Press.

Hinote, Brian P. (2014a). “Life Chances and Health.” Pp. 995–98 in *The Wiley-Blackwell*

Encyclopedia of Health, Illness, Behavior and Society. William C. Cockerham, Robert Dingwall, & Stella Quah, eds. Malden, MA: John Wiley & Sons.

———. (2014b). "Fundamental Cause." Pp. 580–87 in *The Wiley-Blackwell Encyclopedia of Health, Illness, Behavior and Society.* William C. Cockerham, Robert Dingwall, & Stella Quah, eds. Malden, MA: John Wiley & Sons.

———. (2015). "William Cockerham: The Contemporary Sociology of Health Lifestyles." Pp. 471–87 in *The Palgrave Handbook for Social Theory in Health, Illness and Medicine.* Fran Collyer, ed. New York: Palgrave Macmillan.

Hinote, Brian P. & Gretchen Webber. (2012). "Drinking Toward Manhood: Masculinity and Alcohol in the Former USSR." *Men and Masculinities* 15, 292–310.

Hinote, Brian P. & Jason Adam Wasserman. (2012). "The Shifting Landscape of Health & Medicine: Implication for Childbirth Education." *International Journal of Childbirth Education* 27, 69–74.

Hinote, Brian P., William Cockerham, & Pamela Abbott. (2009a). "Psychological Distress and Dietary Patterns in Eight Post-Soviet Republics." *Appetite* 53, 24–33.

———. (2009b). "The Specter of Post-Communism: Women and Alcohol in Eight Post-Soviet States." *Social Science & Medicine* 68, 1254–62.

Hochbaum, Godfrey M. (1958). *Public Participation in Medical Screening Programs: A Sociopsychological Study.* Department of Health Education & Welfare, Public Health Service Publication no. 572. Washington, DC: U.S. Government Printing Office.

Hodges, Laura J., Gerry M. Humphris, & Gary MacFarlane. (2005). "A Meta-Analytic Investigation of the Relationship between the Psychological Distress of Cancer Patients and their Carers." *Social Science and Medicine* 60, 1–12.

Hoffman, Diane, Anita Tarzian, & Anne O'Neil. (2000). "Are Ethics Committee Members Competent to Consult?" *Journal of Law, Medicine & Ethics* 28, 30–40.

Hu, Frank B., Meir J. Stampfer, Eric B. Rimm, JoAnn E. Manson, Alberto Ascherio, Graham A. Colditz, et al. (1999). "A Prospective Study of Egg Consumption and Risk of Cardiovascular Disease in Men and Women." *Journal of the American Medical Association* 281, 1387–94.

Hume, David. (1739 [1978]). *A Treatise of Human Nature.* L. A. Selby-Bigge, ed.; P. H. Nidditch, rev. Oxford: Oxford University Press.

Hummer, Robert A., Daniel A. Powers, Starling G. Pullum, Ginger L. Gossman, & W. Parker Frisbie. (2007). "Paradox Found (Again): Infant Mortality among the Mexican-Origin Population in the United States." *Demography* 44, 441–57.

Iedema, Rick, Arthas Flabouris, Susan Grant, & Christine Jorm. (2006). "Narrativizing Errors of Care: Critical Incident Reporting in Clinical Practice." *Social Science & Medicine* 62, 134–44.

Institute of Medicine. (2000). *To Err Is Human: Building a Safer Health System.* Washington, DC: National Academies Press.

James, Janet Wilson. ([1979] 2001). "Isabel Hampton and the Professionalization of Nursing in the 1890s." Pp. 42–84 in *Enduring Issues in American Nursing.* Ellen D. Baer, Patricia D'Antonio, Sylvia Riker, & Joan E. Lynaugh, eds. New York: Springer Publishing Company.

Johanson, Richard, Mary Newburn, & Alison MacFarlane. (2002). "Has the Medicalisation of Childbirth Gone too Far?" *British Medical Journal* 324, 892–95.

Johnson, Richard W. & Anthony T. Lo Sasso. (2000). "The Trade-Off between Hours of Paid Employment and Time Assistance to Elderly Parents at Midlife." The Urban Institute. www.urbaninstitute.org. Accessed November 15, 2015.

Jonsen, Albert R. (2007). "How to Appropriate Appropriately: A Comment to Baker and McCullough." *Kennedy Institute of Ethics Journal* 17, 43–54.

Jonsen, Albert R., Mark Siegler, & William J. Winslade. (2010). *Clinical Ethics: A Practical Approach to Ethical Decision-Making in Clinical Medicine*, 2nd edition. New York: McGraw Hill.

Jost, Timothy S. (2012). "A Mutual Aid Society?" *Hastings Center Report* 42, 14–16.

Kagan, Sarah H. (2008). "Ageism in Cancer Care." *Seminars in Oncology Nursing* 24, 246–53.

Kaiser Commission. (2013). "Health Coverage by Race and Ethnicity: The Potential Impact of the Affordable Care Act." Kaiser Family Foundation. Retrieved January 19, 2016. http://kff.org/disparities-policy/issue-brief/health-coverage-by-race-and-ethnicity-the-potential-impact-of-the-affordable-care-act/

Kane, Carol K. (2015). "Updated Data on Physician Practice Arrangements: Inching Toward Hospital Ownership." *Policy Research Perspectives*, American Medical Association. http://www.ama-assn.org/ama/pub/advocacy/health-policy/policy-research.page.

Kaptchuk, Ted J. & David M. Eisenberg. (2001). "Varieties of Healing. 1. Medical Pluralism in the United States." *Annals of Internal Medicine* 135, 189–95.

Karp, David. (1996). *Speaking of Sadness: Depression, Disconnection, and the Meanings of Illness*. New York: Oxford University Press.

Kasl, Stanislav & Sidney Cobb. (1966). "Health Behavior, Illness Behavior, and Sick Role Behavior." *Archives of Environmental Health* 12, 246–66.

Kasprzyk, Danuta & Daniel E. Montaño. (2007). "Application of an Integrated Behavioral Model to Understand HIV Prevention Behavior of High Risk Men in Rural Zimbabwe." Pp. 149–72 in *Prediction and Change of Health Behavior: Applying the Reasoned Action Approach*. Icek Ajzen, Dolores Albarracin, & Robert Hornik, eds. Hillsdale, NJ: Erlbaum.

Kasprzyk, Danuta, Daniel E. Montaño, & Martin Fishbein. (1998). "Application of an Integrated Behavioral Model to Predict Condom Use: A Prospective Study among HIV High-Risk Groups." *Journal of Applied Social Psychology* 28, 1557–83.

Keeley, Bethany, Lanelle Wright, & Celeste M. Condit. (2009). "Functions of Health Fatalism: Fatalistic Talk as Face Saving, Uncertainty Management, Stress Relief, and Sense Making." *Sociology of Health & Illness* 31, 734–47.

Kevles, Bettyann H. (1997). *Naked to the Bone: Medical Imagine in the Twentieth Century*. Cambridge, MA: Perseus Publishing.

Kevles, Daniel J. (1995). *In the Name of Eugenics: Genetics and the Uses of Human Heredity*. Berkeley and Los Angeles, CA: University of California Press.

Khatri, Naresh, Gordon D. Brown, & Lanis L. Hicks. (2009). "From a Blame Culture to a Just Culture in Health Care." *Health Care Management Review* 34, 312–22.

Kiatpongsan, Sorapop & Michael E. Norton. (2014). "How Much (More) Should CEOs Make? A Universal Desire for More Equal Pay." *Perspectives on Psychological Science* 9, 587–93.

Kirk, Stuart A. (2004). "Are Children's DSM Diagnoses Accurate?" *Brief Treatment and Crisis Intervention* 4, 255–70.

Kleinman, Arthur M. (1973). "Medicine's Symbolic Reality: A Central Problem in the Philosophy of Medicine." *Inquiry* 16, 206–13.

———. (2013). "From Illness as Culture to Caregiving as Moral Experience." *New England Journal of Medicine* 368, 1376–77.

Kleinman, Arthur, Leon Eisenberg, & Byron Good. (1978). "Culture, Illness, and Care: Clinical Lessons from Anthropologic and Cross-Cultural Research." *Annals of Internal Medicine* 88, 251–58.

Knight, Bob G., Gia S. Robinson, Crystal V. Flynn Longmire, Miae Chun, Kayoko Nakao, & Jung Hyun Kim. (2002). "Cross Cultural Issues in Caregiving for Persons with Dementia: Do Familism Values Reduce Burden and Distress?" *Ageing International* 27, 70–94.

Kolata, Gina. (2015). "Rise in Deaths for U.S. Whites in Middle Age." *New York Times*. November 3, 2015. A1.

Kolata, Gina & Sarah Cohen. (2016). "Drug Overdoses Propel Rise in Mortality Rates of Whites." *New York Times*. January 17, 2016. A1.

Korp, Peter. (2008). "The Symbolic Power of 'Healthy Lifestyles'." *Health Sociology Review* 17, 18–26.

Kovner, Anthony R. & James R. Knickman. (2011). "The Current U.S. Health Care System." Pp. 3–8 in *Jonas & Kovner's Health Care Delivery in the United States*. Anthony R. Kovner & James R. Knickman, eds. New York: Springer.

Kravitz, Richard L., Ronald M. Epstein, Mitchell D. Feldman, Carol E. Franz, Rahman Azari, Machael S. Wilkes, et al. (2005). "Influence of Patients' Requests for Direct-to-Consumer

Advertised Antidepressants: A Randomized Controlled Trial." *Journal of the American Medical Association* 293, 1995–2002.

Kübler-Ross, Elizabeth. (1969). *On Death and Dying*. New York: MacMillan Company.

Kydd, Angela & Anne Fleming. (2015). "Ageism and Age Discrimination in Health Care: Fact or Fiction? A Narrative Review of the Literature." *Maturitas* 81, 432–38.

Lamorey, Suzanne. (1999). "Parentification of Siblings with Disability or Chronic Disease." Pp. 75–91 in *Burdened Children: Theory, Research, and the Treatment of Parentification*. Nancy D. Chase, ed. Thousand Oaks, CA: Sage.

Lantz, Paula M. (2008). "Gender and Leadership in Healthcare Administration: 21st Century Progress and Challenges." *Journal of Healthcare Management* 53, 291–303.

Lazarus, Richard S. (1993). "Coping Theory and Research: Past, Present, and Future." *Psychosomatic Medicine* 55, 234–47.

Leape, Lucian, Ann G. Lawthers, Troyen A. Brennan, & William G. Johnson. (1993). *Preventing Medical Injury. Quality Review Bulletin* 19, 144–49.

Lecendreux, Michel, Eric Konofal, & Stephen V. Faraone. (2010). "Prevalence of ADHD and Associated Features in French Children." *Journal of Attention Disorders* 15, 516–24.

Levy, Neil. (2002). "Deafness, Culture, and Choice." *Journal of Medical Ethics* 28, 284–85.

Light, Donald. (2000). "Fostering a Justice-Based Health Care System." *Contemporary Sociology* 29, 62–74.

———. (2011). "Historical and Comparative Reflections on the U.S. National Health Insurance Reforms." *Social Science & Medicine* 72, 129–32.

———. (2013). "Comparative Models of 'Health Care' Systems." Pp. 543–57 in *The Sociology of Health and Illness: Critical Perspectives*, 9th edition. Peter Conrad & Valerie Leiter, eds. New York: Worth.

Light, Donald & Alexander Schuller (eds.). (1986). *Political Values and Health Care: The German Experience*. Cambridge, MA: MIT Press.

Link, Bruce. (2008). "Epidemiological Sociology and the Social Shaping of Population Health." *Journal of Health and Social Behavior* 49, 367–84.

Link, Bruce G. & Jo C. Phelan. (1995). "Social Conditions as Fundamental Causes of Disease." *Journal of Health and Social Behavior*, 35(Extra Issue), 80–94.

———. (2000). "Evaluating the Fundamental Cause Explanation for Social Disparities in Health." Pp. 33–46 in *Handbook of Medical Sociology*. Chloe E. Bird, Peter Conrad, Allen M. Fremont, &Stefan Timmermans, eds. Upper Saddle River, NJ: Prentice Hall.

Liu, Hui. (2014). "Gender Paradox (and the Health Myth)." Pp. 629–33 in *The Wiley-Blackwell Encyclopedia of Health, Illness, Behavior and Society*. William C. Cockerham, Robert Dingwall, & Stella Quah, eds. Malden, MA: John Wiley & Sons.

Lloyd-Jones, Donald, Robert J. Adams, Todd M. Brown, Mercedes Carnethon, Shifan Dai, Giovanni De Simone, et al. (2010). "Heart Disease and Stroke Statistics—2010 Update: A Report from the American Heart Association." *Circulation* 121, e46–215.

Loewen, James W. (1995). *Lies My Teacher Told Me: Everything Your American History Textbook Got Wrong*. New York: The New Press.

Loftus, Stephen & Sandra Mackey. (2012). "Interviewing Patients and Clients." Pp. 187–94 in *Communicating in the Health Sciences*, 3rd edition. Joy Higgs, Rola Ajjawi, Lindy McAllister, Franziska Trede, & Stephen Loftus, eds. Sydney, Australia: Oxford University Press.

Loftus, Stephen & Trisha Greenhalgh. (2010). "Towards a Narrative Mode of Practice." Pp. 85–94 in *Education for Future Practice*. Joy Higgs, Della Fish, Ian Goulter, Stephen Loftus, Jo-Anne Reid, & Franziska Trede, eds. Rotterdam: Sense Publishers.

Lovasi Gina S., Malo A. Hutson, Monica Guerra, & Kathryn Neckerman. (2009). "Built Environments and Obesity in Disadvantaged Populations." *Epidemiological Reviews* 31, 7–20.

MacDorman, Marian F., Fay Menacker, & Eugene Declercq. (2008). "Cesarean Birth in the United States: Epidemiology, Trends, and Outcomes." *Clinics in Perinatology* 35, 293–307.

Macintyre, Sally, Anne Ellaway, & Steven Cummins. (2002). "Place Effects on Health: How Can We Conceptualise, Operationalise and Measure Them?" *Social Science & Medicine* 55, 125–39.

Maggs, Christopher. (1993). "A General History of Nursing: 1800–1900." Pp. 1309–28 in *The Companion Encyclopedia of the History of Medicine*. W. F. Bynum & Roy Porter, eds. New York: Routledge.

Maklakov, Alexei & Virpi Lummaa. (2013). "Evolution of Sex Differences in Lifespan and Aging: Causes and Constraints." *BioEssays* 35, 717–24.

Makris, Una E., Robin T. Higashi, Emily G. Marks, Liana Fraenkel, Joana E. M. Sale, Thomas M. Gill, et al. (2015). "Ageism, Negative Attitudes, and Competing Co-Morbidities—Why Older Adults May Not Seek Care for Restricting Back Pain: A Qualitative Study." *BMC Geriatrics* 15, 39–48.

Margerison-Zilko, Claire, Catherine Cubbin, Jina Jun, Kristen Marchi, Kathryn Fingar, & Paula Braveman. (2015). "Beyond the Cross-Sectional: Neighborhood Poverty Histories and Preterm Birth." *American Journal of Public Health* 105, 1174–80.

Markides, Kyriakos S. & Jeannine Coreil. (1986). "The Health of Hispanics in the Southwestern United States: An Epidemiologic Paradox." *Public Health Reports* 101, 253–265.

Martin, Anne B., Micah Hartman, Joseph Benson, Aaron Catlin, & the National Health Expenditure Accounts Team. (2016). "National Health Spending in 2014: Faster Growth Driven by Coverage Expansion and Prescription Drug Spending." *Health Affairs* 35, 1–11.

Martin, Kimberly D. & Lisa A. Cooper. (2013). "Maximizing the Benefits of 'We' in Race-Discordant Patient-Physician Relationships: Novel Insights Raise Intriguing Questions." *Journal of General Internal Medicine* 28, 1119–21.

Marx, David. (2009). *Whack-a-Mole: The Price We Pay for Expecting Perfection*. Plano, TX: By Your Side Studios.

Maslow, Abraham. ([1962] 2014). *Toward a Psychology of Being*. Floyd, VA: Sublime Books.

Masters, James & Pat Cash (2014). "Venus Williams: The Champion Trying to Slam Sjorgen's Syndrome." *CNN*. http://edition.cnn.com/2014/03/20/sport/tennis/venus-williams-sjogrens-syndrome/. Retrieved July 9, 2015.

Matthews, T. J., Marian F. MacDorman, & Marie E. Thoma. (2015). "Infant Mortality Statistics from the 2013 Period Linked Birth/Infant Death Data Set." *National Vital Statistics Report* 64(9), August 6.

Maynard, Alan & Andrew Street. (2006). "Seven Years of Feast, Seven Years of Famine: Boom to Bust in the NHS?" *British Medical Journal* 332, 906–08.

McKinlay, John B. & Sonja M. McKinlay. (1977). "The Questionable Contribution of Medical Measures to the Decline of Mortality in the United States in the Twentieth Century." *Milbank Memorial Fund Quarterly—Health and Society* 55, 405–28.

McNamee, Stephen J. & Robert K. Miller. (2013). *The Meritocracy Myth*. Lanham, MD: Rowman & Littlefield.

Mead, George Herbert. (1934). *Mind, Self & Society*. Chicago, IL: University of Chicago Press.

Meyer, Jan H. F. & Ray Land. (2003). "Threshold Concepts and Troublesome Knowledge: Linkages to Ways of Thinking and Practising within the Disciplines." *ETL Project, Occasional Report* 4. http://www.etl.tla.ed.ac.uk. Retrieved July 15, 2015.

———. (2006). *Overcoming Barriers to Student Understanding: Threshold Concepts and Troublesome Knowledge*. New York: Routledge.

Michaelsen, Larry K. & Emily E. Schultheiss. (1988). "Making Feedback Helpful." *The Organizational Behavior Teaching Review* 13, 109–13.

Midkiff, Hurd & Elizabeth Cordaro. (2012). "Developing Work RVUs for Production-based Physician Compensation Programs." *Healthcare Financial Management* 66, 140–5.

Milgram, Stanley. (1965 [2008]). *Obedience*. University Park, PA: Pennsylvania State University Media Sales.

Miller, William R. & Stephen Rollnick. (2013). *Motivational Interviewing: Helping People Change*. New York: The Guilford Press.

Mills, C. Wright. (1959). *The Sociological Imagination*. New York: Oxford University Press.

———. (1959 [1977]). *The Sociological Imagination*. London: Oxford University Press.

———. (1959 [2000]). *The Sociological Imagination*. London: Oxford University Press.

Moisse, Katie & Dan Childs. (2011). "Venus Williams: What Is Sjorgen's Syndrome?" *ABC News*. http://abcnews.go.com/

Health/w_MindBodyNews/venus-williams-sjogrens-syndrome/story?id=14426884. Retrieved July 9, 2015.

Montaño, Daniel E. & Danuta Kasprzyk. (2008). "Theory of Reasoned Action, Theory of Planned Behavior, and the Integrated Behavioral Model." Pp. 67–96 in *Health Behavior: Theory, Research and Practice*, 4th edition. Karen Glanz, Barbara K. Rimer, & K. Viswanath, eds. San Francisco, CA: John Wiley & Sons.

Morgan Paul L., Jeremy Staff, Marianne M. Hillemeier, George Farkas, & Steven Maczuga. (2013). "Racial and Ethnic Disparities in ADHD Diagnosis from Kindergarten to Eighth Grade." *Pediatrics* 132, 85–93.

Mossialos, Elias, Martin Wenzl, Robin Osborn, & Chloe Anderson (eds.). (2015). *International Profiles of Health Care Systems, 2014*. Commonwealth Fund Pub. No. 1802. New York: The Commonwealth Fund.

Murray, Christopher J. L., Theo Vos, Rafael Lozano, Mohsen Naghavi, Abraham D. Flaxman, Catherine Michaud, et al. (2012). "Disability-Adjusted Life Years (DALYS) for 291 Diseases and Injuries in 21 Regions, 1990-2010: A Systematic Analysis for the Global Burden of Disease Study 2010." *The Lancet* 380, 2197–223.

Murray, Rheana. (2012). "Egg Yolks Almost as Bad for your Heart as Smoking Cigarettes, Says Study." http://www.nydailynews.com/life-style/health/egg-yolks-bad-heart-smoking-cigarettes-study-article-1.1138536. Accessed June 10, 2016.

Murtin, Fabrice & Marco Mira d'Ercole. (2015). "Household Wealth Inequality across OECD Countries: New OECD Evidence." *OECD Statistics Brief*, No 21. June 2015.

Musen, Ken. (1988 [2004]). *Quiet Rage: The Stanford Prison Experiment*. New York: Insight Media.

Nahin, Richard L., Patricia M. Barnes, Barbara J. Stussman, & Barbara Bloom. (2009). "Costs of Complementary and Alternative Medicine (CAM) and Frequency of Visits to CAM Practitioners: United States, 2007." *National Health Statistics Report* 18, July 30. nccih.nih. gov. Accessed July 15, 2015.

National Center for Health Statistics (NCHS). (2015). *Health, United States, 2014: With Special Feature on Adults Aged 55-64*. Hyattsville, MD: U.S. Department of Health & Human Services, Centers for Disease Control & Prevention

Needham, Belinda L., Nancy Adler, Steven Gregorich, David Rehkopf, Jue Lin, Elizabeth H. Blackburn, et al. (2013). "Socioeconomic Status, Health Behavior, and Leukocyte Telomere Length in the National Health and Nutrition Examination Survey, 1999-2002." *Social Science & Medicine* 85, 1–8.

Needham, Belinda L., Judith E. Carroll, Ana V. Diez Roux, Annette L. Fitzpatrick, Kari Moore, & Teresa E. Seeman. (2014). "Neighborhood Characteristics and Leukocyte Telomere Length: The Multi-Ethnic Study of Atherosclerosis." *Health and Place* 28, 167–72.

Neimeyer, Robert A. (2001). *Meaning Reconstruction and the Experience of Loss*. Washington, DC: American Psychological Association.

Noar, Seth M. & Rick S. Zimmerman. (2005). "Health Behavior Theory and Cumulative Knowledge Regarding Health Behaviors: Are We Moving in the Right Direction?" *Health Education Research* 20, 275–90.

Norton, Michael I. & Dan Ariely. (2011). "Building a Better America—One Wealth Quintile at a Time." *Perspectives on Psychological Science* 6, 9–12.

O'Connor, Anahad. (2015). "Coca-Cola Funds Scientists Who Shift Blame for Obesity Away from Bad Diets." *New York Times*, August 10, A1.

Okma, Kieke G. H. (2014). "Changing Health Care Systems of the World." Pp. 905–17 in *The Wiley-Blackwell Encyclopedia of Health, Illness, Behavior & Society*. William C. Cockerham, Robert Dingwall, & Stella Quah, eds. Malden, MA: *John* Wiley & Sons.

Olsen, Laura. (2016). "'It's on the MCAT for a Reason': Premedical Students and the Perceived Utility of Sociology." *Teaching Sociology* 44, 72–83.

Omran, Abdel R. (1971). "The Epidemiologic Transition: A Theory of the Epidemiology of Population Change." *Milbank Memorial Fund Quarterly* 49, 509–38.

Organisation for Economic Co-operation & Development (OECD). (2014). *United States: Tackling High Inequalities, Creating Opportunities for All*. Paris: OECD.

Osterman, Michelle J. K. & Joyce A. Martin. (2014). "Trends in Low-risk Cesarean Delivery in the United States, 1990–2013." *National Vital Statistics Reports* 63, November 5, Centers for Disease Control and Prevention.

Paige, Scott E. (2007). *The Difference: How the Power of Diversity Creates Better Groups, Firms, Schools, and Societies*. Princeton, NJ: Princeton University Press.

Pampel, Fred C., Patrick M. Krueger, & Justin T. Denney. (2010). "Socioeconomic Disparities in Health Behaviors." *Annual Review of Sociology* 36, 349–70.

Paracelsus. ([1951] 1979). *Paracelsus: Selected Writings*. Jolande Jacobi, ed. Princeton, NJ: Princeton University Press.

Parker, Tom & Ron J. Lambert. (2008). *Is That Your Hand in My Pocket?: The Sales Professionals Guide to Negotiating*. Nashville, TN: Thomas Nelson.

Parsons, Talcott. (1951). *The Social System*. New York: Free Press.

Parsons, Talcott. (1951 [1991]). *The Social System*. New York: Routledge.

Pear, Robert. (2015). "Health Spending in U.S. Topped $3 Trillion Last Year." *New York Times*. December 3, 2015. A24.

Pearlin, Leonard I. (1989) "The Sociological Study of Stress." *Journal of Health and Social Behavior* 30, 241–56.

Pearlin, Leonard I., Morton A. Lieberman, Elizabeth G. Menaghan, & Joseph T. Mullan. (1981). "The Stress Process." *Journal of Health and Social Behavior* 22, 337–56.

Pence, Gregory E. (2011). *Medical Ethics: Accounts of Ground-Breaking Cases*. New York: McGraw-Hill.

Penner, Louis A., Irene V. Blair, Terrance L. Albrecht, & John F. Dovidio. (2014). "Reducing Racial Health Care Disparities: A Social Psychological Analysis." *Policy Insights from the Behavioral and Brain Sciences* 1, 204–12.

PepNet2. (2014). *Research Brief: Employment Data for Adults Who Are Deaf and Hard-of-Hearing*. www.pepnet.org. Retrieved June 24, 2015.

Peters, William. (1985). *A Class Divided*. Boston: Public Broadcasting Service.

———. (1987). *A Class Divided: Then and Now*. New Haven: Yale University Press.

Phelan, Jo C., Bruce Link, Ana Diez-Roux, Ichiro Kawachi, & Bruce Levin. (2004). "'Fundamental Causes' of Social Inequalities in Mortality: A Test of the Theory." *Journal of Health and Social Behavior* 45, 265–85.

Phelan, Jo C., Bruce G. Link, & Parisa Tehranifar. (2010). "Social Conditions as Fundamental Causes of Health Inequalities: Theory, Evidence, and Policy Implications." *Journal of Health and Social Behavior* 51, S28–40.

Phillips, Katherine W. (2014). "How Diversity Works." *Scientific American* 311, 43–47.

Porter, Roy. (1997). *The Greatest Benefit to Mankind: A Medical History of Humanity*. New York: W.W. Norton.

Prasad, Vinayak K. & Adam S. Cifu. (2015). *Ending Medical Reversal: Improving Outcomes, Saving Lives*. Baltimore, MD: Johns Hopkins University Press.

Privitera, Gregory. (2012). *Statistics for the Behavioral Sciences*. Thousand Oaks, CA: Sage.

Prochaska, James O., Carlo C. DiClemente, & John C. Norcross. (1992). "In Search of How People Change: Applications to Addictive Behaviors." *American Psychologist* 47, 1102–14.

Prochaska, James O., Susan Butterworth, Colleen A. Redding, Verna Burden, Nancy Perrin, Michael Leo, et al. (2008a). "Initial Efficacy of MI, TTM Tailoring, and HRI's in Multiple Behaviors for Employee Health Promotion." *Preventive Medicine* 46, 226–31.

Prochaska, James O., Colleen A. Redding, & Kerry E. Evers. (2008b). "The Transtheoretical Model and Stages of Change." Pp. 97–121 in *Health Behavior: Theory, Research and Practice*, 4th edition. Karen Glanz, Barbara K. Rimer, & K. Viswanath, eds. San Francisco, CA: John Wiley & Sons.

Quah, Stella R. (2014). "Health and Culture." Pp. 926–34 in *The Wiley-Blackwell Encyclopedia of Health, Illness, Behavior and Society*. William C. Cockerham, Robert Dingwall, & Stella Quah, eds. Malden, MA: John Wiley & Sons.

Rau, Jordan. (2013). "Hospital Ratings Are in the Eye of the Beholder." *Kaiser Health News*. March 18. http://khn.org/news/expanding-number-of-groups-offer-hospital-ratings/.

Reason, James. (1990). *Human Error*. New York: Cambridge University Press.

Reed, Ralph R. & Daryl Evans. (1987). "The Deprofessionalization of Medicine: Causes,

Effects, Responses. *Journal of the American Medical Association 258,* 3279–82.

Reeve, Ron & James Wright. (1996). "Module I: Characteristics and Identification." In *A Continuing Education Program on Attention Deficit/Hyperactivity Disorder.* Ron Reeve, Judy Schrag, Mary Spessard, Ron Walker, Ann Welch, & James Wright, eds. Washington DC: Council for Exceptional Children, Reston, VA. Special Education Programs (ED/OSERS).

Reid, T. R. (2009). *The Healing of America: A Global Quest for Better, Cheaper, and Fairer Health Care.* New York: Penguin.

Reinar, Liv Merete & Peter M. Bradley. (2007). "Evidence-Based Practice and Critical Appraisal of Systematic Reviews." Pp. 365–81 in *Research Methodology in the Medical and Biological Sciences.* Petter Laake, Haakon Breien Benestad, & Bjørn Reino Olsen, eds. London: Academic Press.

Riley, Matilda White. (1987). "On the Significance of Age in Sociology." *American Sociological Review 52,* 1–14.

Ritchey, Ferris. (2007). *The Statistical Imagination.* New York: McGraw-Hill.

Ritzer, George & David Walczak. (1988). "Rationalization and the Deprofessionalization of Physicians." *Social Forces 67,* 1–22.

Rogers, Carl. (1951). *Client-Centered Therapy.* Boston, MA: Houghton-Mifflin.

Rosen, Craig S. (2000). "Is the Sequencing of Change Processes by Stage Consistent across Health Problems? A Meta-Analysis." *Health Psychology 19,* 593–604.

Rosen, George. (1993). *A History of Public Health.* Baltimore, MD: Johns Hopkins University Press.

Rosenbaum, Paul. (2005). "Observational Study." Pp. 1451–62 in the *Encyclopedia of Statistics in Behavioral Science.* Brian Everitt & David Howell, eds. Chichester: Wiley.

Rosenberg, Ellen, Claude Richard, Marie-Thérèse Lussier, & Shelly N. Abdool. (2006). "Intercultural Communication Competence in Family Medicine." *Patient Education and Counseling 61,* 236–45.

Rosenstock, Irwin M. (1974). "Historical Origins of the Health Belief Model." *Health Education Monographs 2,* 328–335.

Ross, Catherine E., John Mirowsky, & Shana Pribesh. (2001). "Powerlessness and the Amplification of Threat: Neighborhood Disadvantage, Disorder, and Mistrust." *American Sociological Review 66,* 568–91.

Rossi, Amanda, Anastasia Dikareva, Simon Bacon, & Stella Daskalopoulou. (2012). "The Impact of Physical Activity on Mortality in Patients with High Blood Pressure: A Systematic Review." *Journal of Hypertension 30*(7), 1277–88.

Roter, Debra L. & Judith A. Hall. (2004). "Physician Gender and Patient-Centered Communication: A Critical Review of Empirical Research." *Annual Review of Public Health 25,* 497–519.

Roter, Debra L., Judith A. Hall, & Yutaka Aoki. (2002). "Physician Gender Effects in Medical Communication: A Meta-Analytic Review." *Journal of the American Medical Association 288,* 756–64.

Rothman, Sheila M. & David J. Rothman. (1984). *The Willowbrook Wars: Bringing the Mentally Disabled into the Community.* New York: Harper & Row.

Rushton, Jerry L., Kathryn E. Fant, & Sarah J. Clark. (2004). "Use of Practice Guidelines in the Primary Care of Children with Attention-Deficit/Hyperactivity Disorder." *Pediatrics 114,* e23–28.

Sanger-Katz, Margot. (2016). "Medical Debt Often Crushing Even for Insured." *New York Times.* January 6. A1.

Savitt, Todd L. (1978). *Medicine and Slavery: The Diseases and Health Care of Blacks in Antebellum Virginia.* Chicago, IL: University of Illinois Press.

———. (1982). "The Use of Blacks for Medical Experimentation and Demonstration in the Old South." *The Journal of Southern History 48,* 331–48.

Scambler, Graham. (2014). "Illness Experience." In *The Wiley Blackwell Encyclopedia of Health, Illness, Behavior, and Society.* W. C. Cockerham, R. Dingwall, & S. R. Quah, eds. West Sussex: Wiley-Blackwell.

Schaefer, Gabrielle, Heidi Matus, John H. Schuman, Keith Sauter, Benjamin Vekhter, David O. Meltzer, et al. (2012). "Financial Responsibility of Hospitalized Patients Who Left Against Medical Advice: Medical Urban Legend?" *Journal of General Internal Medicine 27*(7), 825–30.

Schneider, Joseph W. (1978). "Deviant Drinking as Disease: Alcoholism as a Social Accomplishment." *Social Problems* 25, 361–72.

Schoenthaler, Antoinette, John P. Allengrante, William Chaplin, & Gbenga Ogedegbe. (2012). "The Effect of Patient-Provider Communication on Medication Adherence in Hypertensive Black Patients: Does Race Concordance Matter?" *Annals of Behavioral Medicine* 43, 372–82.

Schouten, Barbara C. & Ludwien Meeuwesen. (2006). "Cultural Differences in Medical Communication: A Review of the Literature." *Patient Education and Counseling* 64, 21–34.

Schroder, Kerstin E. E. (2014). "Health Psychology." Pp. 1064–85 in *The Wiley-Blackwell Encyclopedia of Health, Illness, Behavior and Society*. William C. Cockerham, Robert Dingwall, & Stella Quah, eds. Malden, MA: John Wiley & Sons.

Schut, Frederik T. (1995). "Health Care Reform in the Netherlands: Balancing Corporatism, Etatism, and Market Mechanisms." *Journal of Health Politics, Policy and Law* 20, 615–52.

Schwarzer, Ralf. (2008). "Modeling Health Behavior Change: How to Predict and Modify the Adoption and Maintenance of Health Behaviors." *Applied Psychology* 57, 1–29.

Shannon, Sarah E., Mary Beth Foglia, Mary Hardy, & Thomas H. Gallagher. (2009). "Disclosing Errors to Patients: Perspectives of Registered Nurses." *The Joint Commission Journal on Quality and Patient Safety* 35, 5–12.

Sharma, Rashmi K., Nidhi Khosla, James A. Tulsky, & Joseph A. Carrese. (2011). "Traditional Expectations versus US Realities: First- and Second-Generations Asian Indian Perspectives on End-of-Life Care." *Journal of General Internal Medicine* 27, 311–17.

Sharpe, Virginia Ashby & Alan I. Faden. (1998). *Medical Harm: Historical, Conceptual, and Ethical Dimensions of Iatrogenic Illness*. Cambridge: Cambridge University Press.

Shi, Leiyu. (2008). *Health Services Research Methods*. Clifton Park, NY: Thomson-Delmar.

Shi, Leiyu & Douglas A. Singh. (2012). *Delivering Health Care in America: A Systems Approach*. Burlington, MA: Jones & Bartlett.

Shryock, Richard H. (1969). "Empiricism versus Rationalism in American Medicine." *Proceedings of the American Antiquarian Society* 79, 99–150.

Siegel, Rebecca, Deepa Naishadham, & Ahmedin Jemal. (2013). "Cancer Statistics, 2013." *CA: A Cancer Journal for Clinicians* 63, 11–30.

Sigerist, Henry E. (1961). *A History of Medicine*. Oxford: Oxford University Press.

Simon, Robin W. & Leda E. Nath. (2004). "Gender and Emotion in the United States." *American Journal of Sociology* 109, 1137–76.

Singh, Hardeep, Eric J. Thomas, & Laura A. Petersen. (2006). "Understanding Diagnostic Errors in Medicine: A Lesson from Aviation." *Quality and Safety in Health Care* 15, 159–64.

Singh, Ilina. (2007). "Clinical Implications of Ethical Concepts: Moral Self-Understandings in Children Taking Methylphenidate for ADHD." *Clinical Child Psychology and Psychiatry* 12, 167–182.

Singleton, Royce & Bruce Straits. (1999). *Approaches to Social Research*. New York: Oxford University Press.

Skinner, Burrhus F. (1971). *Beyond Freedom and Dignity*. New York: Bantam/Vintage.

Skinner, Celette S., Jasmin Tiro, & Victoria L. Champion. (2015). "The Health Belief Model." Pp. 75–94 in *Health Behavior: Theory, Research and Practice*, 5th edition. Karen Glanz, Barbara K. Rimer, & K. Viswanath, eds. San Francisco, CA: John Wiley & Sons.

Skovlund, Eva & Morten H. Vatn. (2007). "Clinical Research." Pp. 213–40 in *Research Methodology in the Medical and Biological Sciences*. Petter Laake, Haakon Breien Benestad, & Bjørn Reino Olsen, eds. London: Academic Press.

Smedley, Brian D., Adrienne Y. Stith, & Alan R. Nelson. (2003). *Unequal Treatment: Confronting Racial and Ethnic Disparities in Health Care*. Washington, DC: The National Academies Press.

Smith, Robert C. (1996). *The Patient's Story: Integrated Patient-Doctor Interviewing*. Boston, MA: Little, Brown and Company.

Smith-Morris, Carolyn M. (2004). "Reducing Diabetes in Indian Country: Lessons from the Three Domains Influencing Pima Diabetes." *Human Organization* 63, 34–46.

Snow, John. (1849). *On the Mode of Communication of Cholera*. London: John Churchill.

Solomon, Sheldon, Jeff Greenberg, & Tom Pyszczynski, T. (1991). "A Terror Management

Theory of Social Behavior: The Psychological Functions of Self-esteem and Cultural Worldviews." Pp. 93–159 in *Advances in Experimental Social Psychology*, Vol. 24, Mark P. Zanna, ed. Orlando, FL: Academic Press.

Sontag, Lisa M. & Julia A. Graber. (2010). "Coping with Perceived Peer Stress: Gender-Specific and Common Pathways to Symptoms of Psychopathology." *Developmental Psychology* 46, 1605–20.

Span, Paula. (2015). "Overtreated Patients, Underwhelming Results." *New York Times*. November 10, 2015. D2.

Spence, J. David, David J. A. Jenkins, & Jean Davignon. (2010). "Dietary Cholesterol and Egg Yolks: Not for Patients at Risk of Vascular Disease." *Canadian Journal of Cardiology* 26, e336–39.

———. (2012). "Egg Yolk Consumption and Carotid Plaque." *Atherosclerosis* 224, 469–73.

Springer, Kristen W., Jeanne Mager Stellman, & Rebecca M. Jordan-Young. (2012). "Beyond a Catalogue of Differences: A Theoretical Frame and Good Practice Guidelines for Researching Sex/Gender in Human Health." *Social Science and Medicine* 74, 1817–24.

Starr, Paul. (1982). *The Social Transformation of American Medicine: The Rise of a Sovereign Profession and the Making of a Vast Industry*. New York: Basic Books.

Stavert, Robert R. & Jason P. Lott. (2013). "The Bystander Effect in Medical Care." *New England Journal of Medicine* 368, 8–9.

Steptoe, Andrew & Mika Kivimäki. (2013). "Stress and Cardiovascular Disease: An Update on Current Knowledge." *Annual Review of Public Health* 34, 337–54.

Stewart, Moira A. (1995). "Effective Physician-Patient Communication and Health Outcomes: A Review." *Canadian Medical Association* 152, 1423–33.

Straus, Robert. (1957). "Nature and Status of Medical Sociology." *American Sociological Review* 22, 200–04.

———. (1999). "Medical Sociology: A Personal Fifty Year Perspective." *Journal of Health and Social Behavior* 40, 1–16.

Sultz, Harry A. & Kristina M. Young. (2014). *Health Care USA: Understanding Its Organization and Delivery*. Burlington, MA: Jones & Bartlett.

Suminski, Richard R., Erin K. Connolly, Linda E. May, Jason Adam Wasserman, Norma Olvera, & Rebecca E. Lee. (2012). "Park Quality in Racial/Ethnic Minority Neighborhoods." *Environmental Justice* 5, 271–78.

Suminski, Richard R., Jason Adam Wasserman, Carlene Mayfield, & Elizabeth McClain. (2013). "Relationships between Perceptions of Environmental Features and Physical Activity." *Perceptual and Motor Skills* 117, 49–64.

Suminski, Richard R., Terry J. Presley, Jason Adam Wasserman, Carlene Mayfield, & Elizabeth McClain. (2014). "Playground Safety is Associated with Playground, Park, and Neighborhood Characteristics." *Journal of Physical Activity & Health* 12(3), 402–08.

Szasz, Thomas S. & Marc H. Hollender. (1956). "A Contribution to the Philosophy of Medicine: The Basic Models of the Doctor-Patient Relationship." *AMA Archives of Internal Medicine* 97, 585–92.

Tajfel, Henri. (1979). *Differentiation between Social Groups: Studies in the Social Psychology of Intergroup Relations*. London: Academic Press.

Tannen, Deborah. (1991). *You Just Don't Understand: Women and Men in Conversation*. New York: Ballantine Books.

Tarzian, Anita J. (2013). "Health Care Ethics Consultation: An Update on Core Competencies and Emerging Standards from the American Society for Bioethics and Humanities' Core Competencies Update Task Force." *American Journal of Bioethics* 13, 3–13.

Taylor, Eric. (2004). "ADHD Is Best Understood as a Social Construct: Against." *British Journal of Psychiatry* 184, 8–9.

Taylor, Erin Fries, Timothy Lake, Jessica Nysenbaum, Greg Peterson, & David Meyers. (2011). *Coordinating Care in the Medical Neighborhood: Critical Components and Available Mechanisms*. White Paper. (Prepared by Mathematica Policy Research under Contract No. HHSA2902009000191 TO2). AHRQ Publication No. 11-0064. Rockville, MD: Agency for Healthcare Research & Quality.

TeamSTEPPS. (2013). *TeamSTEPPS Pocket Guide 2.0*. Rockville, MD: Agency for Healthcare Research and Quality.

Thomas, Rae, Sharon Sanders, Jenny Doust, Elaine Beller, & Paul Glasziou. (2015). "Prevalence of Attention-Deficit/Hyperactivity Disorder: A Systematic Review and Meta-analysis." *Pediatrics* 135, e994–1001.

Thompson, Lee. (2004). "Long-term Care: Support for Family Caregivers." Long-Term Care Financing Project. Washington DC: Georgetown University Health Policy Institute. http://hpi.georgetown.edu/ltc. Retrieved July 8, 2015.

Timimi, Sami. (2004). "ADHD Is Best Understood as a Social Construct: For." *British Journal of Psychiatry* 184, 8–9.

Tolbert Coombs, Alice A. & Roderick K. King. (2005). "Workplace Discrimination: Experiences of Practicing Physicians." *Journal of the National Medical Association* 97, 467–77.

Tosh, Karen. (2007). "Nineteenth Century Handmaids or Twenty-First Century Partners?" *Journal of Health Organization and Management* 21, 68–78.

Tseng, Chin-Lin, Orysya Soroka, Miriam Maney, David C. Aron, & Leonard M. Pogach. (2014). "Assessing Potential Glycemic Overtreatment in Persons at Hypoglycemic Risk." *JAMA Internal Medicine* 174, 259–68.

Turner, R. Jay. (2010). "Understanding Health Disparities: The Promise of the Stress Process Model." Pp. 3–21 in *Advances in the Conceptualization of the Stress Process: Essays in Honor of Leonard I. Pearlin*. William R. Avison, Carol S. Aneshensel, Scott Schieman, & Blair Wheaton, eds. New York: Springer.

Twaddle, Andrew. (1969). "Health Decisions and Sick Role Variations: An Exploration." *Journal of Health and Social Behavior* 10, 105–15.

U.S. Central Intelligence Agency (CIA). (2016). *CIA World Factbook*. https://www.cia.gov/library/publications/resources/the-world-factbook/. Accessed January 31, 2016.

United States. (1978). *The Belmont Report: Ethical Principles and Guidelines for the Protection of Human Subjects of Research*. Bethesda, MD: The Commission.

Unwin, Brian K. & Anthony F. Jerant. (1999). "The Home Visit." *American Family Physician* 60, 1481–88.

Vallée, Manuel. (2010). "Biomedicalizing Mental Illness: The Case of Attention Deficit Disorder." *Advances in Medical Sociology* 11, 281–301.

———. (2011). "Resisting American Psychiatry: French Opposition to DSM-III, Biological Reductionism, and the Pharmaceutical Ethos." *Advances in Medical Sociology* 12, 85–110.

van Ryn, Michelle & Jane Burke. (2000). "The Effect of Patient Race and Socio-economic Status on Physicians' Perceptions of Patients." *Social Science and Medicine* 50, 813–28.

van Schaik, Sandrijn M., Bridget C. O'Brien, Sandra A. Almeida, & Shelley R. Adler. (2014). "Perceptions of Interprofessional Teamwork in Low-Acuity Settings: A Qualitative Analysis." *Medical Education* 48, 583–92.

Varul, Matthias Zick. (2010). "Talcott Parsons, the Sick Role, and Chronic Illness." *Body and Society* 16, 72–94.

Volpe, Fernando M. (2011). "Correlation of Cesarean Rates to Maternal and Infant Mortality Rates: An Ecologic Study of Official International Data." *Pan American Journal of Public Health (Revista Panamericana de Salud Pública)* 29(5), 303–08.

Vyt, Andre. (2008). "Interprofessional and Transdisciplinary Teamwork in Health Care." *Diabetes/Metabolism Research and Reviews* 24, S106–09.

Wachter, Robert M. (2016). "How Measurement Fails Us." *New York Times*. January 17. SR5.

Wailoo, Keith. (2001). *Dying in the City of the Blues: Sickle Cell Anemia and the Politics of Race and Health*. Chapel Hill, NC: The University of North Carolina Press.

Waitzkin, Howard. (1985). "Information Giving in Medical Care." *Journal of Health and Social Behavior* 26, 81–101.

Waring, Justin J. (2005). "Beyond Blame: Cultural Barriers to Medical Incident Reporting." *Social Science & Medicine* 60, 1927–35.

Wasserman, Jason A. & Brian P. Hinote. (2012). "The End of Modern Medicine: The Evolution of Disease and Transformations in Medical Practice." *Journal of Healthcare, Science and the Humanities* 2(2), 145–56.

Wasserman, Jason A. & Leon S. Dure IV. (2008). "The Social Psychology of Amateur Ethicists: Blood Product Recall Notification and the Value of Reflexivity." *Journal of Medical Ethics* 34, 530–33.

Wasserman, Jason A., Richard Suminski, Juan Xi, Carlene Mayfield, Alan Glaros, & Richard

Magie. (2014). "A Multi-level Analysis Showing Associations between School Neighborhood and Child Body Mass Index." *International Journal of Obesity* 38, 912–18.

Wasserman, Jason A., Shannon L. Stevenson, Cassandra Claxton, & Ernest F. Krug. (2015). "Moral Reasoning among HEC Members: An Empirical Evaluation of the Relationship of Theory and Practice in Bioethics." *Journal of Clinical Ethics* 26, 108–17.

Wasserman, Jason Adam. (2014). "On Art and Science: An Epistemic Framework for Integrating Social Science and Clinical Medicine." *Journal of Medicine and Philosophy* 39, 279–303.

Wasserman, Jason Adam & Brian P. Hinote. (2011). "Chronic Illness as Incalculable Risk: Scientific Uncertainty and Social Transformations in Medicine." *Social Theory & Health* 9, 41–58.

Wasserman, Jason Adam, Jeffrey Michael Clair, & Ferris Ritchey. (2005). "Racial Differences in Attitudes Toward Euthanasia." *OMEGA: Journal of Death and Dying* 52(3), 263–87.

Wasserman, Jason Adam, Michael A. Flannery, & Jeffrey Michael Clair. (2007). "Razing the Ivory Tower: The Production of Knowledge and Distrust of Medicine among African Americans." *Journal of Medical Ethics* 33, 177–80.

Wasserman, Michael R. (2015). "Geriatric and Primary Care Workforce Development." Pp. 99–116 in *Healthcare Changes and the Affordable Care Act.* James S. Powers, ed. Cham, Switzerland: Springer International Publishing.

Webb, David A. & Jennifer F. Culhane. (2002). "Time of Day Variation in Rates of Obstetric Intervention to Assist in Vaginal Delivery." *Journal of Epidemiology and Community Health* 56, 577–78.

Weber, Max. (1904 [1949]). "Objectivity in Social Science and Social Policy" in *The Methodology of the Social Sciences.* E. A. Shils & H. A. Finch, eds. and trans., New York: Free Press.

———. (1946). "The Distribution of Power within the Political Community: Class, Status, Party." In *From Max Weber: Essays in Sociology.* H. H. Gerth & C. Wright Mills, eds. Oxford: Oxford University Press.

———. ([1922] 1978). *Economy and Society.* 2 vols. Berkeley, CA: University of California Press.

Wedge, Marilyn. (2012). "Why French Kids Don't Have ADHD." *Psychology Today.* www.psychologytoday.com. Retrieved July 9, 2015.

Wehner, Mackenzie R., Kevin T. Nead, Katerina Linos, & Eleni Linos. (2015). "Plenty of Moustaches but Not Enough Women: A Cross-sectional Study of Medical Leaders." *British Medical Journal* 351, h6311.

Weinstein, Neil D. (1988). "The Precaution Adoption Process." *Health Psychology* 7, 355–86.

Weiss, Gregory. (2013). "Uninsured in America." Pp. 339–47 in *The Sociology of Health & Illness*, 8th edition. Peter Conrad & Valerie Leiter, eds. New York: Worth.

Weiss, Gregory L. & Lynne E. Lonnquist. (2015). *The Sociology of Health, Healing, and Illness.* New York: Taylor & Francis.

Welch, H. Gilbert, Lisa M. Schwartz, & Steven Woloshin. (2011). *Over-Diagnosed: Making People Sick in the Pursuit of Health.* Boston: Beacon Press.

Wendt, Claus, Lorraine Frisina, & Heinz Rothgang. (2009). "Healthcare System Types: A Conceptual Framework for Comparison." *Social Policy and Administration* 43, 70–90.

West, Candace & Don H. Zimmerman. (1987). "Doing Gender." *Gender and Society* 1, 125–51.

White, Herbert P. (2011). "Health Care Costs and Value." Pp. 257–76 in *Jonas & Kovner's Health Care Delivery in the United States.* Anthony R. Kovner & James R. Knickman, eds. New York: Springer.

Whitworth, Judith A., Paula M. Williamson, George Mangos, & John J. Kelly. (2005). "Cardiovascular Consequences of Cortisol Excess." *Vascular Health and Risk Management* 1, 291–99.

Willems, Sara, Stéphanie De Maesschalck, Myriam Deveugele, Anselme Derese, & Jan De Maeseneer. (2005). "Socio-economic Status of the Patient and Doctor-Patient Communication: Does It Make a Difference?" *Patient Education and Counseling* 56, 139–46.

Williams, Hants, Leigh Ann Simmons, & Paula Tanabe. (2015). "Mindfulness-Based Stress Reduction in Advanced Nursing Practice: A Nonpharmacologic Approach to Health Promotion, Chronic Disease Management, and

Symptom Control." *Journal of Holistic Nursing* 33, 247–59.

Willis, Leigh A., David W. Coombs, Patricia Drentea, & William C. Cockerham. (2003). "Uncovering the Mystery: Factors of African American Suicide." *Suicide and Life Threatening Behavior* 33, 412–29.

Witkop, Bernhard. (1999). "Paul Ehrlich and His Magic Bullets—Revisited." *Proceedings of the American Philosophical Society* 143, 540–57.

Wong-Baker FACES Foundation (2015). Wong-Baker FACES® Pain Rating Scale. Retrieved July 7, 2015 with permission from http://www.WongBakerFACES.org.

Woolcock, Michael & Deepa Narayan. (2000). "Social Capital: Implications for Development Theory, Research, and Policy." *The World Bank Research Observer* 15, 225–49.

Woolfe, Steven H. & Laudan Aron, eds. (2013) *U. S. Health in International Perspective: Shorter Lives, Poorer Health*. Washington, D.C.: The National Academies Press.

World Health Organization (WHO). (2011). *Global Status Report on Noncommunicable Diseases, 2010*. Geneva, Switzerland: World Health Organization.

———. (2016). *Global Health Expenditure Database*. http://apps.who.int/nha/database. Accessed January 16, 2016.

Yach, Derek, Corinna Hawkes, Linn Gould, & Karen Hofman. (2004). "The Global Burden of Chronic Diseases: Overcoming Impediments to Prevention and Control." *Journal of the American Medical Association* 291, 2616–22.

Zborowski, Mark. (1952). "Cultural Components in Responses to Pain." *Journal of Social Issues* 8, 16–30.

Zimbardo, Philip. (2000). "The SPE: What it Was, Where it Came from, and What Came Out of it." Pp. 198–213 in *Obedience to Authority: Current Perspectives on the Milgram Paradigm*. Thomas Blass, ed. New York: Psychology Press.

Zola, Irving. (1966). "Culture and Symptoms – An Analysis of Patients' Presenting Complaints." *American Sociological Review* 31, 615–30.

Zola, Irving Kenneth. (1973). "Pathways to the Doctor: From Person to Patient." *Social Science and Medicine* 7, 677–89.

Zwarenstein, Merrick, Scott Reeves, Ann Russell, Chris Kenaszchuk, Lesley Gotlib Conn, Karen-Lee Miller, et al. (2007). "Structuring Communication Relationships for Interprofessional Teamwork (SCRIPT): A Cluster Randomized Controlled Trial." *Trials* 8(23), online, Open Access. doi:10.1186/1745-6215-8-23.

Note: Italicized page numbers indicate tables and figures.

A

acceptance, 181
access:
  to health care, 115, 118; measuring, 277; quality of insurance coverage, 276; rates of uninsurance, 277–78
  safe physical activity, 148
Activities of Daily Living (ADL), 53
African American (race), 113–18, 125, 127, 128
age, 301
  inequalities: age *55–64* cohort, 100–7, *105–7*; cohort flow, 101; collectivities, 100; life course, 101; older adult populations, 108
  social influence on clinical communication, 202–3
Agency for Healthcare Research and Quality, 42
alcoholism, 153, 154, 157–58, 165
American health care delivery system. *See* U.S. health care system
American Heart Association (AHA) statement, 126–27
American Medical Association (AMA), 115, 228
anger, 141, 181–83
anxiety, 111, 139, 141, 182n5, 188, 192
Asch, Solomon, 11–12
attention deficit hyperactivity disorder (ADHD), 179
  definition, 166
  diagnosis in adult and children: effect on own identity, 170; degree of disease, 171; home and school settings, 166; interviewing process, 166; medicalization, 169–71; rate of, 167; treatment benefit *vs.* degree of abnormality, 171–72, *172*
  identifying, 169
  neurological conditions, 167
  prevalence rates: between cultures and classes, 165; in France, 169; lower, 168, *168*
  symptoms, 166
autism spectrum disorder, 174–75, 182

autonomy, 253, 255
Awakenings (1990), 34

B

bargaining, 181–83
Beecher, Henry K., 248
beneficence, 253, 254
beneficent ageism, 203
bioethics, 72–73
  clinical ethics: case study, 265–66; social psychology of, 263–65
  emergence, 247–50
  origin, 245
  practical, 260–63
  principles: autonomy, 253, 255; beneficence, 252–54; consequentialist approaches, 252; deontological reasoning, 251; dilemmas in health care, 255–56; justice, 252–55; moral reasoning, classic paradigms of, 254–55, *255*; nonmaleficence, 253–55; right to self-determination, 252; teleological approaches, 251; utilitarianism, 251–52
The Birth of the Clinic, 27
Black, Lewis, 38
Blumer, Herbert, 304
body mass index (BMI), 41, 93
Bruhn, John, 14
Budrys, Grace, 16

C

cardiovascular disease (CVD), 14, 39, 83, 109, 110, 126, 131, 135
Cassell, Eric, 180
casuistry, 256–57
categorical imperative, 251
categoric group, 65
causality:
  attribution of, 110
  covariation, 55–56
  eliminating spurious relationships, 56–58
  logical model, 55, 69
Cesarean section (C-section), 155
Charmaz, Kathy, 185–87
Charon, Rita, 212
child and adolescent mental illnesses (CFTMEA), 169

childbirth, medicalization:
  Cesarean delivery, *155, 155–56*
  classification, 156
  direct-to-consumer marketing
    of drugs, 157
  under physicians supervision, 154
  risks management, 154–55
  technological intervention, 157
  time of delivery, 156, *156*
cholesterol, 35, 38, 41
chronic fatigue syndrome, 179
chronic illness, 32, 41, 42, 88, 100, 164,
    185n8, 187
  clinical practice, 40–43
  diabetes and heart disease, 34
  era, 108, 130, 153, 171, 179n2, 188, 211, 229
  incalculability of, 36, 37
  morbidity and mortality, 132
  physical, 185
  prevalence of, 33
  prevention, 38
  sociological nature of, 148
chronic obstructive pulmonary disease
    (COPD), *159,* 160
cigarette smoking, 38, 83, 107, 131
Clair, Jeffrey Michael, 162, 218
classic experimental design, 59–62
  correlational and cross-sectional
    methods, 65
  preexperimental methods, 66
  qualitative methods, 66–67
  quasi-experimental methods, 64–65
clinical communication:
  basic interviewing techniques
    (*see* interviewing techniques)
  eliciting patient narrative, 220–21
  good communication, 199–200
  micro-level interactions, 201
  motivational interviewing technique, 219
  narrative and art of practice: diagnostic
    information, 199, 210–11; hypothetical
    scatterplot, 210, *211*; long-term illness
    management, 211; patient's illness story,
    importance of, 212–13
  patient–provider communication, 199
  practitioners counseling, 219
  problems of, 201, 218

social influences, 210; ageism, 202–3;
  culture, 208–9; gender, 203–5;
  physician–patient relationship, 201, *201*;
  race/ethnicity, 206–8; SES, 205–6
clinical practice:
  dilemmas of difference, 172–74
  medicalization: ADHD diagnosis as social
    control (*see* attention deficit hyperactivity
    disorder (ADHD)); alcoholism, 157–58;
    childbirth (*see* childbirth, medicalization);
    social process, 154
  power (*see* power)
Cockerham, William, 126
Colpo, Anthony, 38
*The Condition of the Working Class in
  England* (1845 [2009]), 13
constant, 52
contested illnesses, 179
Corporatist model, 289–90
correlational and cross-sectional methods, 65
cost effectiveness, in health care:
  assessment, 275
  by country, *275,* 275–76
  out-of pocket, 274–75
  per capita, 275
  responsible factors, 276
  variety of, 274
cost-shifting, 276n2
Crew Resource Management (CRM)
    strategy, 238
CrossFit, 39
Cruzan, Nancy, 249, 250
culture, 301
  clinical communication, 208–9
  inequalities: definition, 119; effect on health
    and disease, 121–23; healthier lifestyles,
    124; illness behavior, 120; prevalence
    of diabetes, American Indians, 123;
    preventative health behavior, 120; role
    in health matters, 119–20; sick-role
    behavior, 121

D

deafness, 173, 174
death zone, 122
denial, 181
dependent variables (DVs), 52, 56

depression, 108, 110, 111, 139, 141, 181, 183, 187, 188, 190, 192
deprofessionalization of medicine, 226, 228–29
detection bias, *70*
Deutsch, Morton, 235
diabetes, 34, *35*, 39, 41, 106, 108, 109, 123, 124, 126, 131, 132, 153, 192, 212
Diagnostic and Statistical Manual of Mental Disorders (DSM-V), 166
disciplinary power, 159
The Doctor (1991), 33
Durkheim, Emile, 7, 224

E

Elliott, Jane, 11
energy medicine, 42
Engels, Friedrich, 13
Enlightenment, 22, 27
ethical decision-making in health care:
  autonomy, 253, 255
  beneficence, 252–54
  dilemmas, 255–56
  justice, 252–55
  moral reasoning, classic paradigms of, 254–55, *255*
  nonmaleficence, 253–55
  right to self-determination, 252
  in Western cultures: casuistry, 256–57; ethics of care approaches, 258–59; narrative ethics, 259–60; virtue ethics, 257–58
ethics of care approaches, 258–59
evidence-based decision-making, 47, 74
exclusion bias, *70*
exercise, 21, *35*, 38, 39

F

falsifiability, 51
federal poverty level (FPL), 82
Flexner, Abraham, 30, 31
Frank, Arthur, 183

G

Gawande, Atul, 223
gender, 200, 203–5, 301
  inequalities: biological explanations, 109–11; classification, 108; differences, 109; mental well-being, 111; mortality, 112–13;

paradox, 109; sex dichotomously, defining, 108–9; social explanations, 111–12
generalizability, 51, 52
Gerard, Harold, 235
Goldacre, Ben, 49
gross domestic product (GDP), 275

H

Hampton, Isabel, 230
healing:
  arts, 23
  force, 26
  of injury, 43
  premodern, 22–24
health action process approach, 139
health behavior and lifestyles, 129–30
  alternative models: integrated behavior model, 138, *139*; theory of planned behavior, 136, *137*, 138; theory of reasoned action, 136–38, *137*
  associated with chronic illness, 132
  balanced diet, 131
  behavioral practices, *144, 145*
  case study, 149–50
  causes, 133
  definition, 130–31, 133
  epidemiological perspective, 131
  group memberships or collectivities, 144, *144*
  habitus, *144,* 145–47
  health belief model, *136*; cost-benefit analysis, 136; perceived barrier, 135; perceived benefits, 135; perceived severity, 135; perceived threat, 135; self-efficacy, 135; uses, 136
  individual risk factors, 143
  life chances, *144, 145*
  life choices, *144,* 144–45
  micro–macro approaches, 133–35
  prevalence, 131
  process models: cost-benefit analysis, 143; health action process approach, 139; precaution adoption process model, 139; process of change, 141–42, *142*; transtheoretical model, 139–41, *140*
  socialization experience, 144, *144*

health care, 301
American, 14–16
grief in, 181–84
history of, 13–14
markets, 291
micro/interactional features, 302–3, *303*
modern medicine: business, 31–32; clinical practice in chronic illness era, 40–43
multidisciplinary approach, 4–8
practice, 147–49
as social institution, 16–17
healthy migrant hypothesis, 118
heart disease, 34, 41, 82–84, 88, 90, 91
heroic medicine, 27
hidden biases, 64
Hinote, Brian P., 126
Hippocratic Oath, 245, 247
human medical error, 240
humoral theory of medicine, 24–26
Hurd, Henry M., 230
hypercholesterolemia, 106
hyperkinesia, 166
hypertension, 62, *63*, 68, 100, 106, 116, 121, 126, 131, 171

I

ideal type, 130, 284, 285, 289, 290
identity, 164, 165, 170, 177, 228
consumer's, 39
and illness: diagnosis, 185; functional impairment, 185; making bodily assessments and subsequent identity trade-offs, 185–86; mental illness, 187; physical illness, 187–88; in social relationships and social functions, 184; stages of grief, 186; surrendering to the sick self, 186
of nursing, 232
race/ethnic, 114
ideology, 17, 86, 273
illness:
chronic, 32, 41, 42, 88, 100, 164, 185n8, 187; clinical practice, 40–43; diabetes and heart disease, 34; era, 108, 130, 153, 171, 179n2, 188, 211, 229; incalculability of, 36, 37; morbidity and mortality, 132; physical, 185; prevalence of, 33; prevention, 38; sociological nature of, 148
definition, 153–54

illness behavior, 120, 121
illness experiences, 195–97
case study, 197
definition, 178–79
vs. disease, 178, 179
etiology, 178
families: caregiving burden, 188–90; stress process model (*see* stress process model)
of patients: breaks free pain, 180; grief in health care, 181–84; identity, 184–88; physical pain in clinical settings, 179–80; social construction, 179; Wong-Baker scale, 180, *180*
incomplete spinal cord injury (ICSI), 53
independent variables (IVs), 52, 55
inequalities:
age, 55–64; cohort, 100–7, *105–7*; collectivities, 100; life course, 101; older adult populations, 108
culture: definition, 119; effect on health and disease, 121–23; healthier lifestyles, 124; illness behavior, 120; prevalence of diabetes, American Indians, 123; preventative health behavior, 120; role in health matters, 119–20; sick-role behavior, 121
gender: biological explanations, 109–11; classification, 108; differences, 109; mental well-being, 111; mortality, 112–13; paradox, 109; sex dichotomously, defining, 108–9; social explanations, 111–12
matrix of, 124–27
race and ethnicity, 113–19
informed consent, 253
institutionalization, 22
integrated behavior model, 138, *139*
interprofessional teamwork:
best practices for: communication, 236–37; coordinated diversity, 236; CRM strategy, 238; educational activities, 234–35; leadership responsibilities, 235–36; self-evaluation and peer feedback, 237; TeamSTEPPS model, 238
bureaucratic model, 242
case study, 244
collaborations models, 241–43

descriptive feedback, 237

just culture practices, 241

medical error: cognitive errors, 239–40; diagnostic errors, 239; forcing functions, 240–41; human error, 240; no-fault errors, 239; preventive errors, 239; reduction strategies, 240; treatment errors, 239

sincere feedback, 237

specialization and complexity, 223–25

specific feedback, 237

usable feedback, 237

interviewing techniques:

closed-ended questions, 215, *217*

eliciting patient narrative, 213, *214*

introductory phase, 214

minimal encouragers, 215–16, *217*

open-ended questions, 215–18, *217*

working phase, 214–15

intuitive knowledge, 23

inverse coverage law, 278

irritable bowel syndrome, 179

J

justice, biomedical ethics, 253–55

K

Kant, Immanuel, 251

Karp, David, 187

Kennedy, Edward, 249

knowledge power, 159–60

Koch, Robert, 27

Kübler-Ross, Elizabeth, 181, 182

L

life expectancy, 33, 34, 109, 112, 118, 280, *282, 283,* 298–300

Locke, John, 251

logical inference, 51, 52

M

Maslow, Abraham, 93

material power, 159

medicalization, 303

ADHD diagnosis as social control (*see* attention deficit hyperactivity disorder (ADHD))

alcoholism, 157–58

childbirth: Cesarean delivery, *155, 155*–56; classification, 156; direct-to-consumer marketing of drugs, 157; under physicians supervision, 154; risks management, 154–55; technological intervention, 157; time of delivery, 156, *156*

social process, 154

medicine, 21–22, 43–44

and healing: humoral medicine, 24–26; premodern era, 23–24

health and disease, 32–33; chronic disease and incalculable risk, 33–34; consequences of risk incalculability, 37–40; epidemiological transition, 34–37

institution of modernity, 26–27; clinical practice, 29; education for medical and allied health professions, 29–31; health care business, 31–32; heroic therapeutics movement, 27; modern medicine development, 27–28

postindustrial shift, 44–45

mental health:

caregiving burden, 193

outcomes, 191, 192

prevalent measures, 111

mental illnesses, 167, 178, 187

methodo-logical approach, 48

Milgram, Stanley, 9–10

Mills, C. Wright, 8–9, 178

mindfulness-based stress reduction (MBSR), 94n1

moral hazard, 294

morbidity, 100, 101, 109, 111–13

mortality, 116

among Hispanics, 118

in Eastern Europe, 126

infant, 118, 119

lower among women, 109

lung cancer, 107, 112

male, 109, 112

NCHS data on, 101

premature, 124

primary sources, 100

rates, 118, 123, 126

statistics, *117,* 123

motivational interviewing technique, 219

mutual aid model, in health care, 284–85

N

narrative ethics, 259–60
National Center for Health Statistics
    (NCHS), 101
national health expenditures (NHE), 274
National Health Service (NHS), 280, 287
neighborhood, 40, 118, 145, 192, 232,
    283, 302
  advantage, 89
  charity-funded ambulatory sites nested
      within, 41
  clinical implications, 94–95
  disadvantage, 91–94, 124
  disorder, 191n9
  exercise-friendly, 146
  face-to-face information, 13
  inner city, 148
  medical, 42
  urban, 148n2
Neumann, Salomon, 13
New York Times (1955), 33
nurse practitioners, 43
nursing, 4, 43, 53, 115, 200, 234, 235, 304
  development, 230–32
  professionalization of, 226
  skilled, 42
  staff, 236, 237
nutrient dense diet, 38

O

obesity, 41, 73, 84, 92, 106, 121, 126, 131,
    132, 140, 146, 153, 191
On the Mode of Communication of Cholera
    (1849), 13
Organization for Economic Cooperation and
    Development (OECD), 275
Overdiagnosed (Welch et al. (2011)), 171
overt biases, 64

P

pain, 205, 216, 254
  analysis of, 120
  back, 203
  chest, 6, 135
  patient's, 218
  physical, 179, 180
  Wong-Baker scale to access, *180,* 180n3
Parsons, Talcott, 164

Pasteur, Louis, 27
patent medicines, 37
patient-centered care, 203, 263, 294
patient-centered communication, 204, 205,
    207, 209, 236, 243
patient-centered medical home (PCMH)
    model, 41–42
patient–provider communication, 67, 124,
    196, 199, 232, 303
patient–provider relationships, 3
Paxil, 157
performance bias, *70*
physical illness, 109, 178, 187, 188, 215
physician assistants (PAs), 43, 230–31
Pilates, 39
political ideology, 285
Porter, Roy, 16
postmarketing, 62
power in clinical practice, 153
  clinical functions: patient encounter,
      161–62; physician encounters, 162–63;
      sick person role, 164–65
  forms: disciplinary power, 159, 160;
      knowledge power, 159–60; material
      power, 158–59
practitioner–patient relationship, 160, 165, 205
precaution adoption process model, 139
preexperimental methods, 66
preventative ethics, 263
preventative health behavior, 120
professionalization:
  features, 231
  of nursing, 226, 231
  process of, 228
professional model, 288–89
professions:
  community of, 225
  deprofessionalization of medicine, 228–29
  development of nursing, 230–32
  interdisciplinary teamwork (*see*
      interprofessional teamwork)
  legally protected practice, 225
  of medicine, 227–28
  problems within, 232–34
  social contract, 226
proton pump inhibitors (PPIs), 68
Psychology Today, 169
Public Health Service (PHS), 248–49

Q

qualitative methods, 66–67
quality of care, 274
  advantages and disadvantages, 283
  cost controls, 280
  infant mortality rates, 280, *281*
  life expectancy at birth for OECD countries, 280, *282*, 283
  low-tech preventative measures, 280
  waiting period, nonemergency care, 278, 280
quasi-experimental methods, 64–65
Quinlan, Karen Ann, 249, 250

R

race/ethnicity, 200, 232, 243, 301
  clinical communication, 206–8
  inequalities, 113–19
racialization, 114n4
randomized controlled trial, 63, *70*
reductionism, 196
Relative Value Units (RVUs), 229
replicability, 51
Report on the Sanitary Condition of the Labouring Population and on the Means of Its Improvement (1842), 13
revealed knowledge, 23
Rivera, Geraldo, 248
Robinson, Edward G., 33
Rush, Benjamin, 27

S

Sack, Oliver, 34
Salmon bias hypothesis, 118
scientific research:
  causality: covariation, 55–56; eliminating spurious relationships, 56–58; logical model, 55
  classic experimental design (*see* classic experimental design)
  definition, 51
  ethics, 72–73
  goal of, 51
  scientific methodology, 52–55
  theories, 51
  thinking critically about, 75
  translation, 67–72
  variables, 51–52, *52*

selection bias, 61, 64, *70*
self-efficacy, 93, 135, 138
self-stereotyping ageism, 203
sensitizing concepts, 304
SES. *See* socioeconomic status (SES)
sick-role behavior, 121
Sjogren's syndrome, 185
Snow, John, 13, 27
social class. *See* socioeconomic status (SES)
social contract, 226
social determinants of health, 79–84, 86, 95, 302, *302*
social epidemiology, 80
social institution, 16–17
socialization, 11, 18, 86, 130, 144–47, 195, 200, 202, 203, 205, 208, 225, 233, 303, 304
socioeconomic status (SES), 99, 130, 200, 205–6, 232, 301
  case study, 96–97
  cause of health and disease: biomedical approaches, 88; health lifestyles, 90; living/working conditions, 89–90; mechanisms, 89; neighborhood advantage, 89; risk factors, 88–89; sense of control, 89, 91; social support, 89–91; stress, 90
  definition, 85
  life chances, 85
  ranking in social groups, 87
  as sensitizing concepts, 304–5
  social interactions, 86–87
  socialization, 86
  in United States, 87–88
sociological imagination, 8–9
  example work: Asch, Solomon, 11–12; Elliott, Jane, 11; Milgram, Stanley, 9–10; Zimbardo, Philip, 10–11
  exercising, 19–20
  reflexive model of social reality, 8–9, *9*
sociology, 4
spiritual fatalism, 115
Stage of Change model, 219n5
Starr, Paul, 227
state model, in health care, 285, 287–88
statistical imagination, 48–51, 74–75
stress, 6, 82, 89, 90, 92–95, 109, 110, 118, 263, 264

stress process model, *191*
  caregiving burden: case study, 192–93; discussion catalysts, 193, *194*; family caregiver role, 193; interventions, 193–95
  personal resources, 191, 193
  physical and mental health outcomes, 190–92
  social resources, 191
stroke, 34, 82–84, *84*
Syphilis, Tuskegee, 249, 253
systematic bias, 63, 69–71

T

Team Strategies and Tools to Enhance Performance and Patient Safety (TeamSTEPPS), 238
theory of planned behavior, 136, *137*, 138
theory of reasoned action, 136–38, *137*
transtheoretical model, 139–41, *140*, 219n5

U

underwater treadmill training (UTT), 53
United States, 111, 118, 119, 121, 122, 126, 127
  age 55–64 cohort, 102, *105*; health care utilization, 106–7, *107*; selected chronic conditions, 106, *106*
  aging population in, 203n1
  life expectancy, 33, 34
  prevalence of: heart disease, 82, *83*; stroke, 83, *84*
  race/ethnic health outcomes, 114, 115
  resident population by age and sex, 102, *103–4*
  women longevity, 109
Unnatural Causes (2008), 123
U.S. health care system, 14–16, 271–73, 301–2
  access: adults and children with no usual source of care, 278, *279*; measuring, 277; quality of insurance coverage, 276; rates of uninsurance, 277, 277–78
  challenges, 297
  complexity, 295–96
  costs: assessment, 275; by country, *275*, 275–76; out-of pocket, 274–75; per capita, 275; responsible factors, 276; variety of, 274
  deal of dissatisfaction, 273
  inequities in, 284
  models, 283–84; comparisons of, 284, *286*; corporatist model, 289–90; mutual aid model, 284–85; professional model, 288–89; state model, 285, 287–88
  patient-induced demand and overtreatment, 293–95
  provider-induced demand and overtreatment, 290–93
  quality, 274; advantages and disadvantages, 283; cost controls, 280; infant mortality rates, 280, *281*; life expectancy at birth for OECD countries, 280, *282*, 283; low-tech preventative measures, 280; waiting period, nonemergency care, 278, 280
utilitarianism, 251–52, 256

V

Viagra, 157
Virchow, Rudolf, 13
virtue ethics, 257–58

W

Weber, Max, 178
Wolf, Stewart, 14
Wong-Baker faces® pain rating scale, 180, *180*
World Health Organization (WHO), 108n2, 275

Y

yoga, 39

Z

Zimbardo, Philip, 10–11
Zola, Irving, 120
Zumba, 39